# ANIMAL MIND
# HUMAN VOICES

# ANIMAL MIND
# HUMAN VOICES

*Nancy Herrick, P.A.*

◆

## PROVINGS OF EIGHT NEW ANIMAL REMEDIES

Hahnemann Clinic Publishing

Hahnemann Clinic Publishing
19775 New Rome Road
Nevada City, California 95959
Telephone and facsimile 530-265-3856



The quotation by Jalaluddin Rumi at the front of this book is from *Rumi: We Are Three,* translated by Coleman Barks, Athens, Georgia: Maypop Books, 1997.

Book and cover design by Lubosh Cech
Illustrations by Hannah Bonner (dolphin, dinosaur); and archive.

1 2 3 4 5 6 7 8 9

ISBN 0-9635368-1-8

Printed in the United States of America

*This book is dedicated to my husband, Roger.*

*I cannot imagine doing any of it without him,*

*for the love we share for our work and for each other*

*is the foundation of all that I do.*

# CONTENTS

# FOREWORD

I did not much believe in modern provings. I was under the impression that the current remedies, if we just knew how to use them, sufficed to cure any patient. And so it was, without much enthusiasm, that I agreed to participate in Nancy Herrick's proving: Lac delphinum. I must admit, I was not at first impressed with the mental, emotional, dream symptoms which developed. What truly impressed me, concrete creature that I am, was that eight people associated with the proving developed pain in the big toe. This humble symptom was the narrow doorway through which my mind entered a new world.

Over the following years, I became an increasingly enthusiastic observer and frequent proving subject. I watched the hundreds of hours of careful study, labor, and integrity which Nancy Herrick brought to each of these provings. Huge volumes of raw data had to be logged and verified with the individual provers. Rather than simply present the raw data, Nancy was convinced that, with deep reflection and study on the exact words of the provers, she would be able to uncover the basic feeling of each remedy. She then delineated this feeling for each remedy in her "Themes" section and exemplified each theme with the words of the provers.

Fears have been expressed (also by myself) that the attempt to synthesize a theme could slant the data of a proving. I have finally come to the conclusion that this rationalist way of thinking is grounded in allopathic research models. The homeopathic method, however, is based upon faith in the prover's (and proving master's) perceptions. Though the importance of the inner state has been disputed, by Hughes and others, homeopathic thought has always been essentially phenomenological. That is, it starts with the premise that inner phenomena have an equal (or sometimes greater) validity to external, measurable events. Certainly this license—to use one's own experience as a means of divining truth—can be (and in some recent provings has been) abused. This leads to results which match the proving master's expectations rather than the substance's true nature. Thus, homeopathy is always dependent upon Hahnemann's "unprejudiced observer." The test of whether a proving is unprejudiced—as with, for example, an espoused "essence" of a remedy—is in its clinical applicability.

Nancy Herrick wrestled with these issues and finally expressed to me her conviction that it is possible for the proving master to act as a vehicle for the meaning of the proving. And so, in many hours of reflection, she has tried to live the inner state of each remedy through and with her provers and to report that state accurately and vividly. The proof that Nancy's methods are reliable and "unprejudiced" is that virtually all of these new remedies are now in use by practitioners and have effected deep cures.

So several years and a complete conversion later, I marvel at the knowledge unfolded in these animal provings. I had accepted the possibility that, for example, a dream of dolphins or swimming might occur during the proving of Lac delphinum. What I did not expect was that the proving would bring out the deepest dilemmas, fears, joys—that is to say the very life of the species—of the animal being proved. For example, the proving of the gray wolf brought out the feeling of imminent death, revealing, shockingly, the inner life of a species on the verge of extinction. Another example is the frustrated, enslaved feeling which came in the proving of Lac equinum—the milk from a noble creature broken to the will of man. In short, each of these provings is a window into the inner life of the animal.

One of the most startling realizations stimulated by these provings is that some of the foremost symptoms which occurred characterize the relationship of the proved species to man. For example, the light and happy feeling in the butterfly proving parallels our instinctive reactions to this living ephemera. In contrast, the feeling of violence and butchering reported during the proving of Lac loxodonta reflects the slaughter of these creatures for their ivory. It appears that our behavior and feelings towards an animal species is integral to the homeopathic use of the substance.

One final realization occurred during these provings: It seems highly likely that human treatment of our cousin species will be reflected in our own pathology. Can we drive the wolf into annihilation without a serious consequence to our own consciousness? Could it be that the rapidly accelerating incidence of deep phobias, anxiety, and depression found in our culture is in part due to our behavior toward the earth? Or, more concretely, can a man whip a dog without tainting or shriveling his own soul?

And so these provings show once again the power of the homeopathic process to reveal the nature of life. May we use this power and these provings as a prism to see inside ourselves, and through seeing, heal.

– Roger Morrison, M.D.

# INTRODUCTION

Homeopathy has sustained and fascinated me for over 20 years. The process of taking a case, giving a remedy, and watching a very ill person bloom into health gives a sense of satisfaction unlike anything I have ever known. But there is something missing. Some cases, no matter how we struggle with them, cannot be solved. Part of the reason for this is that many of the most important medicines have not yet been developed. Foremost among these are the animal remedies, especially the milks of the mammals. We have over 2,000 remedies, and only 14 of them are made from the mammals. Almost 100 years ago, the great homeopathic master, James Tyler Kent, said: "All the milks should be potentized, they are our most excellent remedies; they are animal products and foods of early animal life and therefore correspond to the beginning of our innermost physical nature."

After going to India and being inspired by the work of Rajan Sankaran, I became intrigued by the idea of doing some new animal provings. It soon became apparent that this was a formidable undertaking. Many aspects of the proving process have been difficult—from finding acceptable provers and obtaining the animal substances to organizing the vast amount of material that is developed in the process. Nevertheless, this has been a extremely stimulating and rewarding endeavor. The remedies from Dolphin, Dinosaur, Elephant, Horse, Rat, Butterfly, Lion, and Wolf have already been used successfully based on the informal spread of information from these provings. That is why I believe it is important to formally publish them. Otherwise, the use of these new remedies would remain an arcane and secret practice.

**What Is a Proving?**

A proving is a way of making a new medicine available to the repertoire of remedies used in homeopathy. It involves the documentation and analysis of symptoms that occur when healthy individuals take a remedy. Samuel Hahnemann, the father of homeopathy, determined that when healthy individuals take a substance, they manifest the same symptoms which that substance cures in sick persons. Virtually all homeopathic remedies now in use were proved at one time or another. There is no end to the substances which can be proved. Interest in proving substances is growing even as the science and art of homeopathy reestablishes itself in the forefront of healing arts in the new millennium.

**Methodology of Provings**

The system I use for provings has developed as a result of the work of other provers and my own design. First, eight to twenty people volunteer freely to participate. Preferably they are either homeopathic students, colleagues, or people who are advocates of homeopathy. I do not use any patients or people who are not familiar with homeopathy as provers. Homeopaths make good provers because they are familiar with their own symptoms and are more likely to recognize a new symptom when it comes up. Non-homeopaths are more likely to enter old symptoms in the proving record. I trust homeopaths to record symptoms with accuracy and to appreciate the value of detail, especially that valuable information about mental and emotional states.

Each prover who is a homeopath decides whether or not they want a supervisor. If they want one, I will provide another homeopath to do it. Non-homeopaths must have a supervisor who also takes their baseline case for at least their first proving. Neither supervisors or provers do not know what the substance is.

The substance is selected based on its relative importance to humans—something that people have a strong feeling about one way or another. For example, people love roses; they hate rats.

The remedy is made up into a 30C potency. Each participant, blinded totally as to the substance, is mailed a vial of the remedy. They are also mailed a proving booklet to record each new symptom they experience under the appropriate heading, such as mind, head, stomach, and so on.

All provers start at approximately the same time and day by taking one dose. Some provers will note a symptom that occurs almost immediately upon taking the remedy, while others will note no symptoms whatsoever during the entire proving session. For a period of three weeks, the provers keep notes and detail carefully all symptoms that differ from their usual state. If a supervisor has been assigned to the prover, s/he will phone the prover regularly in order to go over physical symptoms and state of mind as well as the days' experiences.

It is very important that the provers carefully record their emotional state, including dreams and the details of any unusual events that occur in their lives during the entire proving period. Recording details of all kinds is encouraged, especially if there is an acute illness or a crisis, or if important new symptoms occur. If they have no symptoms at all, the provers are asked to repeat the remedy two more times, two days apart. If they have very slight symptoms which dissipate in a matter of days, they are asked to repeat the remedy once, after the symptoms are gone. If they have definite symptoms, they are asked not to repeat the remedy at all but just to watch the symptoms and their general emotional state. Under all circumstances, they are asked to keep their notebooks going and to record each day for three weeks, even if it is only to say "no symptoms." Many times we have seen that symptoms occurred which were so subtle, they were not apparent to the provers themselves until the group meeting, when they saw that other provers had the same symptoms. For example, in the rat proving, many provers felt a strong desire to go out at night—especially to be in the woods in the dark. Virtually none of them thought of this as a symptom in the proving but dutifully recorded it as an activity in their lives. When we got together at the meeting, we were amazed at the consistency of this unique symptom.

The dreams which occur throughout the proving are another extremely important guide to the underlying emotional state of the person who would need this substance. Provers are asked to wake up in the night to record their dreams, but if this is not feasible, they are requested to keep pen and pad by their bed and record dreams within 60 seconds of waking. After this period of time, the dreams are lost to memory in most cases. Some provings bring out an emotional state that is reflected almost solely in the dreams of the prover. For example, in the wolf proving, there were minimal physical symptoms, but the dreams revealed a deep and profound emotional disturbance. Other provings are predominantly physical and have much detailed symptomatology.

If at any time during the proving there is a crisis or any major area of difficulty, I am available any time night or day, and the provers have my home phone number. If I do a proving in another location, I have a local supervisor who is available. It is important to give a feeling of safety and security to provers. The only exception I made to this was in my second proving—dolphin. This entire proving was different in that it was done during a week-long seminar in Hawaii. I was not personally familiar with each of the provers, as I was in my other provings. Also, it was the largest one, with over 20 provers. One prover had long-term symptoms after the proving that she never told me about until over a year later. This was unfortunate and taught me an important lesson about knowing the provers and staying in contact.

Another point that came up during this proving was the use of children as provers. After some debate, we decided to include them. Two sets of parents volunteered. One set gave their daughter the substance in potency and the other merely put it under their child's pillow. Both children had a strong reaction with noticeable behavior changes and many physical and mental symptoms. While this provided a lot of insight into the remedy, I have made a decision not to do provings with children in the future because I feel that the provings are too strong for their comfort level. An interesting point is that several other children, who did not have contact with the remedy but whose parents were provers, also had strong, new symptoms consistent with the remedy. The experiences of these children are not included in these reports.

At the end of three weeks, the proving meeting is held. The provers have been asked not to discuss among themselves in any way their state or symptoms during the proving time. We gather in a quiet room where we will not be interrupted. The session is videotaped, but provers may choose not to be on tape. Each prover in turn reads his booklet and summarizes his or her experience. They may, and do, elaborate a bit. At the end, provers can bring up something they experienced but did not recognize as a symptom until they heard other provers mention it at the meeting. Then they attempt to identify the substance, or at least the kingdom. Finally, I reveal the substance, and we have a discussion about their general experience, the substance, and their feelings about it. At this point, most people who are still experiencing symptoms have a catharsis, wherein the remedy and the symptoms leave them, and they go back to their usual state.

Following this meeting, the challenge of organizing all the material collected from the notebooks and proving meeting begins. This is truly a major job and would be extremely difficult to do without a team.

It is ideal to follow the provers for the next year to identify changes and developments over the long term. However, for the many provers who participate in two or three provings a year, this is not practical. But I do believe it is an excellent practice. Certainly, it is important to follow up on any symptoms that are still active after the end of the proving period of three weeks. Readers will find themselves able to enter into the mind of the animals in this book. The voices of the human provers allow us to "hear and feel" the state of the animals. It is my hope that by doing this, we may heal the animals as we heal ourselves

**Important Things I Learned from Doing Twelve Provings**

1. Treasure your provers. Sensitive provers are gems of unimaginable value to the future of thousands of patients who will be healed by the remedies they have proven. Love them; be kind to them. Do not push them to do a proving if they don't want to, and do not ask them to do too many provings for their comfort level.

2. Select your substance very carefully. Make sure you identify it properly. Many people will offer suggestions, but a proving is a major undertaking. Untold hours of work and effort go into it. Make sure your choice is a good one. If you decide to do a proving that has already been done, do it in a different country or in a different manner.

3. Make rubrics. This adds the proving language to the general lexicon of the

working homeopath. The number of rubrics is secondary to their being accurate and reliable.

4. If you're going to do it, do it right and do it thoroughly. Do only that number of provings you have the commitment to publish. Then publish them. The world needs this information.

# ACKNOWLEDGMENTS

To be a prover and to do a proving properly is not only a gift of time, which is a most precious commodity these days, but a gift of one's body and mind. It requires entering a world of the unknown where any lurking demon may leap out into one's life at any inopportune moment. It is to put oneself at the mercy of the mystery, to surrender to the experience of a variety of mental, emotional, and physical disruptions. It is a gift of magnificent proportions to the healing art. From the bottom of my heart, I wish to thank all the people who committed themselves to do these provings, most of them professionals who are or have been students of Hahnemann College of Homeopathy but some who are devoted, special friends. I do not wish to name any names of these important people because I wish to protect their privacy. They know who they are and the world is grateful. I also wish to thank this same group for spending many extra hours in the videotaping sessions and in the rubric analysis for each of the provings.

My deepest gratitude to:

◆ Rajan Sankaran and Divya Chhabra for their enthusiasm and invaluable suggestions concerning the structure of the proving process. Rajan and Divya's original work in provings was such an inspiration to me that it marked the beginning of my interest in doing provings. I believe it has been the same for many homeopaths around the world. It was Rajan and Jurgen Becker, M.D. who had the original idea of the proving meeting to get the central ideas and to bring about a "catharsis," in order to the help the provers move out of the state of the remedy.
◆ Michael Quinn, pharmacist and owner of Hahnemann Laboratories, for his commitment to all aspects of the complicated pharmaceutical process of making a new remedy. Michael helps whenever he can to gather the substance, identify it accurately, prepare it quickly and perfectly, keep it a secret (for the proving), and then distribute it as a gift to the provers. Often all this occurs at a moment's notice, as with the elephant milk proving.
◆ Marianne Heger, M.D., and Deutsch Homöopathie Union, who generously made up six of the newly proven remedies into high potencies without charge.

DHU is a pharmacy of the highest quality, with the highest ethical standards.
◆ Deborah Gordon, M.D. for her assistance in the beginning stages of this work, for offering helpful ideas around the basic structure of the proving presentations. Deborah also helped with editing and proofreading the book at the end.
◆ Claire Green, N.D. for many hours of very conscientious work on all aspects of Elephant, Horse, and Lion. Claire has been a great help in assisting with rubrics. I am always impressed by the strength of her intellect and her commitment to doing the job right.
◆ Jessica Jackson, L.Ac. for untold devotion to two very special provings: Wolf and Rat. Jessica's deep love of homeopathy and the proving process is evident in all her work. The pure excitement and energy she brought to these provings was infectious and made the process immeasurably more enjoyable. The original idea of the connection between the wolf and the gypsies was Jessica's.
◆ David Warkentin, P.A. for his suggestions on rubrics. His was the excellent idea of listing main rubrics wherever possible and adding sub-rubrics to express the individuality of each substance.
◆ Roger van Zandvoort for his suggestions also on the issue of rubrics. He emphasized that each symptom is important and reminded me that in the original Sulphur proving, only one prover came up with the symptom: "feet warm; sticks out of covers at night."
◆ David Riley, M.D., of New Mexico, for the use of the nicely organized proving journals that he developed in accordance with the guidelines set up with DHU research faculty and Marianne Heger, M.D.
◆ Aimee Zaigon, P.A. for her assistance with Maiasaura and help in collating those themes. Also for her grant-writing assistance.
◆ Lynn Snow for a masterful job in assisting in the dolphin proving. Lynn started this evaluation as part of a research paper and ended up spending many hours reviewing every detail from each prover. One year after the proving, she made phone calls around the world to determine if there were any long-term symptoms. Lynn is another dedicated homeopath and a real gem.
◆ David Penny, D.V.M. for his help in gathering substances, especially the milks, a process sometimes more frustrating than fruitful but at times astonishingly successful, as in elephant's milk.
◆ Pat Tarzian, who did the investigative research on Maiasaura—a challenging task since the material on this dinosaur is difficult to find. Also for her precise, eagle-eyed editing of the final version of the manuscript.
◆ Harianna Chilstrom for her research on *Limenitis bredowii*. She is more knowledgeable about insects than anyone I have ever known.
◆ Lubosh Cech, a talented and precise graphic designer, whose vision of the final book sustained us throughout this process.

◆ George Marks for his untiring willingness to review the animal write-ups. He met this task with his usual easy and cheerful style.
◆ Gloria St. John, who came in at the end of the process and was a real lifesaver with her excellent work of editing and preparation of the manuscript.
◆ Naomi, my wonderful daughter, for her lay person's perspective on editing two provings, and most of all, for the glorious giggles when I needed a break.

◆

Finally I would like to thank my wonderful husband, Roger Morrison, M.D., for his support in all aspects of this work: from his being a sensitive and important prover in three of the provings to his understanding of the untold hours spent on this work. I am especially grateful for his technical support in the endless process of computer, fax and E-mail mishaps and challenges. I love and thank him with all my heart.

◆

Support for this book was partially provided by two organizations. I am extremely grateful for their assistance.

◆ The Homeopathic Community Council for a grant to do three provings, two of which—Wolf and Rat—are in this book.
◆ The Homeopathic Patient's Foundation for funding to do two provings—Elephant and Butterfly—also in this book.

# HOW TO USE THIS BOOK

This book reports on the provings of eight animal remedies. Each animal section contains four parts:

- A description of the animal itself, a brief analysis of the proving, and details about the source of the substance;
- The major themes found in the proving;
- The rubrics for the remedy;
- The provers' journals: reprints of the journals the provers kept during the proving period.

**The Themes**

Each theme is documented with excerpts from the provers' journals. The numbers refer to the prover number assigned to each prover and can be cross-referenced in the provers' journals for that animal.

**The Rubrics**

Both existing and new rubrics have been printed. Following Kent's format, rubrics in plain type mean one prover had the symptom; rubrics in italics mean that at least two provers had the symptom; rubrics in bold mean that at least two provers had the symptom and that at least one patient was cured (long-term) of that symptom.

**Provers' Journals**

Each prover was required to maintain a journal throughout the proving period. These are reproduced in their entirety as written by the prover. Each prover is identified by gender and age (with the exception of the dolphin proving, where greater anonymity was desired). A good way to understand the proving is to read the journals several times.

**The Remedies**

Each of the remedies described in these provings is available in multiple potencies. Please consult the resources section at the end of the book for more information.

You knock at the door of Reality
You shake your thought-wings, loosen
your shoulders,
and open.

–Rumi

# SANGUIS SORICIS

*Blood of the Rat*

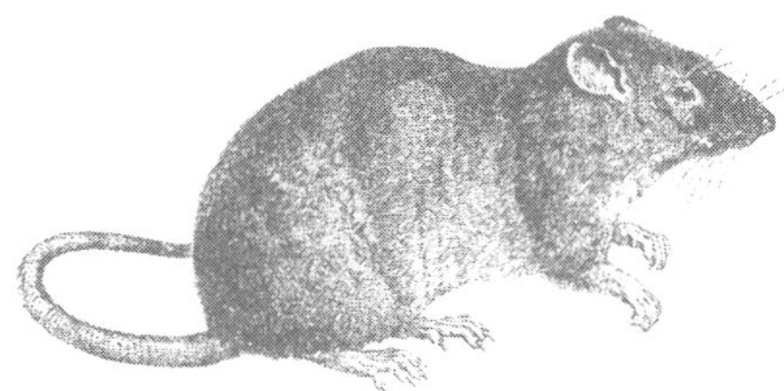

# SANGUIS SORICIS *Blood of the Rat*

Rats are among the most despised creatures on the face of the earth.

They are also among the most abundant. Half of all living mammals are rodents, and rats are among the most prolific of the rodents. One three-month-old female rat can give birth to a litter of 22 rats. Half of the litter will be females, which will in turn give birth in three months. As this process continues, 200,000 offspring will be born in one year—all descendants of the original. The human population on earth roughly equals that of the rat population. Rats, unlike most animals, flourish wherever humans thrive because their basic needs are essentially the same. Both need stored food, shelter, water and a certain amount of protection and privacy.

Rats must gnaw constantly, otherwise their incisors grow too big for their mouths. What they don't eat, such as posts on buildings and foundations, they often chew and destroy. In fact, rats cause destruction wherever they go: They gnaw holes to gain entrance to buildings and shred clothes and furniture to make nests. They also wreak havoc on large amounts of the human food supply—both by eating it and by leaving their droppings in it. They have been known to kill and eat many farm creatures, such as full-grown hens, baby pigs, and lambs. They have even been known to bite the extremities of sleeping adults, especially those with diseases that cause numbness, such as diabetes or leprosy. Perhaps most horribly, they have killed human babies.

The rat used in this proving was a *Rattus Norvegicus,* known as the Norway rat. This strain is considered to be the most feared of all the rodents. The females especially are very violent—far more aggressive than the males. They will jump at and strike each other with their front paws and bite fiercely, inflicting serious wounds. Thus, the origin of the phrase: "fighting like a cornered rat."

Norway rats build underground nests where their young are born and reared. Many have extensive, subterranean tunnels where they live their lives without ever coming to the surface—mating, feeding and foraging underground in total darkness. (**SECRET/HIDDEN**) (**DARKNESS/LIGHT**) They tend to have a short life span because they have many predators. A real old-timer might be two years old.

## Analysis of the Proving

After spending nine months pondering the complexity of this most dramatic proving, I have some thoughts to share. First I want to emphasize that, while these are my ideas on this subject (and Jessica Jackson's, who was very involved in this process with me on this proving), I heartily welcome anyone who is interested to read, study and dwell on the provers' words and then share their insights with me. I would like to know, especially, if anyone discovers other themes in these provings. This can be done by grouping quotations from the provers to substantiate a new idea or theme or by gathering data from cured cases and combining it with data from the proving. This is the main reason I include the entire text of the provers' notes in this book. The search for the core theme is a fascinating and involved process and one which I enjoyed very much. But there is much more to learn about each remedy in this book. Of course, we will also learn a great deal from the results of long-term, cured cases.

The main theme in Sanguis soricis is secrets. Listen to the words of the provers: "Didn't want to be seen...people who sit all day looking out of their secret worlds.... We were having a secret affair. Something about this stuff wants to remain hidden...." These are deep, dark, profound secrets: "not exactly insane but not your everyday, run-of-the-mill...." The second theme is sexuality: "Very sexual and passionate. I wanted men to stare at me. ...in bed with my lover. I'm not a prostitute." I believe that this remedy will be found useful for people whose pathology revolves around a deep secret that involves some aspect of sexuality. They may have buried this secret, as the proving suggests, in a "murky, dark pool" or "subterranean tunnel" in the subconscious. Steven Levine told about a seminar in which he and his wife, Ondrea, invited the participants to meet one of them in an open field and whisper their most painful, long-held secret, a confessional of sorts. He said that eighty-five percent of the secrets revealed were sexual secrets. This is clearly a source of pain and suffering for many people.

One striking theme in this proving is that of the Black Goddess. How does the theme of the Black Goddess relate to rats, sexuality, and secrets? She represents the earth aspect of the feminine. (**BLACK/GODDESS**) She is the destructive energy that kills to bring forth new life, new growth—the raging fire that destroys the forest but is the only power that can open the pine cone to release its seeds. Marian Woodman and Elinor Dickson in *The Fire Within* says: "The Goddess is the life force in matter.... She always carries authority. She guides...and acts with absolute clarity. The death that the Goddess brings is the transformation of the three poisons: lust, anger and ignorance." (**CLARITY**)

Kali is the Hindu name for the Black Goddess. In *Sacret Sexuality,* by A.T. Mann and Jane Lyle, Kali is described as " 'black as the limitless night sky.' " She is thought to represent the deepest and darkest aspect of the divine feminine. She is the embodiment of all that is hidden, mysterious, and sexual. She is the great mother—the patroness of virgins and prostitutes alike. She is fierce in her search for the truth and is the transformer of all that is linked to deception. "Kali dances and laughs with abandon, intoxicated with the mystery she is," say Woodman and Dickinson. (**DANCING**)

The scapegoating of female healers and midwives in the 14th century was largely an attempt to control feminine energy. This impulse later evolved into the witch-hunt massacres of the 1700's. As a result, women learned that hiding their powers of divination and intuition was necessary for survival. (**CLARITY**) This in turn resulted in the suppression of other important aspects of their creativity. One of the most important of these was their sexuality. (**SEXUALITY/SENSUALITY**) A woman could be holy only if she were nonsexual: a cloistered, ascetic nun, for example. Female saints from this period had remarkably severe attitudes towards the body. Long periods of fasting, scourging, and physical chastisement were the rule. Kali was shut away at this point in history.

During this time, only the White Virgin Goddess was allowed to be worshipped. The Black Goddess was exiled into the subconscious, and with the exile came the revenge of the rat—the black plague. (**BLACK/WHITE**) The plague was transmitted from one rat to another via the intermediate host, the flea, which then transmitted it to humans. (**DIRTINESS/CLEANLINESS**) During the mass hysteria of the plague, the only defense of the healthy was to quarantine the afflicted. (**HIDDEN**) Fifty percent of Europe's population perished. In fact, it is estimated that rat-borne diseases have killed more human beings than all wars combined. Only now in the years right before the end of the millennium, do we see a shift in attitudes toward the body, feminine power, spirituality, and the color black. Our capacity for seeing the wholeness in the polarity—male/ female, black/white, sun/ moon—is starting to develop. Only with this willingness to see and accept all that is—as it is— will the Goddess be satisfied.

The number seven which came up in this proving ("..it's very important...seven petticoats") also seems connected to the rat and the theme of the Goddess. In his book, *The Art of Life by Number,* Jerry Terranova states that seven symbolizes an honest inquiry into the self. He says that fear and secretiveness keep us in isolation because we have the belief that there is "some deep dark horrible thing that (we) must keep running from." (**SECRET/HIDDEN**) What we are really searching for is the truth. (**CLARITY**)

**Proving Synchronicities**

Several interesting events occurred in connection with this proving. During the proving meeting, just as we were discussing the core dreams and feelings brought up by the provers, the phone rang. It was a man from a pizza parlor where one member of the group had just gone to place an order. He wanted to ask this woman out on a date. She just happened to be the prover who wrote: "I wanted men to stare at me." Sexuality seemed to pervade this proving.

Another very interesting confirmatory of the proving was an event that happened to Jessica Jackson. A few days after the proving, she was at an antique fair where she met a friend who was selling at one of the booths. The friend, unaware of the proving, said she had something special for Jessica and presented her with a small statue of a black goddess figure riding on the back of a large, black rat. In Hinduism the rat is considered the most powerful of the demons. Ganesha, the great elephant-headed God, rides on the back of the rat. The rat has the responsibility to care for its holy charge and look ahead to problems they might encounter.

Another synchronicity occurred during the proving and the analysis when mice invaded our cabin; it took us months to get rid of them. At the same time, squirrels, who are members of the rodent family, chewed through our telephone lines (at a replacement cost of $1500). Meanwhile, a very large rat took up residence in our garage. These were first-time events for us.

The final and most frustrating event was the effort it required to get this proving typed and analyzed. Everything remained hidden. (**SECRETS/HIDDEN**) The computer wouldn't turn on, the printer wouldn't print, and so on. Most amazing of all, when we finally got everything typed and printed, we discovered significant gaps in the typed pages. What was missing? The section of the transcript from beginning to end containing the dreams about the Goddess was simply gone. Does the Goddess wish some of these things to remain a secret? Make of it what you will.

Clearly, rats have had a powerful influence in human history, and our destinies will continue to be intertwined for a long time. Hopefully, with this remedy, part of that influence will be a deeply healing one.

### The Substance

Due to many problems encountered during repeated attempts to obtain the milk of a nursing female rat, we finally gave up and took the blood of a hearty male pet rat (*Rattus Norvegicus*) named Cody. He is tan and white and has a minor problem with sneezing. Otherwise he is healthy and well-loved by his owner. He lives in a clean cage with other rats and is the father of ten offspring born one month prior to the proving. The drop of blood was obtained from a small nick, made by a razor, in his tail.

*Sanguis Soricis* **Themes**

*Blood of the Rat*

- *Secret/Hidden*
- *Clarity*
- *Sexuality/Sensuality*
- *Dancing*
- *Darkness-Light/Black-White*
- *Dirtiness/Cleanliness*
- *Feminine/Goddess/Woman/Mother*

# Secret/Hidden

**#7** Dream: Walking into a building to get away from everyone. Don't want to be seen. I go into the second door on the left and walk into a dark bar with a pool table. There are several rooms, kind of low light. I turn to the left and stoop to enter a low door that I have to get down on my hands and knees to crawl into. It feels like Alice in Wonderland. It is a long, low tunnel, glowing red. I am afraid to close the door behind me as I crawl in. Everything seems a bit distorted, and I realize that I'm afraid to close the door once I'm in there.

**#3** Feeling burdened by social circumstances, wishing for anonymity. Thoughts of homeless people who sit all day looking out of their secret worlds...reminds me of the far-out fancies and realities of the people who live underground in New York City, not exactly insane but not your everyday, run-of-the-mill fancies...wanting to be separate, not merged into regular society.

**#8** Didn't want to be seen, would stay in the shadows.

**#2** Feel like I don't belong or fit in anywhere. All I wanted to do was go off into the woods with the dog. A strong feeling not to be in my everyday life at all. I didn't want to deal with life, society, and work.

**#6** Dream: ...I was with a man I couldn't have as my own partner because he was married to a conservative woman. We were having a secret affair.

**#7** Dream: I am going to a homeopathy meeting on a bizarre walkway way up high on these entangled roadways, way up in the air. Arrive at a huge gym, a stadium really, and it's all very secretive and hush-hush.

**#3** Repeating the proving remedy. Something about this stuff wants to remain hidden, and I want to find out what that is.

## *Clarity*

**#8** A goddess dream where I am suddenly out in an open field way up high. It's a whole expanse that is like tundra, desert, very beautiful but barren. My teacher is beside me holding my hand. We see a huge, huge black woman. She's looking right at me this whole time with these fiery red eyes. My feeling is that I'm being shown clarity and focus. I have no fear, and it has to do with the need for myself not to get caught in illusion or emotionality, that I need to stay clear about what the truth is.

**#4** Thinking I was back at a time when I wasn't able to handle certain things, I ended up able to handle them. I thought: "This remedy is stronger then I am, and it will do what it is going to do, and perhaps I can learn from it in some way." There are certain basic things I got reminded of. I would start thinking of things I thought would bother me, but they didn't. I was able to put them in a certain perspective.

**#7** A little bit removed, not quite detached. I was very clear, able to move through decisions. Able to function quite well. Felt clear about decisions, not involved in dramas. More clarity.

**#3** A greater strength of my boundaries—feeling solid, contracted, unaffected by others' vibrations. Feel well emotionally, stable, Taurean, planted. Feeling like a warrior, sensing great hope for the goodness in the world. Decisiveness. Resolute. Friendly feeling without judging people. Desire for a contemplative lifestyle and life experienced through the observation of coincidences. What would it be like: pure knowing, clear perception?

**#3** Meditation: To know the beauty of the Goddess is to understand mathematics, geometry, and an abstraction from the material world. My mind wants to grasp this knowing.... I know this is her [the Goddess's] fear, to be used and controlled by a purpose not her own.

# *Sexuality/Sensuality*

**#1** I wanted men to stare at me. It was the weirdest thing. I would be driving and looking for men to stare at me.

**#3** Dream: ...yellow-pink-orange sheets puffed high in a bed since my husband is there making love to me.... My husband is making love to another woman, but I don't mind.

**#3** Dream: Foreign men in expensive cars trying to pick me up. One is a judge. "I am not a prostitute!" I say. Actually I'm in bed with my lover, preparing for a trip—someplace I've never been before.

**#3** Heavy, enlarged, relaxed, ponderous. Body feels thick and heavy. Liking the way I look; flushed and rosy.

**#8** ...a vibration in my pelvis..that's new...like I'm sitting on a whoopee cushion, sense of vibration and power. All the energy dropped into my pelvis.

**#6** Dream: ...very sexual and passionate.

**#1** Dream: ...My husband and I were at a party. He was flirting with a friend of mine. Lots of sexual innuendoes going on between the two of them.

**#6** Dream: ...one student who had been driving recklessly ended up in jail. Some of the women in class were talking about him, making flirtatious and sexual comments. Saying how handsome he was and wanting to go visit him in jail.

# Dancing

**#5** Dream: Of black couple, in their early to mid 50's. They go to a very high-class bed and breakfast. It's Victorian, everything done up perfect and they're dressed to the nines. He's got on a black suit with a red handkerchief, a big, gold ring, a pinkie ring with a ruby, and a gold front tooth, just completely duded up. She's in a 1920's style, purple hat that comes down over her head with a little daisy. She's in purple with white velvet gloves. They check in, and they're very like, "ah yes," signing their name in the register, everything very proper. They get into their suite; there's a stereo system. They turn on the stereo system and it's playing music like Benny Goodman. They start dancing, I mean really dancing. This old guy is break dancing on the floor, twirling around and hops up and does one of those things where you roll back and push up, and he lands on his feet; at the end, he slides on the floor on his knees. The woman is dancing, boogie-woogie- woogie, just gyrations. It's playful, but beyond playful because it's un-afraid to totally expose that side of nature, not the least bit inhibited.

**#3** Dream: ...Below are hundreds of primitive natives painted from head to toe and dancing on the surface of the dark water. I wave and hear them say they want to help find the biggest, baddest creature known to walk the globe. They show us reams of religious texts, some religious, some ancient, that relate to the existence of this huge thing. I hear the music of a Middle Eastern, religious song before waking up.

**#3** Dream: ...I climb the ladder next to him and he asks me to dance. In dancing, I fall backwards and he holds me. I can't see how I'll get upright and rebalanced without his assistance, but I'm trying with all my might; enjoying our dance but not wanting to depend on him.

# Darkness-Light/Black-White

**#3** Meditation: Here is the Goddess, wanting to rock us in the cradle of loving kindness, but there is something dark and evil she fears, some force that covets power over us.... There's a glimpse of the darkness in me, wanting to claim her, use her, albeit with the best of intentions; the grasping arises before there's been sufficient—even much of any— awe, devotion—before there's been any wonder....

**#1** Preferred darkness to a lighted house. Reading in the dark.

**#3** Dream: Hot day and going swimming. The pool is murky, dark, and brown. I don't want to go in.

**#6** Dream: I went into the corner of a darkened room in the school with a night light on waiting for everything to calm down. I was trying different night lights to find a softer one.

**#7** Image of a very clear, white space, ready to be decorated, everything was white.

**#8** Dream: These children come out across the horizon, they're black children, look dwarfish, and they're standing there. My sense is that they have a neediness to them, a lack of sense of themselves.

**#1** Delusions: Saw hundreds of small, black bugs running across the floor.

**#5** Dream: Black couple, in their early to mid 50's. They go to a very high-class bed and breakfast. It's Victorian, everything done up perfect and they're dressed to the nines. He's got on a black suit....

**#3** Dream: White-walled, sterile clinic. My associates are simultaneously adjusting me. It feels so good.

**#7** Dream: We are watching a light show where a person way down at the end of the hall would walk up into the front of the light, and as they stand there at the end of the stage, and as they move, their body forms different angles and geometric figures breaking out from the light. There would be shapes they'd create just by moving their bodies and the light hitting it. I thought: "I think I'll go and do that because it's really fascinating."

**#3** Images of black gods and fanning plant limbs.

**#3** Dream: Baby clothes wave at me from a dark closet. Where am I going?

**#3** Dream: A man in all whites, skinhead and thick glasses, is standing on a ladder.

**#3** Dream: The light goes off in the bedroom, and a child is playing hide-and-seek from me in the dark.

## *Dirtiness/Cleanliness*

**#1** Feel dirty all the time; can't bathe or wash my hands enough.

**#3** Dream: ...He tells me to take a shower. It's a huge room with one showerhead. A young guy was there. He idolized my ex. He wanted to help me. He was kind of an idiot-imbecile. I shower, but there's no shampoo, so he pulls the soap dispenser off the wall and brings it to me. My ex calls up and says he'll come wash my back. I say, "Don't bother!" But he explains how "tightly wrapped" everything is, nerves on edge; it needn't affect me he says. "O.K.," I say. Another man comes to shower and only one shower....

**#6** Dream: ...There was one group bathroom. It was crowded and difficult to get in there to brush teeth, etcetera. There was much inconvenience, crowding, disorganization and confusion with getting even the simplest things done.

**#3** Dream: The pool is murky, dark, and brown. I don't want to go in. My husband wants to clean it with a big machine. It goes down into the water while we ride on top of it. He points up to a cloud—the Tiger Cloud, he calls it—and says it would come to rain on the pool to make it clean.

**#3** Averse to bathing. Irritated and impatient with the amount of time it takes to groom myself, washing hair, brushing teeth, etcetera—when will it end.

**#4** Things were taking too much time, e.g. flossing teeth.

## Feminine/Goddess/Woman/Mother

**#8** Dream: ...out of the left-hand side [of the horizon] comes a huge, huge black woman with a really fierce face and long, curly, dark hair. She's wild, she's absolutely wild. She walks over and as she walks, the earth is shaking. Her feet are so big that, as she takes a step, she steps on one of these children. I hear the sound as the bones are being crushed under her foot. She takes another step and steps on the head of the second child. I hear the sound of the skull being split....

**#3** Dreams or feelings for Mother, not so specifically my mother but some sense of Mother as universal, my Mother, I am Mother, Everything is Mother.

**#1** I felt very feminine today, more so than usual. I felt more aware of being a woman. I enjoyed being a mom, being womanly. I felt blessed.

**#3** Dream: Of meeting a friend for lunch. While waiting for a table, many women arrive—they're not waiting—and enter to take all the seats. My friend and I are separated. Someone's holding seats by placing high-heeled shoes on the floor at each place. I find a place but am crowded in by women I don't know....

**#3** Meditation: Here is the Goddess...."What does she want?"

**#3** After taking the remedy: Image of the Goddess [appeared to me]—startled and wide-eyed!

**#5** Dream: Of a woman wearing petticoats and it's very important, she's wearing a series of seven petticoats, one inside the other.

**#8** Sense of vibration and power in my pelvis. [Female prover]

**MIND**

ABRUPT
speaks bluntly
ANXIETY; conscience, of
mistakes, over past
*AVERSION; society*
AWARENESS; heightened
body, of
pelvis, of
connection of herself to everyone in the room
feminine, womanly awareness of
*CLARITY*
COMPANY; aversion to, agg.
solitude, fond of
*separate from society, desires to be*
CURSING, swearing
DARKNESS, desire for
DELUSIONS, imaginations
animals, of
bugs, of; small and black running across floor
dinosaur; missing his mate, he is an old
insects; sees
diminished
small, he is
dirt, dirty
he is
homeless people
hunted, she is being
hunter, he is a
images, phantoms, sees
image in minds eye
black gods with fanning plants, of
*Goddess, of a*
homeless people, of
looking at her, everyone is
past, of events long
past anxious thoughts and things are present
reliving his past, he is

DELUSIONS (cont.)
- *separated; world, from the, that he is*
- smaller
  - he is
- stare, something about her makes others
- weather is a purification rite of Mother Nature

DESIRES; clean diet, a
- watched, to be
  - by men, in a woman

DETACHED
- warrior-like fierceness, with

DIRTINESS; aversion to, especially of the hands

DREAMS
- affair, extramarital
- anger
  - she cannot find car and thinks it is towed
- animals, of
  - scorpions
  - spiders
- anxious
- baby clothes waved at her from dark closet
- *child, children; about*
  - black
  - kidnapped, being
  - playing hide and seek in the dark
  - playing with
- coition; of
  - husband is making love to another woman, her man
  - saying, "I promise not to dominate you in bed any more."
- colored; white
  - everything was
  - walled, sterile clinic
- clothes; baby clothes waved at her from dark closet
- creature; existence of the biggest, baddest to walk the earth
- dancing
  - primitive natives, on surface of dark water
  - uninhibited
- danger, of
- dirty
- everything is the universal
- flood, of
- *Goddess, of the*
- hell
- jealousy

kidnapping, of
child, of a
men
old, lost and alone
watching her
light, of
mother, of
numbers, of
seven
seven petticoats, one inside the other
seven subsidiaries
*people, of*
*black*
woman, huge, wild with fierce face
pool, dark and murky
prostitute, men thought she was a
reading, about
what another person points to, but can't see it
religious songs, of singing, Middle Eastern
robbers
empty her wallet leaving contents strewn about
sexual innuendoes between her husband and a friend
shoes, high-heeled
singing
religious songs, Middle Eastern
truth, being shown the
violence
watched, being
water
flood, of a
*wild*
women
huge, black with wild and fierce face
DULLNESS, sluggishness, difficulty of thinking and comprehending
ESTRANGED; society, from
FEAR
controlled by a purpose not her own, being
looked at
*HIDE, desire to*
shadows, stay in
IMPATIENCE
grooming herself
*INDIFFERENCE, apathy*
business affairs, to
*duties, to*

*INDOLENCE; aversion to work*
company, with aversion to
heaviness of limbs, with
INDUSTRIOUS, mania for work
IRRITABILITY; noise, from
LIGHT; shuns light
reading in the dark
LONGING for; anonymity
LOOKED at; cannot bear to be
desire for men to look at her
MEDITATION
MEMORY; active; past events; for
REMORSE
indiscretion, over past
*SECRETIVE*
SENSITIVE, oversensitive; odors, to
sensual impressions, to
SIT; inclination to
and stare
SLOWNESS; morning on waking
purpose, of
SPACED-out feeling
STARING, thoughtless
THOUGHTS; past, of the
TIME; passes too slowly, appears longer
WANDER; desires to; night
home, and ranges in woods

## VERTIGO

*MOTION; from*
*WALKING; while; agg.*

## HEAD

EXPANDED sensation
cone, like a, going upward
with sensation of energy in pelvis

## HEAD PAIN

GENERAL; forenoon; 11 a.m.
sleep; amel.; from
sleepiness with

LOCALIZATION; Forehead
        - forenoon; agg.; 11 a.m.
        - eyes; above; left
    - Sides; left
            - extending; neck, to
    - Temples; left

CUTTING, darting, stabbing
        - Temples
            - left
                - moves to right
            - extending to; temple to temple

PULSATING, throbbing
    - Forehead

## EYE

PAIN; General; left
            - headache, with left sided
        - *headache; during*

STYES
    - left eye

## VISION

ACUTE
    - details, for fine
    - see even in darkness, seems to

## EAR

PAIN; General
        - right
        - morning
            - waking, on
        - lying; ear, on; agg.

## HEARING

ACUTE
    - heartbeat, sound of

## NOSE

CORYZA
    - air; open; agg.
    - constant
    - wind, from; cold, dry

## EXTERNAL THROAT

PULSATION; Carotids

## STOMACH

PAIN; General
        eating; agg.; after

## ABDOMEN

DISTENSION; sensation of
PAIN; General; afternoon; agg.; 3 p.m.
        constipation; from
    cramping, griping
        flatus; from
    cutting
        right
        afternoon
VIBRATION and power, sensation of, in pelvis while sitting

## RECTUM

*CONSTIPATION*
DIARRHEA
*HEMORRHOIDS*

## STOOL

BLOODY
    pure blood

## FEMALE

ITCHING; Vagina
*SEXUAL; desire; diminished*

## COUGH

MIDNIGHT; agg.; after; 3 a.m.
BARKING
    night
SLEEP; wakens from

## CHEST

CONSTRICTION, tension, tightness; Heart
grasping sensation
hand, like a, around her heart

## BACK

STIFFNESS; Cervical region
left
stretching amel.
waking on
stretching amel.
waking on
extending; arm, down; right

## EXTREMITIES

CRACKED skin; Fingers
cuticles
ERUPTIONS; Foot
Hand
desquamating
foot
hand
NUMBNESS, insensibility; Upper Limbs
right
TINGLING, prickling
Hand
palm
Foot
sole

## SLEEP

*INTERRUPTED*
RESTLESS
SLEEPINESS; headache; during
SLEEPLESSNESS; midnight; before; 2 a.m., until
WAKING; frequent
every; two hours

## SKIN

DRY
*ITCHING*
    bathing; amel.
THICKNESS, sensation of, and heavy

## GENERALITIES

AIR; open; desire for
BATHING, washing; aversion to, dread of
COLD; air; aversion
EATING; after; agg.
EXERTION, physical; amel.
EXPANSION; sensation of
FOOD and drinks; dry food; desires
    *meat; desires*
    farinaceous food, starchy; desires
    sweets; agg.
        aversion
        desires
*HEAVINESS; externally*
*SLUGGISHNESS of the body*
WEAKNESS, enervation, exhaustion, prostration, infirmity
    afternoon; 2 p.m.; 3 p.m., until

EDITOR'S NOTE: *Punctuation, abbreviations, and individual stylistic nuances of the original journal entries have been preserved wherever possible.*

**Prover #1 · Female · 31 years old**

**Day 1**

◆ I didn't feel anything, so I took it again the next day; I didn't wait. Then I had a strong reaction.

**Day 2**

◆ The second time I took it, I felt lazy; calm on the outside but tense inside.
I went to a burrito shop to get dinner and while I was waiting there, my right arm got numb. It kind of felt like I had slept on it, and I felt like I couldn't move it. Then I had this feeling like I had been there for a long time. I kept thinking, "God, what's taking people so long, I've been here forever." I started having like a panic attack. I couldn't catch my breath, and I was thinking, "What's going on here?" I felt like everybody was staring at me. There was a man sitting there, and I turned around and looked at him, and he just looked at me. I kept staring at him, as if to say, "Yeah, what are you looking at?" I would never do that.
When I got to the car, I had only been there for about ten minutes. I thought I had been there for at least a half hour.
◆ The other thing that happened, I was standing there waiting, and I felt like I was getting really small. All of a sudden I felt small.
◆ My energy level was poor. I actually took a two and a half hour nap that day, and I was still tired. I felt very lackadaisical about everything. I knew I had to get up and do my papers and do some stuff, but I didn't want to do it and I didn't care. I knew I had to do it, but it wasn't bothering me at all; I'm just not going to do it.
◆ I had a headache that day at around eleven o'clock which was right in my forehead from temple to temple. It was a dull throbbing pain. My eyes hurt; they felt achy. The headache lasted for about an hour and it left.

**Day 3**

◆ The next day I continued to feel like people were staring at me. I was also staring at other people. I got to the point where I was really paranoid about people staring at me. The other strange thing about it was, even though I didn't want people to stare at me, I wanted men to stare at me. I would be driving and looking for men to stare at me.
◆ My hearing was really very strong and sensitive. I had turned the phone off.
I was in the other room and I heard it ringing. I went in there and answered the phone and

there was somebody there and I heard it ring. My hearing has been really great since then.
◆ I was actually in the house, and our neighbors are all on the property line so they are fairly close, but I heard their kids in their house playing. I thought it was my kids in the other room, but it was actually their kids!
◆ That night I woke up at 3 a.m. coughing, a dry nonproductive cough that sounded kind of like a bark. I coughed for about a half hour and then it stopped and I just went back to sleep. It just woke me right up, and I coughed and it was gone.

**Day 4**
◆ I felt very feminine today, more so than usual. I felt more aware of being a woman. I enjoyed being a mom, being womanly. I felt blessed. I was just taking everything in. For instance, I noticed our apricot tree; I went into this type of meditation about how the apricots feel, how they smell. It got very sensual. How they would taste and what it felt like to pick them. The whole thing was very involved.
◆ Colors seemed brighter to me. I was also very determined and efficient.
Energy level was O.K., but I had a very definite lull period in the afternoon throughout the proving, especially between 2-3 p.m.
◆ I preferred to have the lights off in the evening. Normally have all the lights on in the house, but I noticed that I wasn't doing that at all. I was even turning off my kids' night light. I said "oh forget it, they don't need it." Even reading in the dark.
◆ My hearing is great. Woke up the following morning with a terrible stiff neck on the left side. Worse turning left, better turning right and stretching. It felt better in the evening. My skin got very dry and itchy. The skin on my foot peeled.
◆ Unrefreshing sleep felt extremely tired, almost hungover. When I first woke up, took me almost a half hour to an hour, then seemed to be O.K. after that.

**Day 5**
◆ Snappy today. If things don't go the way I want them to, I get mad. I'm efficient and getting things done. In the morning, between 6 and 10 a.m., was kind of spacey. Husband even asked me, "What are you on?" because I was kind of out of it.
◆ General energy level was still low. I feel sluggish, like I'm in mud, but I'm also restless at the same time. I was pacing back and forth like I'm caged. Restless, but still felt kind of sluggish at the same time.
◆ My nose was watery. Clear coryza, almost continuous. Worse in wind and outside. Had a lot of vaginal itching. Sex drive was O.K. but not great.
◆ Dream: My husband and I were at a party. He was flirting with a friend of mine. Lots of sexual innuendoes going on between the two of them. I asked him if he was attracted to her, and he said, "Yes, I'm attracted to her face." I felt hurt and jealous in the dream, but I didn't say anything.

**Day 6**
◆ I worked the night before and I was very busy. The woman I was working with at the hospital tried to have me take over a lot of her duties to her patients. Normally, I really wouldn't say anything and just kind of do it, but that night I went up to her and said, "No, you're gonna have

to do your own work." I left and left her at that. She ended up having to do her own work.
◆ I still feel efficient. I can handle things, whatever they may be.
◆ I had a delusion that I saw hundreds of small black bugs running across the linoleum in the bathroom.
◆ I felt that everyone is staring at me. Fear that everyone is looking at me.
◆ Nose continuing with the watery coryza. I desired starch. I actually wanted to eat Bisquick dry. I was looking at this Bisquick thing, thinking: "God, that looks good."
◆ My abdomen feels bloated, feel like I'm just about to start my period.
◆ Skin remains dry and itchy.

**Day 7**
◆ I feel heavy and sluggish. I don't like it. I'm irritable and have no energy.
◆ My nose is still running.
◆ Skin dry, peeling on my hands now and on my feet.

**Day 8**
◆ I have been very blunt lately. I'm straight to the point. When talking to someone I know and I didn't like the subject matter, I said: "Listen, I don't really care. I don't feel like talking about this, and I don't give a shit." This is very unusual for me.
◆ I still have very low energy. My head, I felt dizzy and shaky off and on throughout the day, especially when I was moving or walking.
◆ I had a friend actually call me up and say, "Please drink some coffee," and I said, "No, I need to find out what happens," and she moaned.
◆ On one hand I kind of liked being blunt, and on another I didn't. I have a brother I've been talking to who's going through some things, and I was almost too blunt, I think. I kind of sent him over this edge that I shouldn't have.
On that hand it wasn't good. I also noticed I was swearing a lot and that's kind of still stayed with me [laughs]. I keep trying to lose that part.

**Day 9**
◆ Much less irritable. More patience today. In a better mood overall. Feel more calm.
I feel dirty all the time. I can't bathe enough or wash my hands enough.
◆ Energy level is still poor but a little bit better.
◆ Hearing very sensitive to noise. Noise bugs me.
◆ Sex drive low.

**Day 10**
◆ I feel restless and agitated, like I'm in hurry to do everything.
◆ Abdomen bloated and uncomfortable last two nights from 9 p.m. to about 10:30 p.m. Some cramps.
◆ Sex drive remains low and I'm not liking that.

**Day 11**
◆ I still feel like people are staring at me, especially men. I want men to stare at me.

It's this weird thing; I look for men to look at me. I have been swearing a lot during the whole proving.
◆ More vaginal itching.
◆ Skin wasn't so dry this day.
◆ Sleeping O.K., but energy level is still low. I feel lazy.
After this, things started to go down a little bit.

**Day 12**
◆ I'm grouchy and have a short fuse. Irritable.
I started my period today, first time I've had it since February, menses normal, moderate flow, lasted five days, moderate cramping, nothing unusual other than it actually started. No other dreams except that one, and I normally remember my dreams.
◆ (PD: what would you say was the strongest feeling you had?)
The overall feeling: I had an irritable-grouchy feeling, and was tense.
Strange paranoia about people staring at me, me staring at people and being really aware of that. It was very strange. It was a paranoid feeling. I thought: "What are they looking at? I must have something on me."
◆ Overall I didn't like it because of the grouchiness. I was very grouchy and short and I'm normally not with my kids. This swearing thing; if my kids did something, I was trying to hold it under my breath, but I would just swear in front of them. I would have to go in the other room. I had a shelf in my bathroom fall on me. I came out and said to my husband: "God thanks for checking on me to make sure I was O.K.," and he said: "I knew you were O.K., I heard you" because I was in there swearing up a storm. I usually swear once in a while but not like that.

## Prover #2 · Female · 44 years old

**Day 1**
◆ Foot is a little sore since just started breaking in orthotics.
◆ Dreams: I woke up at 2:15 with a dream of a robber. I dreamt that I was in some house with stairs. He left my wallet all over the place and things were strewn apart. He had taken money and credit cards. I was worried because the next day was Monday, and I wouldn't be able to take care of it. I get so busy at work. That was my main worry; for a whole week I wouldn't be able to make the calls and wouldn't get it taken care of, and I'd lose all my money. I was really scared and have never had this dream before. I was afraid of the robber being in the house, not so much about the money, but I felt scared he would return again while we were home. I woke up scared.
◆ Restless night is sleep but woke up feeling O.K. and ready to go, Monday can be hectic. My sleep has been interrupted since taking this remedy. I'd sleep lightly and wake up every couple of hours.
◆ I had a dull earache on the right. I woke up with it and it hurt to lie on it. Didn't last very long, it happened a couple of times. It happened the next day. I haven't had this

for a few years and thought it was a really odd thing to come back, but I thought it seemed related to the remedy.
◆ Localized itching in middle of back, lasted two weeks, can drive me nuts.

**Day 2**
◆ I felt spacey, forgetful, and just want to sit still; not much umph. I didn't want to go to work, and generally I can go to work pretty well. I came home from work and wanted to space out. I did not have much motivation. Overall, I do not feel well, spacey and out of it.
◆ My right shoulder started aching a lot for two days. I've had a little bit of bursitis, but not for a long time. On the third or fourth day, my fingers started aching a little bit on the right hand. That didn't last but a day or two. I've never had that before. The shoulder a little bit, but not the fingers.
◆ Stomach—I started to have more gas, which is unusual in general. It lasted three or four days, and I think I craved sweets for a day or two. We had cake at work and I had little willpower. I like to eat the icing.
◆ 8 p.m.—After talking to a few of my friends who were depressed, needed reassurance and were taking care of a sick child, I went to work out for awhile. Exercise almost always perks me up, just clears the head. Then came home and got a phone call from another down-in-the-dumps friend and finally cleaned the house.
◆ The highlight of the day was we came in third place in our dance on Saturday and won a special mug and someone brought me mine today as an award for hard work. It was fun.

**Day 3**
◆ Did not take further remedy because the spacey feeling and forgetfulness and lack of motivation made it difficult to work. I was pretty tired and run-down.
Every day I would write that I felt really groggy, fuzzy and restless at night.
The remainder of this day I was less tired and the groggy or fuzzy feeling improved.
Went to work out in the evening to work it off and felt better.
◆ Shoulder and ear are fine, no recurrence of discomfort and no new symptoms.
◆ Right foot still bothers me with too much activity, no other specific symptoms developed during the night.

**Day 4**
◆ Overall things are fine, have lots to do but am not overwhelmed.
My energy seems pretty good.

**Day 5**
◆ General—Energy O.K., busy day at work.
◆ My mood was fairly level, a little sad, and no real excitement for awhile. Things are pretty routine, but feel like I don't belong or fit in anywhere. All I wanted to do was to go off in the woods with the dog. It was a really strong feeling. I would look up at the mountain, and it was kind of funny because I knew it was the remedy, but it was a very strong feeling not to be in my everyday life at all. I didn't want to deal with life, society, work and all the hassles. Everything felt overwhelming. I just wanted to go into the

woods. Very strong, this attraction to the woods. I wanted to hang out there, live there and get away from everything.

◆ GI—I had a sharp pain in the right lower quadrant for a few hours. It began around 3 p.m. and was very uncomfortable, constipated (NS) and had lots of gas. Finally around 6:30 and 7:30 p.m., I had a bowel movement and released gas and felt better by 8:30. I had noticed that my bowels had changed. Besides the gas, I became a little more constipated, which is unusual. My bowel movements started changing; I wouldn't have one for a day, than I would have two. This was different.

◆ Dream: I woke up around 1:45 a.m. and dreamt that our clinic was robbed. I went there one night and saw a car in the parking lot and no one in sight. I went downstairs to investigate and upon returning to the main floor saw my wallet and its contents strewn on the floor. Heard voices and hid while calling the police on a cellular phone ( I do not even own one). I woke up feeling disturbed and once again anxious and like I did not fit in anywhere.

**Day 6**

◆ Fair, weary, would like a break. I feel alone and disillusioned and tired of working so hard.

◆ Hamstring pain (OS) returned and I had trouble sitting. Also, last week before the remedy, I experienced stiffness in right fourth and third digit at PIP joint.

This returned today in fourth PIP joint.

◆ It's as if this remedy took a bunch of my old symptoms which had improved and brought them out again.

**Day 7**

◆ Went for a run with a good friend and our dogs. She helped me work through an issue about growing apart from a friend of mine. At first the issue reinforced my feeling of being isolated and left out (except for work), but after our conversation, I felt worlds better and was able to process the situation and not hold onto it.

◆ Unfortunately, I still am stiff and my knees and right foot hurt more than ever. Seems like I've lost anything I gained with therapy and previous remedy, less energy, eyes still itchy, medial aspect.

◆ Overall after one week on this remedy, I feel it was a setback. It made me tired, spacey, forgetful, lackadaisical, inefficient and caused most old symptoms to return (eyes itchy, urinary frequency, stiffness and discomfort in hamstring right and left, and marked difficulty sitting for over 30 minutes). Also interfered with sleep; would wake up every two hours.

**Day 8**

◆ Beginning to feel more relaxed. This is Memorial Day weekend. I have time to work on cases and get stuff done. Planted flowers today. It is a sign and a hope for spring. Finished my cases and busy work, yeah!

◆ Energy—Pretty good, seems like the effect of the remedy wore off.

Appetite—pretty good.

No dreams remembered.

◆ Sleep—fairly good, stayed up late reading a book.
◆ GI—urinary frequency. Second bowel movement of day, which is unusual at night, I had bright red blood. This was another reason why I antidoted the remedy. The blood poured right out and I've never had that either before or after. It surprised me. It was not associated with constipation. I thought, I have to get rid of this. It wasn't clotty and I didn't have a hemorrhoid or anything to attribute it to. It was bright red blood, just that one bowel movement, one evening.

**Day 9**
◆ I woke up a little groggy, tired, mild, dull headache, no real zip since took the remedy. I am much more forgetful. Relaxing day, I do not feel like working. This is unusual and a pretty big pain considering I have tons of work this week and homework and an out-of-town conference. I feel a little overwhelmed.
◆ Right foot especially sore. I was kind of stiff today and did not run well.
Vague headaches, mid-forehead, which made me sleepy; felt better after sleep.
◆ At the end of this day, I felt the need to antidote because it was so difficult to function, specifically care for patients or even to get up in the morning. I did not have my usual enthusiasm for life and felt dull, blunted, with lack of energy. My sleep has been greatly affected and I wake up every two hours or so.

**Day 10**
◆ Although remedy was antidoted, I will mention some different symptoms (specifically new):
◆ My period began 6/5 with no cramps, no breast tenderness, usually I'll have a little of this. Also, insomnia premenstrual, which has been a chronic problem, was much worse; in fact my sleep pattern is way off since taking the remedy, waking frequently and sleeping too lightly. Also, became very dizzy twice at beginning of menses while exercising (running)—never had this before.
Many old symptoms that had been improved with homeopathy returned.
◆ Still have itching mid-back.
◆ My overall feeling was fuzzy and groggy, not sharp and not motivated. If I felt like that all the time, I would want to take Prozac. It was a distinct departure from my usual state.

**Day 11**
◆ Mind Emotions—no real change today, relaxing day, family celebration of grandparents' 50th wedding anniversary, and we drove to the valley Saturday and home Sunday.
◆ General—I was tired after the event, driving and staying up with an old friend.
I felt kind of weary, went to bed a little earlier.
◆ I was O.K. before I started this. The experience wasn't very positive. It made me feel fuzzy and groggy the next day right off the bat. I antidoted on day eight because I didn't feel with the program. I felt very lazy. Normally I would be able to stay up late and do my homework and plod through things, but I just didn't have it. The thing that made me feel better was if I went out for a run or walk. I felt better with exercise. It would clear my head, but generally my head was fuzzy.

**Prover #3 · Female · 41 years old**

**Day 1**

◆ 9:35 p.m.—1 capful of substance.

◆ 11:30 p.m.—heavy, enlarged, relaxed and sleeping heavy on my back, without a pillow, a pillow is too high, Images of black gods and plant limbs crossed or fanning. I sense my vital force taking inventory at the usual trouble spots, my lower abdomen, right leg, a tricky tooth...big, heavy, ponderous.

◆ 4:30 a.m.—dreams or feelings for Mother, not so specifically my mother, but some sense of Mother as universal, my Mother, I am Mother, everything is Mother.

**Day 2**

◆ Dream: Of impatience. Clients wanting to come in and shoot the breeze. There is an elderly fellow lazing around on the treatment table. I tell him, irritably, that he has to leave, make an appointment and come back. I go to lunch with my telephone, only imagining I would use it too far from the base. Had lunch in a fancy house turned into a restaurant. I'm drinking a beer—a beer! I never drink beer at lunch. A good-looking guy is watching me as my chair, with me in it, begins to wander. I meet a child and play with her until I realize time's awasting—where's my lunch? I'll be late for my next appointment.

◆ Dream: One hot day and I decide to go swimming. The pool is murky, dark, and brown. I don't want to go in. My husband wants to clean it with a large motorized piece of equipment; it goes down into the water while we ride on top of it—then we are riding down Center St., going and coming back. He points up to a cloud—the tiger cloud he calls it—and says it would, could come rain on the pool to make it clean. At the corner, a man waves at me. I don't know him, but my husband tells me his story—neurological problems and a singer with a blues band.

◆ Dream: A family in my office—the entire family. This family is chaotic and out of control: The kids don't behave, the father has no power and the mother is mindlessly controlling. They've been to the zoo. I ask no one in particular since I'm finishing up a chart: "What was your favorite animal?" When he says, "foxglove," I'm confused and wake up.

◆ My body feels heavy, especially my head. I'm more sensitive to sound; irritable from it. Scratching myself feels so pleasurable. Mantra comes very slowly.

Slowness, especially at the beginning of a task. Image of the goddess—startled, wide-eyed! Getting dressed: keep it simple, make it direct, something of the soldier's uniform, wanting it ironed, crisp!

More interest in the finer details of things—how they are close up.

Massage: my skin feels thick, body feels thick, heavy.

◆ Feeling heavily weighted by my circumstances in society, wishing for anonymity where no one knows me; longing for something unfamiliar but too heavy to get there. In spite of this feeling, I'm having pleasant and cheerful conversations with acquaintances I might usually shun because their energies are so demanding. Rather than being sucked by them, I'm sensing a greater strength of my boundaries—feeling solid, contracted in myself, unaffected by their vibrations.

◆ Killed a bunch of ants this morning making their way into the house. Normally would have ignored them or sprayed with citrus stuff, but couldn't bear the thought of its smell so I stamped on them with my feet—this is either a symptom of lack of feeling or adverse to odors? Anyway, found one crawling on my neck at last appointment, and I'm feeling every little hair that touches my neck or face with great sensitivity now.
Not inclined to wear makeup as usual—looking flushed, rosy without it, liking the way I look.
◆ Husband says I was irritable and "jerky" in my sleep like I used to do—meaning I was rocking, rocking my hips like I used to do to get to sleep when I was upset. (A friend or family member?) wants me to write about playing the piano which she's never heard me do, nor has my husband: "I didn't know you could play piano?" I think it's a coincidence because I've wanted to learn "That's Amore" for some time and finally got the music today.
◆ I'm skeptical about having much response to the remedy so far. My skin has been more sensitive, the itching has gotten worse. Left-sided pain is worse and more focused in the left eye, temple. The heaviness seems to persist—could it be the relaxation from the intensified Tai Chi? Generally, I'm feeling very well emotionally, stable, Taurean, planted.
◆ Irritated and impatient with the amount of time it takes to groom myself, washing hair, conditioning hair, shaving, braiding, brushing my teeth—when will it end? I usually don't do these things this late but am already in bed asleep—why am I still awake? Why is there more yet to do? Bathing has decreased the itching plus reminded me of circulatory phenomenon at Tai Chi and working no harder—it seemed—than I could feel my pulse hard and fast at my carotids. While in the hot bath I could hear my heart beat. Tonight a friend said: "Let's do some bitterness exercises." "Bad name," someone said. "Bitter is good for the heart," I said, remembering the five flavors of Chinese medicine. In fact the exercises are bitter cause they hurt like hell. Still, I love this practice; driving 15 miles each way four times a week to get there. Tonight I told my friend I would much like to treat the kids he works with who are incarcerated (it might have been me were I a teenager now). It's complicated but I've put it out there to see what happens—drove away from class feeling like a warrior for one moment or two and sensing the (great hope for) goodness in the world. Shit more grooming to do....
◆ Dream: I'm coming home late, driving a Porsche, parking below a window lit up with yellow pink orange sheets puffed high in a bed since my husband is there making love to me, but I am down here just entering the house, tall doors, modern lines, high-glossed enamel in different peach colors. I don't belong here, this isn't my kind of house—the light goes off in the bedroom and a child is playing hide and seek from me in the dark. He's making love to another woman but I don't mind. This isn't the life for me.
◆ Dream: I'm returning from a trip and can't find my car—it's a huge parking lot. It's very upsetting, unable to find my car. I think they've towed it and I begin to get angry.

**Day 3**
◆ Mornings are not so good. Slow to start, then get some little thing accomplished and all's underway. Some sense of overdoing it, not enough sleep and more appointments than usual today. Odd weather for May, rainy and cold; chills me. Can't say I'm markedly affected by the proving—considering another dose for tonight yet I'm generally feeling so well, I don't want to mess with it.

◆ 2 p.m.—I'm beginning to wonder—if I'm proving this substance how do I stay in this state?! There's so little indecision or irresolution—things come simply, directly: now this, now that, do this, O.K. no problem, no internal dialogue arguing about the decision. I might even say that in general, the internal dialogue has mellowed and relaxed—not so noisy and contrary, maybe not so discriminating— (if I were to be discriminating about it)! Feeling especially friendly in a gentle, easy way; less judgmental with acquaintances and carefree. Feeling very open and revealing with client I really enjoy—cracking jokes with her and laughing with her when I might have been more reserved before.
◆ 7 p.m.—Now I'm definitely in an altered state: absolutely no desire for sweets and after helping (family member or friend) out with her huge plate of syrupy strawberry waffles, now I'm feeling a bit nauseous or queasy from it. Driving afterwards: I must have air, some anxiety about not getting enough air in—opening windows, turning on the fan—and it's cold—don't want cold. The weather has been a bizarre series of extremes today—all in one day: wintry cold and rainy, then warm and sunny and raining—the humidity stifling to me—now it's cold and the dark clouds are returning.
After astrology class: I can see explanations for the slowness, the longing for anonymity or invisibility, as well as the greater ease socially—explain in the motions of the planets but the thought arises: This is occurring at the proving, so the substance, if it's never been proved before, has a relationship to the current motions of the planets; the synchronicity of the proving and universal events. It comes to mind that life might be so simple and quite directly experienced by observing the multidimensional—are they fractals?—coincidences as they occur. I imagine we'd still eat and groom ourselves but the contemplative lifestyle would be rich with wonders, beyond comparison to the American routine, far beyond waffles with strawberries and cream—bringing me to the inspiration, come over me tonight, to clean up my diet—free of caffeine, alcohol and sugar, the addictive substances remaining. The thought of sweets makes me queasy—so what an opportune time!
◆ Also coincidental with this proving—at least today—is the remarkably weird weather—like a purification rite by Ma Nature: wet, cold, hot, dry, windy all in a day. Can't say much about the emotive aspect to this stuff—feels pretty detached—at the movies with (friend, family member) and I didn't let myself cry as usual—it came up but right away "but it's just a corny movie," lump went down, no tears came out. Very at ease in class tonight, even though I was dropping stuff and holding things up in a Sulfuric pursuit of a never-found quote on a very esoteric point. "Oh well," not self-conscious, nor guilty for it, but "so here's a stop in the action for a moment" and then the dance goes on. Slowing things down again... the speed returns soon enough back to the American 90's. I worried or anyway thought (worry is not it!) of high speed crashes on the freeway home. Started a prayer but it was so slow coming out my mind went to something faster. On the way to class tonight I saw the tiger cloud of my dream—the cloud to come clean the murky pool.
◆ Dream: Meeting for lunch with a friend and while waiting for a table, many other women arrive—they are not waiting and enter in to take all the seats—my friend and I are separated—someone's holding seats by placing high-heeled shoes on the floor at each place. I find a place but am crowded in by women I don't know: Two are homeopathic

students from India. I'm reading a bookmark they have brought with them. The cafe is in a bookstore and in the stacks a Finnish man, young and an employee, is saying in a loud voice to someone, presumably a woman unseen behind the shelves, "I promise not to dominate you in bed anymore." Strange place for a conversation like that I think. Back at the office, more like a white walled sterile clinic, my associates are simultaneously adjusting me and it feels so good. The clinic fills up with people. We're waiting for something to begin. A man in all whites, skinhead and thick glasses (an image of a doctor or professor?) is standing on a ladder. I climb the ladder next to him and he asks me to dance. In dancing, I fall backward and he holds me. I can't see how I'll get upright and rebalanced without his assistance, but I'm trying with all my might; enjoying our dance but not wanting to depend on him.

**Day 4**

◆ 9:10 a.m. Taking another capful of the remedy. There's something about this stuff that wants to remain hidden and I want to find out what that is.

◆ Dream last night just remembered of a bird like an eagle but not. It was standing in the clinic like a patient so we went to administer to it, finding it had something in common with the eagle but more of a gull's beak, bright yellow and it was very placid, yielding and dull.

◆ Meditation: this a feminine energy, ancient and powerful but afraid, afraid of being taken over. Here is the Goddess, wanting to rock us in the cradle of loving kindness but there is something dark and evil she fears, some force that covets power over us. We are so familiar with its form and feeling we can't recognize it; its omniscience is like the air we breathe; we can't see it but it's integral to us now. To know the beauty of the goddess is to understand mathematics, geometry and an abstraction from the material world. My mind wants to grasp this knowing, to apply it to my clients and their needs and with a sick feeling, I know this is her fear, to be used and controlled by a purpose not her own—there's a glimpse of the darkness in me, wanting to claim her, use her, albeit with the best of intentions, the grasping arises before there's been sufficient—even much of any—awe, devotion and before there's been any wonder "what does she want?"

◆ Now there's masculine energy, like an old man separating strands of my hair with withered fingers, staring at the microscopic life on my head. He's lost and alone like the old men I treat who've hung on past their wives' deaths, confused as to why, and cut off from real living, apart from the feminine, apart from their mates, but still hanging on. What would it be like: pure knowing? Clear perception. I look upon presented ideas through the medium of my mind—what's beyond—or how shall I cleanse the medium? Heavy and ponderous like an old dinosaur missing his mate.

11:20—very sensitive to the smells of last night's cooking; not my cooking, not my smells, I don't like it.

12:00—eating, like grooming, seems to take so much time and energy-all that chewing, swallowing, digesting, assimilating. How primitive! (Air and light and water should be enough.) Textures and tastes all mix together undifferentiated and lacking any excitement, no enjoyment of flavors.

Two phone calls in the last hour without ever hearing it ring—concentrating on a drawing

nothing else coming in; can't get in; totally absorbed.
9:30 p.m.—Really don't think I'm getting much into this stuff. It seems if I could just sit and watch my mind I might get glimpses of it, but somehow it's just not translating into the external work-a-day world. I think of ascetics because of the detachment from food (haven't had sugar, alcohol or caffeine today!) and appearances. I think of homeless people who simply sit all day looking out of their secret worlds, if they're looking out at all. I don't see many homeless people living where I do, but in my town this week, there was a man standing against a wall, completely still and closed in to himself. I really wanted to greet him! But he never looked up from his meditation when I tried to catch his eye. My own meditation after repeating the remedy this morning reminds me of the far-out fancies and realities of the people who live underground in NY—from the *Utne Reader* article; not exactly insane but not your everyday, run-of-the-mill fancies.
Wanting to be separate, not merged into regular society.
Looking back; memories of what was: a midwestern thunderstorm, a car I used to have. Maybe sentimental. Maybe nostalgic. More detached than either of those descriptions.
◆ Dream of taking care of my little brother—a child in the dream. We're in a metropolitan place with tremendous tall signs covered with advertisements. He's wanting to learn to read the signs but there are so many and all together its difficult to see what he's seeing to read it. Suddenly he takes off, after something he wants and I can't see him, I'm afraid he'll be kidnapped.

**Day 6**

◆ Feeling very lazy today—don't want to garden, don't want to see anybody, just want to sit and stare. Having some crazy ideas that go round and round and then some odd detail catches my eye and I've forgotten what I was thinking, completely absorbed with what that thing is—what is it called—what does it do—e.g. something on electrical poles....
◆ Smells evoke the most emotional response I'm aware of. That and the irritability with noise. One smell is sickening and irritating—another smell is so pleasant and familiar can't get enough of it, e.g. can't stand the smell of cooking food; love the smell on my hands, like linseed oil; can smell my husband's genitals from six feet away.
Slept from 2-5 p.m. this afternoon. Very happy, no can't say happy, but a great sense of relief that no one is home and no one came home till after 8, which was easy on me. Much better alone, but lazy.
◆ Thoughts seem to vanish—what was I just thinking so intently about. Image of a road coming up to hit me in the face on falling asleep.
◆ Dream: Foreign men in expensive cars trying to pick me up—one is a judge. I am not a prostitute! My sister(?!) calls me on the phone—she's screaming, thinks I'm dead. Actually I'm in bed with my lover, preparing for a trip—someplace I've never been before. I go to the Father's room to find out more. He's sleeping and shouldn't be disturbed—baby clothes wave at me from a dark closet. Where am I going?

**Day 7**

◆ Sat my usual 30 mins and 15 more—this morning—8:05 want to keep sitting—no, don't want to do anything is what I want. Sitting with this remedy hasn't been connected

really—dull, lumpish, thoughts of my house partner who's moving soon, of all the things she's wrecked, her lack of respect for other people's stuff, just does what she wants even if it means trashing someone else's thing—Lac felinum would be good. I'd rather do something violent than give her a remedy. Yell at her...some yoga would feel good—I don't want to do anything—lying around or just sitting feels fine. Sensitive to smells, earth smells are strong, odor of plant and herbs, familiar, sort of comforting. Man-made smells are awful.
1:45 p.m.—not a lot of time differentials—was it this morning, was it last night, what does it matter, had the idea that bathing may antidote this proving, while I begrudgingly took a bath because I smelled.
◆ Realizing one thing that does feel very pleasant and good lately is cuddling with my family, the three of us in a bundle—it's just heaven.
◆ Still no caffeine, alcohol or sugary things—but I ate meat for lunch, first meal I've really enjoyed since this proving. Maybe the bath did antidote!

**Day 8**
◆ Thoughts of past mistakes, thing I wish I hadn't done. Feeling I could just sit and wait for the world to come to me—it would be much safer—less chance of doing the wrong thing. Feeling guilty about these memories. Why did I ever...? Canceled my last appointment today without guilt! Another expression of the laziness I'm feeling. Don't want to do anything.
◆ Thoughts seem obsessive—round and round on a single subject of no great importance. Some realization of "karma," of my wanting something to happen so much that I haven't honored certain things I should have. In all those things I did not honor I am reaping the same effect on myself.
Understanding and practicing devotion seems paramount because it is so sadly lacking.
◆ Dream: At my husband's: a broken down place with locks I can't lock and hinges all spring loose. A community shower across the yard. I am angry for having come to this place. I dig my fingers into his shoulders. I hit him across the back. He tells me to take a shower. It's a huge room with one showerhead. A young guy was there. He idolized my ex. He wanted to help me. He was kind of an idiot/imbecile. I shower but there's no shampoo so he pulls the soap dispenser off the wall and brings it to me. My ex calls up and says he'll come wash my back. I say, "don't bother," but he explains how "tightly wrapped" everything is, nerves on edge. It needn't affect me. O.K., I say. Another man comes to shower and only one shower, I want to finish before he does but I'm stopped up at the edge of a cliff. Below are hundreds of primitive natives painted from head to toe and dancing on the surface of the dark water. I wave and hear them say they want to help find the biggest baddest creature known to walk the globe. They show us reams of religious texts, some religious, some ancient, that relate to the existence of this huge thing. I hear the music of a Middle Eastern religious song before waking up
◆ Drank coffee this morning—wanting to have some initiative, some motivation-justifying it by thinking I might measure the contrast between before antidote and after. I was only high on coffee after without much discriminating awareness. I did feel more emotive, more feelings about circumstances—more like myself in that way. Is it detachment that

the remedy has or a lack of feeling? Before the coffee I wanted to cancel all my plans for the day, not see anyone. Stay home. Do nothing. Obsess in mind, imagine.

**Day 9**

◆ Some thoughts after the proving: Definitely affected cravings—none for caffeine, not even the characteristic withdrawal headache from quitting; no desire for sugar—even an aversion. All these desires returned with my usual left-sided headache.

But what really sets me down to write now is this—I saw a king snake on the road and pulled over to watch its serpentine moves, to see it coil in reaction to a passing car then carry on across the road—watching it move into the grass. I suddenly thought, "Darn, I should have grabbed it," brought it home to live in our yard, to protect us from rattlesnakes—and then I remember the proving, the feeling of having to grasp, to possess, to own something of nature, to use it for my own purpose without regard for its purpose.

**Prover #4 · Male · 50 years old**

**Day 1**

◆ I took it at night before going to bed. While the pills were dissolving under my tongue both hands started to really hurt, all over, cramps, but they weren't cramps. They just started to hurt. I would have spit them out but I figured it was too late. I turned to my partner and said it's working, and it's not going to be so good, and it wasn't. I didn't like it at all. It made me feel out of sorts, I put irritable down for mind/emotional but it wasn't really irritability or anger, out of sorts is a better description. I just felt like I didn't want to feel this way, crummy.

◆ I had a lot of gastrointestinal complaints, gas flatulence, bloating. This was reminiscent of how I was in medical school, with that kind of pressure and always working. When I would get tired, I would get a lot of stomach-aches and complaints. That came back, it was just like reliving those years. That was a common theme, I felt like I was reliving my past, and I didn't like that because a lot of business that I had gotten out of the way started to come back.

**Day 2**

◆ I was always in a hurry, not for any particular reason. Things were taking too much time. When getting ready in the morning, there was too much to do in the morning, for some reason. Maybe I'll floss every other day. It was taking too long to get everything started in the day.

◆ I had a lot of wandering pain, leg hand elbow, but very familiar kind of pains. I wasn't sure if it was the remedy or just me. Nothing happened that was uncharacteristic of me, just things that hadn't happened in a long time.

◆ I had to go to party that my group put on for office girls of surgeons. This was to get the office girls to call you for the surgery, a salesman type of thing which I despise, but I went. I was pretty sociable and I mingled well. I didn't think I was able to do it but I did it pretty well. Another theme of the remedy was that I seemed to be able to do O.K. Even though I would think I was back at a time when I wasn't able to handle certain things, I ended up being able to handle them. So that was good.

**Day 3**

◆ I was always worse eating, which is awful for me because I love to go out and eat, but I couldn't. If I didn't have a stomachache I'd get one, or I'd get bloated or already be bloated. I had a lot of that stuff.

◆ I had a dream but I can't remember, I tried but I couldn't.

◆ I had hemorrhoids, like I had some time ago, constipation diarrhea kind of things. Stool has been somewhat abnormal since I took the remedy, not as regular as usual.

◆ Started craving meat, haven't done that in years. Wanted hot turkey sandwich, was going to have one but never got around to it, but I was planning on this sandwich.

**Day 4**

◆ I felt separate from people. I felt at a party that I was being cold-shouldered, which I was, but I really felt it. I felt that again at other times, which brought my mind back to other times in my life when I felt like that. I did a lot of that. Driving down street and see certain way that light hit something and would remind me of something in my childhood. I didn't mind. I thought this remedy is stronger than I am and it will do what it is going to do and perhaps I can learn from it in some way.

**Day 6**

◆ I had dinner with a friend and his wife. I felt badly for not being more successful, an old feeling, like when I dropped out of high school as a teenager.

◆ I realized that I'm still here, like the Paul Simon album, I'm still crazy after all these years. I realized that I became aware that I was still here even though a lot of years have gone by since I was sixteen or twenty. There are certain basic things still there that I got reminded of, but I figured it was O.K., I'm still standing kind of still, very basic.

**Day 7**

◆ I feel very much like I'm reliving my past, many aches and pains that remind me of the past. I have been thinking of the past, what my life used to be like, things I don't want to relive. A person I don't want to be, but I AM. I think I can learn from this remedy.

I would start thinking about things that I thought would bother me but they didn't. I was able to put them in a certain perspective. It wasn't unpleasant and there were moments when I suspected that it could have turned unpleasant but it didn't. I thought that was good.

◆ I have felt physically pretty strong and mentally somewhat energized, focused. After all these years, I find that more is still in there. It's nice getting reacquainted, getting in touch.

◆ I got a sty in my left eye, I had one of those years ago. This was unusual for me. I had been bike riding all day, felt that my eye was irritated. Partner said it was a little red. When got home it was a sty, it was all ready to be ruptured. I thought that was kind of quick to find a sty that was ready to rupture. Woke up in the morning and it was already gone. That was fast, a sty to come and go so quickly.

**Day 9**

◆ I caught cold, my summer cold, which lasts a long time when I get them. It cleared up quickly, surprisingly fast. I had a stuffed nose with drainage, sore throat, went into chest. Still a little hoarse but main symptoms cleared up.

**Prover #5 · Male · 42 years old**

**Day 2**

◆ The day after the remedy, I had a dream that I was a corporate lawyer involved with a company. I was trying to protect the company from conflict of interest by creating subsidiaries, one subsidiary inside the other, seven of these. It was very important that it had to be seven.

**Day 4**

◆ Dream: There was a black couple, in their early to mid 50's. They go to a very high-class bed and breakfast place, it's Victorian, everything done up perfect and they're dressed to the nines. He's got on a black suit with a red handkerchief, a big gold ring, a pinkie ring with a ruby, and a gold front tooth, just completely duded up. She's in a 1920's style purple hat that comes down over her head with a little daisy. She's in purple with white velvet gloves. They check in and they're very like, "Ah yes," signing their name in the register, everything very proper. They get into their suite, there's a stereo system. They turn on the stereo system and it's playing music like Benny Goodman. They start dancing, I mean really dancing. This old guy is break dancing on the floor, twirling around, and hops up and does one of those things where you roll back and push up, and he lands on his feet; at the end, he slides on the floor on his knees. The woman is dancing, boogie-woogie-woogie, just gyrations. It's playful, but beyond playful because it's unafraid to totally expose that side of nature, not the least bit inhibited.

◆ Dream: A woman wearing petticoats, and it's very important, she's wearing a series of seven petticoats, one inside the other.

◆ Dream: I have to go to hell; not all that upsetting. There are three levels, I only have to go to the first level of hell. I am relieved because this is the level of annoyance, not really torture, it's not painful. It's more like there's more mosquitoes than usual. It's not really bad, so I'm really relieved. I got out pretty good, all things considered.

**Day 8**

◆ I repeated the dose about six days later to see if I'd get anything else.

◆ Dream: A flood on our street. I'm going down our street, working out a plan so everybody can get out of the street safely. It's just enough danger to enjoy it, not enough to be really scared. I enjoy the drama.

◆ That night I write, my right knee is killing me. That whole week up until now my neck had been extremely stiff. Often I will have some stiffness in my neck, but this is more than usual. Especially for sleeping at night, especially sleeping on the left side, never had this symptom before. I had to switch to an orthopedic pillow because I'd be sleeping on my side and have this terrible cramp and stiffness that would go down my right arm. It was altogether unpleasant and hasn't stopped yet.

## Prover #6 · Female · 41 years old

It didn't effect me at all in my daily life. Usually after I take a remedy I feel something, some little buzz or something. I had a dream the night I took it, but I don't know if it's related because it's not that far-fetched from something I could have on my own.

**Day 1**

◆ Dream: A homeopathic school with a dormitory. Most of the people in our class were there. It was somewhere in England or France because there were old stone buildings, cobblestone streets and windy roads. A lot of new students. Some new male students got drunk and drove school vehicles around campus. We had a real campus with real vehicles, dorms and big rooms. It was at night, they were driving around, fast and reckless, doing a lot of damage. Eventually the police were called. One student who had been driving recklessly ended up in jail. Some of the women in class were talking about him, making flirtatious and sexual comments. Saying how handsome he was and wanting to go visit him in jail. This same man had made woven metal and wicker furniture which the school had purchased. During all the reckless drunken activity, I was trying to find a place that was safe and quiet, away from all the craziness. I didn't like what was going on, wasn't comfortable with it, and didn't feel safe. I went into the corner of a darkened room in the school with a night light on waiting for everything to calm down. I was trying different night lights to find a softer one. After all the reckless driving was over, the chase scene, I went to where my suitcase was. We had all come from far away. Looking for food in my suitcase. Trouble and confusion getting to the food, finding it, getting it put together so I could eat it. I fed someone else in the class who was also hungry. There was one group bathroom. It was crowded and difficult to get in there to brush teeth, etc. There was much inconvenience, crowding, disorganization and confusion with getting even the simplest things done.

**Day 3**

◆ Dose 2 taken.

Then waited four days and took the remedy again because I didn't notice anything.

**Day 7**

◆ Dream: Very sexual and passionate dream, more so than my dreams usually are. I was with a man I couldn't have as my own partner because he was married to a conservative woman. We were having a secret affair. My mother and I were at their house with this man's real children and real wife. As if we were living there or visiting. When we were with them, all the conversations were friendly; it was a platonic relationship with this man. I was being socially appropriate but knowing we were suppressing our real desires. We were all eating as a group or family at a table. I was being kind in offering assistance, help or services in more of a platonic or business-like type of way, but still those underlying desires were there.

**Prover # 7 · Female · 44 years old**

**Day 1**

◆ 6:50 a.m.—took four pellets, and actually during the first half hour my lower lip started to tremble, I thought that was really fun, I thought oh this is good, this is going to be really strong. It only trembled for about a minute and then it stopped, and I couldn't feel anything or notice anything for the rest of the day and that night and as I was going to sleep it wasn't quite a dream but in that state between being awake and going to sleep I had an image of a wounded deer falling down on his knees.

◆ I too would wake up many times during the night, which isn't usual, I can usually sleep throughout the night and I couldn't quite catch dreams. It felt like I was trying to solve problems but they were elusive, I couldn't quite get a hold of stuff.

**Day 2**

◆ My stool was very hot and I had had spicy food the night before so I don't know if it was from that or not, and I actually had, I think it was the next day, I had the same spicy chicken and I had a flare-up of a hemorrhoid that I've had in the past, and I don't know if it's connected. Spicy food can do that. It's been over a year since this has happened.

◆ Body sensations were regular, not feeling much actually. My mind felt active, like I was moving from one thing to the next but I was slow for many of the days—tired and yawning.

◆ Dream: Of a scorpion hanging on a long stick, most of my dreams were just images, they didn't have a sequence of a story line.

◆ A mild headache over the left eye, just right on the surface, not enough to do anything about, kind of dull.

**Day 3**

◆ Dreams: Images, one was in a very clear white space, like a room, but everything was ready to get decorated, but everything was white. We had the paints and everything ready to do but the space was very clear and white, and we were getting ready to do something. Then the next dream there were these musical instruments and they were all set up getting ready to play. That's interesting, I didn't put those two together. And then the next dream all my cousins were gathered getting ready to take a photo. That's interesting, my cousins all gathering for a photo in front of their house.

**Day 4**

◆ Still a mild headache. Afternoon and also for many of the days tired and yawning.

**Day 5**

◆ Dreams: Again were elusive, trying to get the details, they would leave real fast, usually I can catch more of a dream and write it down.

◆ Dream: So I'm at a party up on a hill in the country and I'm trying to get somewhere but I want exact directions but I can't get the exact directions, then I walk into a child's library, I also had a lot with children it seemed, looking for something, I'm not sure what. I'm looking for something in this child's library, wanting directions. I'm asking someone and they won't give me the details and it seems elusive again, and like there is this plan that these people are going to go on this hike with these directions and then it doesn't happen, and I wake up in the middle of the night thinking it's morning already, so I was waking several times during the night.

◆ Then I wake up in the morning at 8:35, Thursday morning with a slight headache, sneezing, a little bit of pain in the left lower leg just below knee on inside—upon walking, it didn't last very long.

**Day 6**

◆ Dream: Adolescent girl in dorm room with sliding door, which is open. Creepy man comes to the window—he is scared away by friend coming in at just the right time.

◆ Tired, yawning, sneezing. Basically I'm not feeling much.

**Day 7**

◆ 6:30—Took 15 more pellets. That dull headache kind of persisted in there, it was a slight, slight headache inside—dull, generalized, behind forehead.

**Day 8**

◆ I got my period today—so irritability and tiredness are coming with this.

◆ Can't catch any dreams—very elusive—almost like they're not there.

No new symptoms.

**Day 9**

◆ Dream: Interviewing children, I don't remember what it was about, but it was questioning children.

◆ Dream: Conference with parents and teachers, in this huge hall, big hall. There were a lot of buildings in my dreams, and a friend and I, in this huge hall, were watching a light show where a person way down at the end of the hall would walk up into the front of the light, and as they stand there at the end of the stage and as they move their body, it forms different angles and geometric figures kind of breaking out from the light. Someone would go off and another person would go on, there would be these shapes they'd create just by moving their bodies and the light hitting it. I thought: I think I'll go and do that because it's really fascinating

◆ A lot of the time I forget I'm taking the remedy, I would just feel so regular.

**Day 10**

◆ Dream: I am being shot up into the air and I kind of float down—it's scary because it's so high but it seems to be O.K. because it keeps happening and I just float down and actually it's kind of nice 'cause I can just drift, and I know I could fall but somehow I just drift down and am O.K.

◆ 10:40—stuffy nose

◆ Period starts to get heavy.

**Day 11**

◆ Dream: 6:30 a.m.—taking law boards. Obviously someone else thought they were a lawyer—too hard. Then taking medical boards—don't know the answers, anxious—after I see my uncle and aunt—she alludes to the fact that he is drunk—making silly and somewhat lewd comments....I guess this is the same dream or another one that night but I'm looking for a place to go. I ask help from a fellow student. I can't understand what he is saying. I'm feeling confused, unprepared for the exams, lost, not knowing where to go.

◆ Cats kept coming in and out all night. Partner had just gotten home from trip. I felt trapped by cats scratching and clawing—must fix it so they can't get on roof. Relations with my children have been good, smooth, fun and close.

◆ Heavy day of my period today.

**Day 12**

◆ 7:30—took 15 more pellets of the remedy for the third time, can't remember if it's the morning or evening.

◆ 10:00—feeling a bit anxious in tummy and confused in mind.

◆ Slight wave of nausea that passed, that must have been at night.

**Day 13**

◆ Dream: 6:15—here's a bizarre dream: My friend that I watched the same light show is demonstrating to a group of kids how to do a rectal exam; but she wasn't doing it on somebody, she was using a plastic balloon and her finger and was showing them how to do a rectal exam.

◆ Forgot I was taking the remedy—nothing happened, and then I just mark (on the paper) it's interesting that I mark because I didn't have any of this itchiness, but my son on that Tuesday or Wednesday came down with a terrible rash that lasted a week, it was awful. We thought it was from some grasses in a field, and it would flare up between 3-5 each day and I never even thought to mention it until everybody talked about rashes, and sometimes you say there are associations. It was awful. It lasted a long time, and he's only now just healing. He took this remedy, Sanguinaria. It seemed to help. Heat and hot and sunlight really seemed to affect it, the rash came out all over his body and then the only places it stayed, I realized after two or three days, were places still exposed to the sun, so around his neck, his face, his arms from his sleeves down. The first couple days he was wearing pants and then at the end of the week he was wearing shorts and all of a sudden the rash started coming out on his legs. I started to put two and two together, and then he went swimming on Sunday where he had nothing on but his bathing suit and the rash came out on his back, and I said, "O.K., out of the sun," and it was those hot days, it was awful, but it's on the mend. But the rash, after two weeks, is still all over, it's just not itching, it's starting to dry out. Interrupted sleep at night, couldn't catch dreams.

**Day 14**

◆ It seems to be mostly dreams that I'm catching, I have a dream that I'm going to a homeopathy meeting—on this bizarre walkway way up high on these entangled roadways way up in the air. Arrive at a huge gym, a big stadium really, and it's all very secretive and hush-hush. There was a lot of this hiding and secrets somebody else had.

**Day 15**

◆ Dream: Driving down by meadow to the water's edge and I look out, the plain goes right down the grassy field to the water's edge and I think it's a lake or ocean, and there are cars and trucks driving back and forth on the water parallel to the land. Somebody else had these people doing things on the water, and I was just amazed, this huge semi-truck went by driving on top of the water, I thought: "How can this big semi-truck float?" I thought it had special pontoons on its front and back wheels—why didn't it tip over—then I realized it was a flooded highway, that they were actually driving on the highway, but it looked like an ocean to me.

**Day 16**

◆ Dream: Big house, visiting a good friend of mine whom I had actually just seen the weekend before back in Ohio. Her sister and cousin are coming by, we're about to go on an adventure, a big caravan adventure, and this woman I haven't seen in a while. I write down that she's her usual haughty, self-absorbed self in the dream.

**Day 17**

◆ Dream: Walking into building to get away from everyone—don't want to be seen—go into second door on left—walk into a dark bar with a pool table—several rooms, kind of low light. I turn to the left and stoop to enter a low door that I have to get down on my hands and knees to crawl into and it kind of feels like Alice in Wonderland—it is a long low tunnel—glowing red—I am afraid to close the door behind me as I crawl in, everything seems a bit distorted and I realize that I'm afraid to close the door once I'm in there. That's the last dream I remembered.

**Day 18**

◆ And I was just trying to think about it before coming today, and I realized I hadn't been paying much attention to the tiredness, and usually I get regular exercise and I realize I have gotten literally no exercise since I took the remedy; unusual for me, I haven't gone for walks or gone for runs, and I was thinking it was, "Oh I'm busy," but I realize I haven't gotten any regular exercise and I haven't had the urge to do it, or not felt inspired to do it.

◆ I noticed a pimple on my left cheek—unusual.

**Day 19**

◆ Proving Meeting—wrote down to mention my son's rash and something about feeling a little bit detached; felt that some, but I was very clear, still able to move through the decisions I was making, I was actually able to function quite well, but I felt clear decisions and I wasn't getting involved in the dramas, and there were a lot of dramas going on, but I wasn't wrapped up in them and I seemed to have a little bit more clarity than the people around me on these issues as everyone was getting pushed. It didn't quite feel like detachment but it's something a little bit removed; maybe that's what it is that felt familiar when I heard others talking about that.

People finding me funny.

◆ Oh yeah, I completely forgot an appointment; I was going to meet someone and I just didn't go, which is very unlike me, although I have to say that recently I'm forgetting more than I used to, and that's very disconcerting.

◆ No sexual desire.

◆ Overall, it was interesting how many people kept retaking the remedy. I've only done this once before, but it was really strong and I didn't have to retake it; there was so much going on, it was very unclear what was remedy and what wasn't, but there is a strong feeling of similarities.

**Prover #8 · Female · 37 years old**

As I listen to everybody, I realize that the remedy had a lot more effect on me than I realized at the time.

◆ In the house that I live in, there was someone who was in their dying process and died during the course of this. After working all day, I would be up most of the night with this person often, was very exhausted because of that. Also, got the sense that my body was so heavy in the start of this, as soon as I took the remedy. It was as if I couldn't contact myself physically so I would have these urges to go out in the woods late at night. I'd go out toward the evening and I'm used to doing these long runs and I couldn't get my body to do it, and I was of course making it all because I've been working so hard, but that was very similar.

◆ Interestingly, when the remedy was passed out, I held it in my hand, which I do with things, and as I held it I felt an immediate sense of expansion. At the same time all my energy dropped down to my pelvis. My soles and palms were tingling. As I was holding it, there was a sense of expansion at the top of my head, like a cone going upwards. That has really stayed. Every time I took the remedy, that would return.

◆ I took the remedy when I got home; there was the same occurrence, just more heightened. I forgot and I let the remedy go through the x-ray machine at the airport. I felt a significant difference before and after. I called the clinic and they said it doesn't effect anything, but that wasn't my experience.

◆ The interesting overall theme was a detachment emotionally but a clarity at the depth of my person that I had not contacted before. That expressed itself during my meditation there and the retreat we had at the house, of an experience where as I was working with my breath, I had an awareness of the connection of myself, not just to the meditation teacher but to everything in the room, and to as far as I could let my senses expand, very strong.

◆ Also a vibration in my pelvis, while I'm meditating especially, but in general that's new. It's like I'm sitting on a whoopee cushion, sense of vibration and power.

◆ It was very interesting too when my friend was dying and died; my ability to stay completely focused on what had to happen and wondering why I was so detached from the situation. I was very present for him, it wasn't as if I was spaced-out at all. There was a warrior-like fierceness to it. That was also true with my dealings with patients. Even now I don't feel suppressed emotionally but I feel slightly detached.

◆ Dream: It was a goddess dream where I'm suddenly out in an open field way up high. It's a whole expanse that is like tundra, desert, very beautiful but barren. My teacher's beside me holding my hand. These children come out across the horizon, they're black children, look dwarfish, and they're standing there. My sense is that they have a neediness to them, a lack of sense of themselves. I'm feeling peaceful. Out of the left-hand side comes a huge, huge black woman with a really fierce face and long curly dark hair. She's wild, she's absolutely wild. She walks over and as she walks the earth is shaking. Her feet are so big that as she takes a step she steps on one of these children. I hear the sound as the bones are being crushed under her foot. She takes another step and steps on the head of the second child. I hear the sound of the skull being split, the sensitivity to hearing. She's looking right at me this whole time with these fiery red eyes. My feeling is that I'm being shown clarity and focus. I have no fear and it has to do with the need for myself not to get caught in illusion or emotionality, that I need to stay clear about what the truth is.

◆ I had episodes of a stabbing pain through my temples that would start at the left side and go to the right. When I took the remedy, that sense in my pelvis maintained itself. Here was this buzz and an awareness of my pelvis that I hadn't had before. Some constriction through my chest that felt like a hand was around my heart, that lasted a few hours after I took the remedy and then dissipated.

◆ I took the remedy three times, three days apart.

◆ The cuticles on my fingers are cracking and bleeding which they never do. Had an outbreak for the first time in a long time of herpes, on my left buttock. I have had this before. Itching in the middle of my back; only thing that felt good was to be out in the yard and lie on the ground and just scratch, like a dog. When the moon was full, I pulled all the blinds up in my room, had all the lights out. I didn't want any bright lights. A very acute sense of hearing. I just wanted to be outside roaming around, late at night. I was having difficulty sleeping until about 2 a.m., I could go to sleep about 2 a.m. I did roam around a little too; I would go out and walk around and take in the night air. I went out at night when the moon was full. Didn't want to be seen, would stay in the shadows. There was no fear at all, not worried about anything. Wanted to stalk, didn't matter what, but what was important was the experience of being that focused, and just the hunt.

◆ The other significant thing in terms of interactions was this sense that people were somehow after me for something. That I was almost being hunted. Slight paranoia to it. I just wanted to be out, wanted to be free of all that. There was too much neediness in the house, my friend dying and all these other people reacting to it.

# LAC LOXODONTA AFRICANA

*Milk of the Elephant*

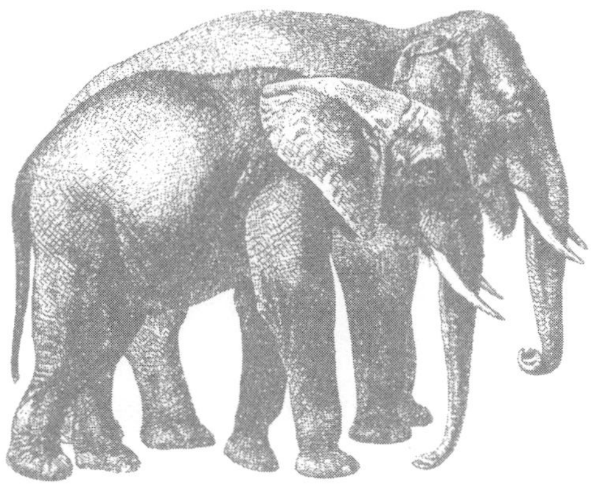

# LAC LOXODONTA AFRICANA
## *Milk of the Elephant*

The African elephant is a magnificent, gentle giant whose life is characterized by its extraordinary sense of community and cooperation. The African elephant is distinct from its smaller counterpart, the Indian elephant, an animal that is highly trainable and tamable, while the African elephant is neither.

The basic family unit of the elephant is the cow-calf group led by the elder matriarch, plus her grown female daughters and their young. The cousins and sisters of the matriarch and their offspring may also be part of the family unit. This family will range from 10 to 24 members. Except for the occasional female who may leave this family to become the leader of a new one, this clan of females will remain together for their entire lives.

Male elephants, however, lead a very different life. For the first four years, they are nurtured and watched over by their mothers. After this period, the young males assume a more tentative position in the family group. They may be allowed to remain until they are about 10 years old. However, as they become older, they grow more rambunctious—ramming and butting each other and causing great havoc. The mothers, solicitous of their new calves, are apt to boot out the wild, young ruffians at any time. Some males, however, are allowed to remain for another six years or so. Regardless, at some point the male goes off on his own for a solitary life of bachelorhood. Their solitude is occasionally relieved by spending an evening with other males in a small, temporary herd. Other than this, their life is spent eating prodigiously and searching for females in estrus.

Once a year mature males will go into *musth*. This is an Urdu word for "intoxicated," and truly, it is a state of hormonal intoxication. Their testosterone levels go up fifty fold, and their behavior becomes dangerous and unpredictable. All the other males, even the largest and most dominant, will give them plenty of room especially if there is an estrus female nearby. Females, on the other hand, are especially attracted to the *musth* male and will make every effort to solicit his sexual attentions. When the mating occurs, the entire family goes wild around the couple, bellowing, rumbling, and stomping. It is an all-out party atmosphere, and everyone gets in on the act. (This is very similar to wolf sexual behavior and the ensuing tumult that occurs in the wolf group during a mating episode.)

Another major celebration occurs yearly in the life of the elephant tribe. After the drenching downpour of the rainy season, there comes a time of lush green grasses, and the savanna is rich, vibrant and loamy. Suddenly and inexplicably, clans of all the different elephant kinship groupings (all the family members that have broken off from the original cow-calf group) come together. As many as 2,000 arrive at this festival. When they meet, it is with obvious rejoicing. (**POSITIVE EMOTION**) There is the most outrageous kissing, caressing, urinating, defecating, screaming, and trumpeting imaginable. The elephant clans socialize and browse for days, and then they separate for another year.

Elephants live to be about 60 to 70 years old. While most other animals are born with the brain 90 percent developed, elephants are born with only 35 percent of their brain development complete. This leaves plenty of room for growth and learning new information and may explain why the elephant is known for having such a prodigious memory, such an extraordinary ability to add new information to the memory banks. The quality of this memory may be cyclic rather than linear and is vital to elephants because it allows the elders, who have experienced many dry seasons, to remember where the best water holes may be and where to find the only remaining food. It may be the only factor that makes the difference between life and death for the entire clan during the worst of the droughts. Memory may be related to the theme of timelessness that came up over and over again in the proving. (**TIMELESSNESS**) One prover said, "I get this timeless, ancient feeling."

The adult male elephant is approximately 20 to 24 feet long and weighs between 12,000 and 20,000 pounds. The adult female is about 20 feet long and weighs between 5,000 and 10,000 pounds. Elephants eat enormous amounts. They will go through approximately 500 pounds of food daily. (**FOOD**) Most of their food consists of grasses and trees with berries and flowers thrown in for dessert.

One of the most outstanding characteristics of the elephant is its devotion to its young. The mother stays in constant contact with her calf for the first six months and never lets it out of her sight. The entire herd is ever watchful of the calf's every move. With the slightest hint of danger, all calves are quickly herded into the center and the adults form a protective barrier around them. The matriarch may charge an intruder or the entire herd may stampede if necessary. Under all conditions, even when there is extreme danger to herself, the female will fiercely protect her young. All this maternal devotion to the young is very similar to dolphin behavior. Wolves have much more paternal involvement in the raising of the young, in addition to maternal care.

On the savanna, elephants live near water holes in the dry season and travel during the wet season. Elephants love water and will bathe and play and loll in it for many hours. (**WATER**) They especially love muddy water, which will protect their surprisingly delicate skin from little parasites and from the sun.

Elephants provide an invaluable service to the entire animal population during the dry season by locating and digging with their tusks into the deepest water holes, thus exposing water to the surface for all animals to drink.

Elephants are highly affectionate creatures. The whole family moves as one, and the merest whimper from a calf causes them to stop and patiently wait until the problem has been solved before moving on. From playtime to the moments of greatest danger, elephants will be in constant physical contact with one another—touching, nudging, caressing, and even kissing by putting their trunk tips in each other's mouths

It could be said that the elephant is the true king of the jungle because even the lions retreat when the elephant arrives. However, elephants are so gentle when they are not being threatened, their behavior is unlike that of most kings this planet has ever known.

### The Elephant Today

One of the greatest tragedies to befall the jungle was the coming of the dreaded ivory poachers. Poaching went into full swing in the 60's and 70's, and over 100,000 elephants were maimed and slaughtered each year. Kenya alone lost one-half of its elephant population. Poachers were often local farmers turned mercenaries, who discovered they could make more money selling the tusks of one bull elephant than they could earn in 12 years of hard work on the farm. The poachers in many cases did not or could not fully kill the enormous elephant—all they could manage was to get the elephant down and quickly saw off the tusks. Many times, the elephant family would watch as their matriarch or bull was attacked for his or her large tusks. The elephant would then slowly and painfully bleed to death. In 1990, the Convention in International Trade in Endangered Species banned the selling of raw ivory. While poaching is now outlawed, it is unfortunately still rampant in Africa today. Poachers hope that someday the sale of ivory may again become legal.

Sadly, as a result of this brutal practice, almost all elder elephants have died at the hands of the poachers. This memory seems to be held in a sort of morphogenetic resonance in the consciousness of elephants in all corners, and zoos, of the globe. In Africa, it means that most elephants have experienced the trauma of seeing their wise ones viciously murdered. It has also left them without knowledgeable leaders. This was strongly revealed in the proving of elephant's milk, which produced many images of brutal beatings, violence, blood, and gore.

Elephants still can and do band together, but now it is often in scattered groups that have no family ties and are made up of deeply disturbed and frightened creatures. In a recent report from Africa, it was noted that there has been a surge of sudden and unprecedented attacks on white rhinoceroses by young male elephants. These elephants are using their enormous strength and power in uncontrolled violence against a vulnerable neighbor. Since the rhinoceros is also in some danger of extinction, there has been an official response to these attacks and the African government is making some efforts to stop the killing of the elephant matriarchs and to keep the youngsters in some sort of family grouping. It seems that one of the important functions of the elephant family is to teach these potentially dangerous youngsters how to behave properly and to use their strength appropriately. Without the benefit of the matriarch and the elderly bull's wisdom and guidance the young males have become wanton killers. This is a lesson we can learn from the animal kingdom. It seems that these enormous creatures have equally enormous emotional and social needs.

The future of the 650,000 remaining elephants is questionable. They have to live in limited space in parks and reserves that are being defoliated quickly by their voracious appetite and tendency to tear up trees by the roots. These parks are surrounded by tribal villages and farms where the elephants are clearly unwanted intruders, and they are sometimes shot for stomping on the farmers' gardens. It is a difficult social, moral and ecological problem.

### Analysis of the Proving

I found myself very surprised initially at the violent images that were coming out of the elephant proving. This was not at all what I had expected (although every proving has been full of the unexpected). It was only after I understood the current conditions in which the elephant lives that I understood how accurate the themes of **HOMELESSNESS, BRUTALITY, VIOLENCE, MURDER** and **NOT ENOUGH FOOD** have proved to be. Of course this is not the state of a healthy, wild elephant. The more natural state is also in the proving, with a lot of interest in **AIR, WATER, FOOD, FEEDING OTHERS** and a feeling of **POSITIVE EMOTIONS** and **TIMELESSNESS. THEORIZING ABOUT THE SUBSTANCE** was another theme and seems to indicate a quality of intellectual awareness in elephants.

It may be that in the near future, the only elephants to be found will be in zoos and formal "wild" parks, where people pay to ride through and observe animal behavior. As this possibility comes closer to reality, more and more humans will take on elephant energy (thus the theme, **PEOPLE AS ANIMALS**) and will need the remedy Lac loxodonta africana.

**The Substance**

A calf was born to an 18-year-old African elephant, Donna, at the Oakland Zoo in California in the spring of 1996. Unfortunately, the calf had an untreatable and severe deformity and had to be destroyed. At the same time, another African elephant had a calf but was completely uninterested in nursing her, and she was being hand-fed by the zoo keepers. Suddenly many people in different fields saw an opportunity to study, analyze and use Donna's breast milk. The biggest problem was in obtaining it. As a newspaper article said, "So, how do you breast-pump an 8,000-pound elephant?" The answer appeared to be, "Carefully."

First, Donna was isolated and then two of her legs were chained to fence posts. A trainer then crawled underneath her and put the suction cups on her nipples. The cups were subsequently attached to an electric breast pump. Donna appeared to take it all with a great deal of equanimity. The trainer said her own state of mind under the four-ton creature was not so relaxed, but she was so grateful to be able to get the milk for the new calf, it was worth it.

Meanwhile, Dave Penny, our wonderful, local, homeopathic veterinarian saw the golden opportunity to get the milk for a proving. He jumped in his car in the middle of a workday, drove to the zoo, and then zoomed to the Hahnemann Clinic Pharmacy with the tiny sample still warm and fresh. Michael Quinn immediately triturated it and then potentized it to a 30C for the proving. This was real teamwork.

Donna, herself is a basically healthy animal with some arthritis and a slight stiffness in her movements. She was wild and captured in Africa. She tends to be aggressive with other cows and is a dominant cow but very good with people. The proving of her milk reveals the deep inner story of the experience of the African elephant in the modern world.

*Lac Loxodonta Africana* **Themes**

*Milk of the Elephant*

- *Murder/Brutality/Violence*
- *Suffering/Homeless*
- *Air/Water*
- *Food/Feeding Others/Not Enough Food*
- *Positive Emotions*
- *People As Animals*
- *Theorizing about the Substance*
- *Timelessness*

# *Murder/Brutality/Violence*

**#1** I walked along the beach at sunset, and I kept thinking about the whales and dolphins and sharks and how few there are now compared to before our slaughtering of them started.

**#8** Dream: Nightmare of a military guy who was involved in nuclear war planning, and he sequentially murdered people whom he knew. I did not actually observe the murders, but they involved brutally bashing in skulls with a garden trowel. He was partially disabled and walked with a limp. He was nuts, diabolical, and there was a feeling of vengefulness in the murders. Someone else caught on to him and saw a bed filled with a pool of blood, so I have confidence he was about to be stopped. Not sure what I was doing there but felt endangered myself. He was crafty and completely ruthless. On waking I was not sure if I was a witness or actually in the story, but I was scared and was trying to figure out how to get him but not having any success.

**#4** Dream: Someone I do not know but am friendly with and I am helping him with some task. I feel he is dangerous and should not be trusted and then he turns on me and we fight using our fists. He has so much hate. I am forced to protect myself and I hit him with a broomstick ruthlessly, and he breaks his wrist and falls down. He is defeated. I think to give him Anacardium and wish someone would give it to him. The feeling is: "I do not want to fight but I have to or I will die." A friend who becomes a foe. A white trash male: scared, violent, fighting, bloody. I am scared but at the same time ruthless.

**#7** Dream: My beloved son goes off to the Crusades and he comes back half nuts, crazy on this wild stallion that is vital and beautiful and untamed. It comes running at me in this field and I have this stake and I plant it in the ground and the horse impales itself and dies. My son is very upset.

**#5** Dream: I was going to sea in an open boat. Some people walk to get off the boat willingly. A well-to-do passenger is afraid his friend is conspiring to kill him. The wealthy man kills his friend but tries to make it look like an accident: He got stuck in the air duct and died. They were anxious to cover it up and buried his body quickly.

**#4** Went to a restaurant and while we were waiting a man was pushing his way through the line. I said: "You can get by me," and he answered rudely and smugly, "Are you confident about that?" I felt a very violent aggressiveness inside, like I wanted to hurt him, kick his ass. It surprised me.

# Suffering/Homeless

**#1** ...I was listening to choral music and thinking of whales and sad about them being hunted to extinction. I started crying. Thinking about animals and our natural world in general. This is an old worry of mine but the thing with the deep sea and whales is definitely new.

**#5** Dream: At an AA meeting, in order to check in must put your tie tack in a special rack. I could not get my tie pin stuck on in the right way. They were looking for a wanted man, and he was trying to get out of the building. He befriended a bunch of homeless people, and they were to transport him to prison, but his family is in the car, and we cannot drive away because the car is stuck in the building.

**#3** Dream: My mother asked me for a remedy for herself, and I realized the remedies I had given her had worked. Her suffering is old age and stoicism.

**#4** In the restaurant I got up to go to the bathroom and the light was strange and faces seemed to come out at me. The people in the restaurant seemed stranger than normal. Plates of meat and dead carcasses—strange, anguished, unconscious people—so ugly, broken, old, diseased. Like a low realm of life.

**#4** Dream: Two old clients came and one is deeply depressed and suicidal. He is broken, from a low-class, sick, white family. The mother has been sick with cancer for 20 years, and he was her caregiver and confidant, since the father was detached from the family. Everyone in the house was suicidal. I woke and viewed the whole family a different way. Lots of suicidal feeling. Dark, sick unrecoverable.... Broken, white, low-class impoverished: no way out, damaged feeling.

**#4** Dream: (On a train) we pass my stop but it is too late to get off. Pass my old landlord's house, and there are picketers protesting against him. Lower class, poor and downtrodden fighting for redemption.

## Air/Water

**#2** Felt very tall and high off the ground. Looking far down as though looking far down to the ground. Felt very airy, high in the air. In motion, but stillness.

**#2** Dream: I was lying in bed and the air felt delicious and breezy, and I insisted on having the window open so I could feel the air—an amorous feeling.

**#1** Dream: I had a powerful dream about being underwater and suddenly realizing that I could breathe underwater and being delighted because I had finally come home.

**#2** Dream: The pilot overshot the runway and we landed in water, and I watched the jet twist and we were submerged underwater. I unbuckle and I am free. The key thing for me was being in air though we were sitting on water.

**#1** I was almost asleep when twice, I woke up with a start because it seemed like my right hand was lying in a puddle of water. Of course, it wasn't, but the sensation was so real.

**#1** Feel kind of dull in general—felt relaxed and fuzzy and dull as though in a pool of water where all the stimuli come to you through water. A pleasant sensation.

**#3** The creek on my property flooded, and I had to go out and pull plants out from it.

**#5** Dream: A window with a number of panes lying over a container of water. Eventually the panes became broken and one could see the water below.

## Food/Feeding Others/Not Enough Food

**#1** I felt a sudden need to eat—not because my stomach was growling or I wanted to taste something I like —but because I had a physical sensation in my body of being unwell from not having eaten for a while. This was not my usual irritability or mild nausea feeling. It was deeper, like hunger of the cells of my body. It is hard to explain.

**#2** Dream: My mother was in the hospital, and my father was there and some concern about eating, what we would eat.

**#2** Dream: 15 people at a gathering, a homeopathic group, and I was supplying food and feeding the group. One person ate a falafel, and I realized I had nothing left to feed them all.

**#2** Dream: D. and I had to prepare dinner for everyone—a large group. We were there only two nights, and I realized we were the only ones providing food. Usually there are five nights and each family has a turn. Someone borrowed some sesame seeds. The plate was overflowing with sesame seeds: all large and gooey, an overabundance.

**#5** Dream: I take some crackers, shaped like fish, in a pita bread, but when I realize it is someone else's, I return it to them. I realize they do not have enough food.

**#3** Bought salmon that was so beautiful. Rubbed oil on it for a long time. Into radishes. Kept walking to the fridge looking for something, and it was not there. Did this hourly. Ate ice cream. Stuck head and hand into freezer and laughed and stayed there for a while.

**#4** Dream: (Some boys and I) are on a train (and) going fast, and I want to take care of this boy and his companions. I feed them with food from my mother's kitchen, but they are greedy and grab it. White trash, broken, desperate, hungry, poor.

**#5** Dream: Eating takeout and there was not enough food.

## *Positive Emotions*

**#5** Dream: Something about going to a gambling casino and sure I would win, confident of my ability; air of detachment.

**#5** More emotional and sentimental, grateful for my marriage. Taking things more personally, more vulnerable. Loving feeling.

**#7** Felt clear, calm and centered, almost floating, singing and cheerful.

**#2** Still feels calm, high. In that ponder state it was a calm, still, peaceful feeling; even if I was in motion, I felt still.

**#3** Feel great—SPRING! Expansive feelings. Excited about my work, very creative. Writing is the best it has been. "Stuff is happening." It feels as if some big planetary change has occurred. Projects I had worked on for years suddenly resolved without me doing anything. Easy: three big projects suddenly resolved.

**#8** Beautiful sunny day. Went hiking in the mountains and felt ecstatic and out of my body, blissful and at peace. Good change of pace.

**#8** Yesterday went for a run and felt very peaceful and happy. Sat for a minute and it was very sweet, a period of not having to do anything. Communal feeling of hearing birds, smelling flowers and trees.

**#2** While waking up and still emerging from the dream, the dogs were barking and I go out to see (still in the dream state). There is a man in a leather jacket and a motorcycle. He is all happy and says he almost hit a cow in the road and asks me if it is my cow. He assures me he did not hit the cow and is very upbeat. I go walking down the road in my jammies. Felt happy and fun and not upset about being wakened.

**#3** Big party with drumming. Ecstasy.

# People As Animals

**#1** As a child I had what nowadays would be called a near-spiritual experience that went as follows: I was swimming underwater lengths—back and forth, back and forth, mesmerized by the rhythm of breath and swimming. I got to the point where I could breathe underwater. This experience really happened as a child and has never recurred. (Memories during this proving that were stimulated by a similar dream.)

**#1** ...I described myself in the process of pupating. Changing careers felt like changing from a caterpillar to a butterfly.

**#2** Vultures flying above me and they seemed high up, and I was watching them and I felt I had become them, as though I was in their body and flying with them. Felt the downward movement. Being a bird in the sky. I was playing tennis when this happened. I was leaping into the air joking, "I've got wings."

**#3** A friend made a big thing about my mustache. Said I looked like a walrus and I could dive underwater and bring up brine shrimp in my mustache; and they laughed too much.

**#5** Dream: ...there is a rustic fireplace.... I am disgusted by a cow or elk with two horns that is in the fire. Then it transforms to a human face. Theme of two again: two horns.

**#8** Dream: A woman friend had an orifice in her abdomen and she passed a stone.... This transitioned to a series of globular shapes, slightly furry like kiwis, the size of grapes. Then a tubular thing came out and it turned out to be a weasel. Shocking and disturbing. It got up and moved around. Feeling of fascination and disgust. Someone in the dream said it was a skunk but looked more like a weasel.

**#3** Dream: D. was a shiny bug in a fly's armpit. (A parasite on a fly.)

**#4** Dream: Two teenage girls naked, with a poodle. They seemed homeless, broken and yet surviving. One girl is emaciated and had large anus hole. The feeling is she had been abused, broken, tormented, no hope, doing what she had to do to live. She had an animal look in her eyes, no trust. Weary, hungry, frightened, jumping around like a primate.

## *Theorizing about the Substance*

**#1** Really aware of my heartbeat. Like my whole body had changed into a big, soft bag with my heart beating in the middle of it. The shape that comes to mind is one of those shark purses or stingray eggs. I think they are actually shark eggs that sometimes wash up on beaches. They are shiny black on the outside and light on the inside. I live on a boat and had a feeling of ocean swells. So my first thought was that this remedy was made from a sea creature.

**#2** I was sure I was a butterfly the whole proving. I do not know if I am responding to husband or not? [He was doing a proving of the butterfly, Limenitis bredowii, while she was doing Lac loxodonta africana.]

**#3** I own a lot of snake paraphernalia and I noticed it more. Picked up a romance novel while at grocery store (never before had done this), and the first line on the book jacket is that a guy gets a poisonous snake in his mouth and it killed him. I am concerned that I might be creating energy here—undue, so I will resist snake stuff.

**#3** Called the proving director: "Don't even think about the proving remedy around me, I am feeling strongly intuitive." I was sure the remedy we were proving was Puff Adder snake.

**#7** I wondered if the remedy was a mineral like a halogen.

# Timelessness

**#1** I am beginning to notice a strange sense of fuzziness where time seems to stop. The fuzziness is detached, almost hypnotized feeling. I'll be driving or writing and going through the motion but not mentally aware, kind of robotic. Not mentally aware, almost in remote control, and time seems to have stopped, as though I have been doing this thing forever. Time stops flowing the way it usually does. This sense comes and goes quickly. It is like a vacuum.

**#1** The main feeling of the last two weeks has been one of being intermittently spaced out. It is neither pleasant nor unpleasant. It is kind of like being in a time warp because my perception of time changes, slows down incredibly.

**#2** Feel filled with air—stare for long periods of time. It was as though there was a spaciousness in me where I could leave and do something like that. Time warp feeling and timeless feeling. Staring and pondering but not pondering about anything specific. I felt I was reflecting a lot. If there was a potential conflict, I could see it, but I did not feel it, sense of being unaffected by these conflicts.

**#4** My son in bed with me and I get this timeless, ancient feeling. Quiet—Deep state of timelessness, present ancient state, staring out the window at the mountains. Feel free and a lot of space around me. No history, no self but self, only peace. It feels like my cured state but does not last.

## MIND

ANCIENT; feeling
ANXIETY; pains, from
AWKWARDNESS
CURSING; swearing, curses; desire to curse
DELUSIONS; imaginations; air, airy; filled with; sensation as if
high in the
that he is hovering in
body, body parts; hand; puddle of water, in;
lighter than air
separated, body and thoughts are
clothing, clothes; not wearing
faces, sees; hideous
come out at him
*floating in air*
hunger, of; cells starving
motion, in; downward
yet feels still
naked; he or she is
people; sees
disagreeable, sees
sea; that he is immersed in
starved; cells being
tall, taller; he is
DESPAIR
DREAMS; amorous
animals, of
cattle
dogs
dogs; ear enlarged
elephants, riding on
elk
fetuses
fishes
horses
lions
rats
skunks

DREAMS; animals, of (cont.)
turtles
weasels
whales
wolves
body, body parts; penis detachable
cars, automobiles, of
child, children; abused
starving
colored; vivid
computers, broken
cooking, of
crimes
concealment of
disease
disgusting
emotions; without
evil, impending
helpless in presence of
extinction
feeding people
fetuses
fighting
food
groups
haircut
homeless; people are
homeopathic remedies
hopeless
hungry, people are
impoverished, people are
jet airplane; exploded
jet airplane; water; submerged in
mothers; old age
motorcycles
murder
violent
patients; suicidal
people, of; desperately poor
people, of; hungry
police; pursued by
relatives; dead
relatives; frail health, of
ship; going to sea in

suffering of; others of
swimming; water, in
tools; beating, with
tools; repair, using for
trees, of
*unremembered*
*vivid*
walking; nature, in
water
weaving
wonderful
DULLNESS; sluggishness, difficulty of thinking and comprehending
EUPHORIA
alternating with weariness
FUZZY; unfocused
LIGHTHEARTED
LIGHTNESS; feeling of
LOQUACITY
alternating with detachment
MISTAKES; makes, talking
wrong words, using
writing, in
confounding letters
MOOD; changeable, variable
PROSTRATION; mental exhaustion, brain fag
QUARRELSOMENESS; scolding
QUICK; to act
QUIET; disposition
REFLECTING
SADNESS; despondency, depression, melancholy
SPACED-OUT; feeling
THEORIZING; proven substance, about
TIME; loss of conception, of
*passes too quickly, appears shorter*
timelessness
TORPOR
TRANQUILITY; serenity, calmness
conflict, amid
WEEPING; tearful mood; tendency; despair, from

### VERTIGO

DESCENDING; as if
HEADACHE; with
LOOKING; downward

### HEAD

PAIN; forehead
        left
        left to right
        right
        extending to neck
        extending to neck; right
    vertigo, with
    waking, on
    chilliness, with; 3-6 p.m.
    perspiration, with; 3-6 p.m.
    shivering, with; 3-6 p.m.
PERSPIRATION; forehead
        left

### EARS

EARS; itching

### EYES

DISCHARGE; yellow
        lids, on; morning
STARING
TIRED; sensation

### VISION

ACUTE
COLORS; green; stripes
SQUINTING

### NOSE

CORYZA
ITCHING

## MOUTH

ITCHING; palate

## FACE

EXPRESSION; scowling
PAIN; bones; malar
    left

## THROAT

ITCHING
PAIN; sore
    evening
TENSION; left side

## STOMACH

ANXIETY
  waking, on
APPETITE; *capricious*
  *diminished*
  *increased*
EMPTINESS
  afternoon
ERUCTATIONS
  breakfast, after
    dinner, after
  foul
NAUSEA
PAIN; burning
    waking, after
  drawing
    upward
TENSION

## ABDOMEN

DISTENTION
EMPTINESS
PAIN; drawing; upward

## RECTUM

DIARRHEA
FLATULENCE

## STOOL

LOOSE

## KIDNEYS

PAIN; right
    morning; 5-8 a.m.

## FEMALE

BUBBLE; water or air in vagina; as if
MENSES; *early*
    *heavy*
    *clots*
SEXUAL DESIRE; decreased

COUGH
DRY

## CHEST

AWARENESS; heart's beating; body is soft bag, as if
CONSTRICTION
PAIN; pressing
        sitting stooped
        standing aggravates
PALPITATION; tea, after
PERSPIRATION; axilla, right

## BACK

PAIN; cervical region
    dorsal region
        scapula
            left
    crampy
        dorsal region, scapula
            left
        sacral region
    straightening of the back

## EXTREMITIES

- CRAMPS; thigh
- HAND; sensation, in puddle of water
- PAIN; fingers; third
    - joints
    - left
- RESTLESS
    - hands
    - feet
- TREMBLING; legs
    - afternoon
- WEAKNESS; legs
    - afternoon

## SLEEP

- CATNAPS; *refresh*
    - afternoon
- *DEEP*
- FALLING ASLEEP; difficult
    - thoughts; rush, flow of
- REFRESHING
- RESTLESS
- SLEEPINESS; morning, waking, on
    - afternoon; 3-4 p.m.,
- WAKING; frequent
    - morning; dawn, at
    - 3 a.m.

## GENERALITIES

- MORNING; waking, on
- EXERCISE; aversion to
- FOOD and drinks
    - alcohol; desires, increased
    - chocolate; desires
    - fish; desires
    - fruit, fresh juicy; desires
    - indistinct, knows not what; desires
    - melons; desires
    - salmon; aversion
    - spices; aversion
    - sweets; desires

FOOD and drinks (cont.)
    tea; aversion
    vegetables; desires
        cucumber
        radishes
    wine; desires
    yogurt, kefir; desires

HEAVINESS; internally
    externally
LASSITUDE;
    lie down;
        before dinner, must
        5 p.m.
PAIN; cramping
SHIVERS; as if air blew over me
STOOP SHOULDERED
WATER; playing in; amel.
WEARINESS
    afternoon
    8-9 p.m.

## JOURNALS ............................................................ *Lac Loxodonta Africana*

EDITOR'S NOTE: *Punctuation, abbreviations, and individual stylistic nuances of the original journal entries have been preserved wherever possible.*

**Prover #1 · Female · 32 years old**

A lot going on: leaving job of 10 years and new one starts in 2 weeks.

**Day 0**

◆ Took the remedy at 10 p.m. Really aware of my heartbeat. Like my whole body had changed into a big soft bag with my heart beating in the middle of it. The shape that comes to mind is one of those shark purses or sting ray eggs. I think they are actually shark eggs that sometimes wash up on beaches. They are shiny black on the outside and light on the inside. I live on a boat and had a feeling of ocean swells. So my first thought was that this remedy was made from a sea creature. Deep sea experience. Totally immersed in the sea. Otherwise no symptoms, I slept deeply and peacefully without dreams which is unusual for me.

**Day 1**

◆ The next day at noon I saw stripes or bars of green on my white shirt mostly from my left eye. Only lasted five minutes.

◆ Later in the evening: Out to dinner with a friend and she went to the bathroom. All of a sudden I had the feeling the room was filled with water and the customers were submerged—a deep sea restaurant. Then I began to remember fragments of a dream I think I had—about being underwater and suddenly realizing that I could breathe underwater and being delighted because I had finally come home. It was a powerful dream. As a child I had what nowadays would be called a near-spiritual experience that went as follows: I was swimming underwater lengths—back and forth, back and forth, mesmerized by the rhythm of breath and swimming. I got to the point where I could breathe underwater. This experience really happened as a child and has never recurred. Finally the waiter brought us a fish dish instead of the eggplant dish we had ordered. I was also reading a Lawrence van der Post book of whaling stories—horrific!

◆ Shape recurring in mind's eye: hollow shape with pointy ends. Filled with eggs: skate or shark egg container.

◆ Menses started that day 2 days before the full moon, a little early for me. I also noticed a huge ring or corona around the moon tonight.

**Day 2**

◆ Slept well. Next night dreamt of weaving shop in Thailand where the women were weaving with single strands of silk. Speaking of silk it came up in my language a few times yesterday. I described myself in the process of pupating. Changing careers felt like changing from a caterpillar to a butterfly.

◆ My heartbeat still reverberates around my body when in bed. Last night my body still felt like a big soft bag—dark on the he outside, light on the inside. I woke at dawn, unusual for me, but went back to sleep. Feel kind of dull in general—felt relaxed and fuzzy and dull as though in a pool of water where all the stimuli come to you through water. A pleasant sensation.

◆ Left upper palate really itchy. Lasts five minutes.

◆ Mild sore throat in evening.

◆ Argument with doctor at work. I held my ground, did not mince my words. This happens very rarely.

**Day 3**

◆ Do not recall dreams and this is unusual.

◆ Eyes really goopy and crusty this morning. Great chunks of tan-yellowish stuff in them.

◆ During breakfast it was storming outside, I was listening to choral music and thinking of whales and sad about them being hunted to extinction. I started crying. Thinking about animals and our natural world in general. This is an old worry of mine but the thing with the deep sea and whales is definitely new.

◆ I noticed that when writing I am making mistakes, also in speech. I wrote the number "3" backwards and could not figure out for a second what was wrong with it. In speaking I noticed I was using a word and I was going to say "further" in a sentence early on, and therefore out of context. Or I used a word I had already spoken again but out of context.

◆ A moment of itchy palate on left side again.

**Day 4**

◆ My sleep is different. Usually when I wake up I have a sense of having slept. The last 3 days it feels my sleep has been very deep sleep and I don't remember or sense that I was asleep. Still no dreams.

◆ Spoke briefly to proving director. She said to take another dose so I will do that tonight. (I told her I wasn't having many physical symptoms and primarily this shark/ ocean thing).

◆ Again a sharp, itchy feeling in left upper palate, near back tooth. Only lasted a few minutes.

◆ The quality of my period is also different. Instead of smooth red blood it is dark blood with bits in it that were almost clots.

◆ Took another dose at 1 a.m. before gong to sleep.

**Day 5**

◆ Sleep as previous nights, snippets of dream where I am in New Zealand bemoaning the development of the town I used to live in.

◆ This morning I was stretching and got cramp right upper leg. I remembered that 2-3 nights

ago while changing position in bed, my right buttock muscle cramped up.
◆ Also, since the beginning of this proving I've had a very mild itchy throat and an occasional dry cough.
◆ Afternoon: feeling quite tired and listless. I drove to my usual stomping ground for a walk, got out of the car, got back in, I just could not be bothered. Usually I *love* walking in nature. Almost overwhelming, I went to bed at 5 p.m. I can't find the mental energy (or physical for that matter) to do much more than sit in a chair.
◆ 7:30 p.m. Energy has picked up a little (mentally). Physically I still have a tired, heavy feeling in my body. I hardly did anything today—practiced singing and laundry that is it.
◆ Food cravings for fresh fruit and vegies.
◆ Between 8 and 9 p.m. I had another short episode of overwhelming tiredness. It came over me, I noticed it, and then few minutes later I was back to writing letters and it wasn't until a while later that I was consciously aware of being alert again and I became almost euphoric and had a very productive letter writing evening. I also noticed that I am not getting hungry in the same way that I used to. At about 4:30 p.m. I felt a sudden need to eat—not because my stomach was growling or I wanted to taste something I like —but because I had a physical sensation in my body of being unwell from not having eaten for a while. This was not my usual irritability or mild nausea feeling. It was deeper like hunger of the cells of my body. It is hard to explain.

**Day 6**
◆ Slept deeply again, I did have some dreams which I cannot remember. I am beginning to notice a strange sense of fuzziness where time seems to stop. The fuzziness is detached, almost hypnotized feeling. I'll be driving or writing and going through the motions but not mentally aware, kind of robotic. Not mentally aware, almost in remote control and time seems to have stopped as though I have been doing this thing forever. Time stops flowing the way it usually does. This sense comes and goes quickly. It is like a vacuum.
◆ I also feel like I am coming down with a cold. Slight runny nose, slightly irritated throat—all my usual cold symptoms except I should not be getting a cold right now.
◆ It still seems like I am alternating between bursts of energy or talkativeness or activity and this strange remote control feeling—a twilight of consciousness.
◆ Less interested in food.
◆ Driving past a sign at twilight and a word leapt out in 3-D, the name of an Italian restaurant.
◆ Felt my posture is more curved and hunched over than usual.

**Days 7 and 8**
◆ Nothing significant.

**Day 9**
◆ I have noticed that I am having a really hard time getting out of bed in the morning. When the alarm goes off I am in deep sleep and it seems impossibly early. I lie in bed for half an hour or so before I get up.
◆ Energy is low and I feel listless and melancholic today. Depressed about the state of

the world. Feeling really wiped out. Took a short nap and felt much better afterwards. Still craving fruits and fresh veggies—big salads with lots of different veggies.
◆ I've noticed a sensation of a bubble of fluid or air in my vagina—this has been since early in the proving. Sex drive is zero!
◆ Legs felt weak and trembly in the afternoon. I still feel hunched over and also feel like I am scowling a lot. I am constantly relaxing my mouth and trying to look what I imagine to be less severe.
◆ Mood really labile: go from happy to really depressed or hopeless in a matter of minutes just sitting in the car driving!

**Day 10**
◆ Beautiful, warm, sunny day. Usually on a day like today I'd leap at the chance of getting lots of exercise in the outdoors but still feeling pretty lazy about it although I did go for a bike ride and a walk up a favorite trail to smell the narcissus. I had a singing recital in the afternoon so was in my usual state of anxiety but it went well. Then afterwards I got really depressed and I don't know why. It was the same rapid flip like I wrote about yesterday. While driving the car at 65 mph it felt like I was hardly moving at all.
◆ Mood flipped between the fuzzy and really aware states. Wanted to take naps, really tired, so took two short naps during the day. Felt better after them. Both of these are new symptoms. I usually don't take naps, and when I do they are long and deep and I feel like death when I wake up which is why I avoid them.
◆ Heartbeat all through body again.

**Day 11**
◆ It took me a long time to fall asleep—bizarre thoughts that I can't remember. And something else weird: I was almost asleep when twice, I woke up and with a start because it seemed like my right hand was lying in a puddle of water. Of course, it wasn't, but the sensation was so real.
◆ Dream: Of being at sea in a boat, can't remember the details.
◆ Still feel like I am fighting a low-grade cold. I have not had this little energy in a long time. I feel really wiped out—always ready for nap, I don't know whether this is from the cold I am fighting, my impending job change or the proving. It is probably all three. A friend tonight said I seemed quiet and pre-occupied.
◆ I am farting and craving fresh, juicy things like cucumber and melons.
◆ I walked along the beach at sunset and I kept thinking about the whales and dolphins and sharks and how few there are now compared to before our slaughtering of them started.
◆ Still slow and kind of spacey at intervals. A sort of pall settles over me and I am out for a while and then suddenly it flicks off and I am back.
◆ Desire chocolate, and suddenly and inexplicably not too interested in tea which has always been a very enjoyable morning ritual. It gives me palpitations more easily than it had.

**Day 13**
◆ So greatly tired. Desperately want to take a nap but need to work.

◆ Itchy palate and throat.
◆ Would walk out and be worried I was not wearing pants and look down and see I was and still not trust it; so I looked to others to see their reaction.

**Day 14**
◆ Dreamed about blood sugar???
◆ Clumsy and have noticed that I am having a hard time doing more than one thing at a time.

**Day 15**
◆ Nothing specific I can remember but, I wanted to sort of summarize the proving. The main feeling of the last two weeks has been one of being intermittently spaced-out. It is neither pleasant nor unpleasant. It is kind of like being in a time warp because my perception of time changes, slows down incredibly. Then there was the whole ocean creature thing. Speech and thought seemed slower also intermittently, and I even had more difficulty than usual finding words.
◆Easy cramping of muscles. More anxiety than usual about whether I am fully dressed when in public. I could not trust my senses. Hard to separate what happened to me or someone else if we had talked about something several days before.
◆ Summary: Slower in speech and thought. Hard to find words.

**Prover #2 · Female · 37 years old**

◆ I am sure I was a butterfly the whole proving. I do not know if I am responding to husband or not (who was doing a proving of a different substance concommitantly). The first evening I dreamed about D's mother who had died in September. D. and I both lost our mothers within 4 months, and one died while we were celebrating at N. and R.'s place. A butterfly appeared and we connected this to the spirit of D's mother. We kept the butterfly since it kept coming back. I dreamt of both our mothers being alive to die again, and I awoke feeling this remedy was butterfly. My mother was there and in the hospital and my father was there and some concern about eating, what we would eat. My father was eating in the restaurant, waiting for mom to die. I was deciding whether or not to change my flight reservations. The dream seemed more focused on D's mother dying. (I have never dreamed of her.) I was D's younger girlfriend. He was wandering, lost and distant; he seemed angry with me. The feeling was transformative; so we could process it all again.
◆ Dream fragment: A little boy with two fathers; all of us helping him with luggage. A haircutting scene, it would take seven hours. We were getting reacquainted.
◆ At midnight my 5 year old came down saying his throat is clogged and he can't breath. He was upset and crying and then D. gave him Spongia. He settled down and slept through the night.
◆ Another dream the same night: I was watching a fighter jet and it was doing fancy

moves and then it exploded. Then I was buckling in with others in another plane and we were told if we make it through the critical point (a downward thrusting maneuver of 25 seconds) we will be fine and not explode. The pilot overshot the runway and we landed in water and I watched the jet twist and we were submerged underwater. I unbuckle and I am free. The key thing for me was being in air though we were sitting on water. Feeling of wonderment and yet it seemed normal.
◆ While waking up and still emerging from the dream, the dogs were barking and I go out to see (still in the dream state). There is a man in a leather jacket and a motorcycle. He is all happy and says he almost hit a cow in the road and asks me if it is my cow. He assures me he did not hit the cow and is very upbeat. I go walking down the road in my jammies. Felt happy and fun and not upset about being wakened.

**Day 2**
◆ Felt very tall and high off the ground. Looking far down as though looking far down to the ground. Felt very airy, high in the air. In motion, but stillness. Very calm.
◆ Feels filled with air—stare for long periods of time. It was as though there was a spaciousness in me where I could leave and do something like that. Time warp feeling and timeless feeling. Staring and pondering but not pondering about anything specific. I felt I was reflecting a lot. If there was a potential conflict I could see it but I did not feel it, sense of being unaffected by these conflicts.
◆ Vision: At distant squint through fuzziness, zoom in with crystal clarity. Vultures flying above me and they seemed high up and I was watching them and I felt I had become them as though I was in their body and flying with them. Felt the downward movement. Being a bird in the sky. I was playing tennis when this happened. I was leaping into the air joking, "I've got wings."
◆ Abdomen: feels puffy—extended.

**Day 3**
◆ Dream: 15 people at a gathering, a homeopathic group, and I was supplying food and feeding the group. One person ate a falafel and I realized I had nothing left to feed them all.
◆ Still feels calm, high. In that ponder state it was a calm still peaceful feeling, even if I was in motion I felt still. But slight down side—flat feeling on occasion a need for rest. At 3 p.m. all I wanted to do was rest like in a cocoon. 3-4 p.m., wanting everything to stop.
◆ Increased appetite especially for sweets.
◆ Abdomen feels hollow, big.
◆ Slept very deeply every night. So deep I felt I may not have even gone to bed.

**Day 4**
◆ Dream: At our house in Mill Valley with a group of people above and I was on a deck. I was fluttering around in a short skirt. I was below and they were above and sense of fluttering. Then a sense of riding on an elephant's back descending fast and steeply and it was misty. We did not have rain gear and were not prepared, so we had to hurry back.
◆ Dream fragment: A motorcycle in the house going 144 mph. I got out of the way so it could pass. The police were chasing. Friendly and lighthearted and fun feeling.

**Day 5**

◆ Nothing noted.

**Day 6**

◆ Dream: P. and I were walking out in nature. There are five choices of paths to take. They were thick, dense, intense brown. Colors of nature were important and I was very aware of every detail of the environment. I saw P. later that day (in reality, not a dream) and she had a shirt covered with flowers and butterflies called the butterfly garden. I blurted out "What are you doing wearing that?" She replies, "It's my T-shirt!" Then it dawns on me that she is doing the proving as well and I am amazed at the symbolism. I called later and apologized for screaming at her.

◆ Occasional slight shivers over my body. As though someone blew air over me.

◆ Stomach: less hungry.

**Day 7**

◆ Dreamt but could not remember.

◆ Mood is content, quiet.

◆ Energy: better, more energy than yesterday.

◆ Took remedy again at 9 p.m.

**Day 8**

◆ Dream: About D's mother and his whole family. We were all gathered for a family reunion and the focus was on her and her frail condition. A sister-in-law took her for a walk down the street and I watched them walking. D and I had to prepare dinner for everyone—a large group. We were there only two nights and I realized we were the only ones providing food. Usually there are five nights and each family has a turn. Someone borrowed some sesame seeds. The plate was overflowing with sesame seeds: all large and gooey, an overabundance.

◆ Dream: I was lying in bed and the air felt delicious and breezy and I insisted on the window open so I could feel the air—an amorous feeling.

◆ Energy: good, though tired around 3-4 p.m. I want to rest the whole body.

◆ Vision: acute.

◆ Stomach: increased appetite, especially for sugar, candy.

◆ Abdomen: full.

**Day 9**

◆ Dream: N. and I were in a house or cabin near a lodge. It was N's cabin which should be all by itself but all of a sudden we were in a neighborhood, there were houses all around the cabin. I was surprised to see all the houses in the daylight. A neighbor came in and woke us up. I ended up in a little theater with all these guys. We were drinking and I borrowed $60 from this man. Everyone was laughing because I did not know him. I was late and had to find my way back to the house to see N. and my daughter. They would be worried about me, they did not know where I was. Also something about eating gumballs off a gingerbread house. Lighthearted feeling.

◆ Mood: calm, quiet, not affected by conflict.

◆ The day had a lot of disruptions but the disruptions did not bother me. Keys lost several times in the day: locked in jeep, forgot the keys to a friend's cabin. Had an encounter with an animal. It was dark and I had to go down the road to get a key (though there were two in the car) and there was a large animal, perhaps a bear or mountain lion, and I froze to make a decision of what to do. It seemed timeless and I got the key and figure if I got past the curve I could run. It was stockier than a deer, on all fours, bigger than a dog. I was scared and afraid it would chase me. My legs felt like jelly afterwards.

◆ Occasional brief vertigo and had to hold onto something as I was looking down. Everything below me moves, I feel so dizzy for a few moments. Sense of downward motion.

◆ Stomach: increased appetite for sugar, candy.

**Day 10**

◆ Restless sleep—awakened several times but never really felt awake. Dreamy, deep feeling.

◆ Mood easy, lighthearted, relaxed.

◆ Good energy. At a facial at 3 p.m.a woman wrapped me like a cocoon and I went into a deep sleep and came out rejuvenated.

◆ Rectum: loose stool, tons of jalapeno peppers yesterday.

**Day 11**

◆ Mood: Calm, peaceful.

◆ Energy: increased energy in afternoon, no sleepiness.

◆ Menses started eight days early. Pieces or things came out. Intense, heavy.

**Day 12**

◆ Calm and peaceful.

◆ Lots of energy.

◆ Decreased appetite.

◆ Menses extra heavy.

**Day 13**

◆ Repeated remedy at 9 a.m. (Third dose.)

Intense left-sided headache. Cheekbones ached like a sinus infection. Began left side went bilateral and then to the right side. Went to neck and upper back. Had all day, took Tylenol at 6:30 p.m. Some vertigo before the state left.

**Day 14**

◆ Awakened with intense headache that is all over the head throughout the neck and upper back. Took Tylenol at 8 a.m. Relief for one hour. Suffered all day with this and repeat the Tylenol around 1 p.m. with very little relief. Repeat Tylenol at 4 p.m. Slept for 45 minutes but headache continues. Cheekbones hurting almost like a sinus ache. Feels very cold 3-6 p.m. shivering and freezing. Warmed up with extra clothes and made a

fire. Increased thirst; skin clammy.
◆ Took two extra-strength Tylenol at 9 p.m. and slept all night.
◆ I had felt lighthearted and fun until the third dose.

**Day 15**

◆ Woke up with right-sided headache, down into right side of neck, shoulder and upper back. Relief around 10:30-11:00 a.m. Some tension in my neck. Around 1:00 on tennis court experienced brief vertigo with some head tension.
◆ Rest of the day no pain. Good energy, peaceful and calm.
◆ Decreased appetite and increased energy.

## Prover #3 · Male · 46 years old

**Day 1**

◆ Took remedy and one of my dogs barfed right away.
◆ Left side of throat tight like emotional throat, but no emotions associated with sensation—slight.
◆ Energy low.
◆ Lot of confusion around me, remedy was sent to wrong address so got to me a week late. Got the instruction booklet eight days late. Got three sets of instructions from different places. Not a lot has happened to me as much as what happened to the people around me—the rest of the world got the remedy. Took it TID for three days, I used that set of instructions. I was starting to scream.
◆ The creek on my property flooded and I had to go out and pull out plants from it.

**Day 2**

◆ Working really hard. Search of a friend's name: sent faxes to all the same named people in that country—weird. Feel great—SPRING! Expansive feelings. Excited about my work, very creative. Writing is the best it has been. "Stuff is happening." Actually the symptoms of elation started 3-7 days before I took the remedy. The remedy was sent to the wrong address so the elation started the day I was supposed to take the remedy.
◆ Bought on impulse four Groucho Marx disguises. An impulse to go shopping at Thrifty's—no need to.
◆ Stomach: desires wine.
◆ I own a lot of snake paraphernalia and I noticed it more. Picked up a romance novel while at grocery store (never before had done this) and the first line on the book jacket is that a guy gets a poisonous snake in his mouth and it killed him. I am concerned that I might be creating energy here—undue, so I will resist snake stuff.
◆ A friend made a big thing about my mustache. Said I looked like a walrus and I could dive underwater and bring up brine shrimp in my mustache; and they laughed too much.

**Day 3**

◆ It feels as if some big planetary change has occurred. Projects I had worked on for years suddenly resolved without me doing anything. Easy: three big projects suddenly resolved.

◆ Still noticing snake stuff: books, carvings, etc.

◆ Worked in the creek again: pulling out irises, loved it: helped my chronic back pain.

◆ Called the proving director: "Don't even think about the proving remedy around me, I am feeling strongly intuitive." I was sure the remedy we were proving was Puff Adder snake.

◆ Felt like warm garlic butter in my veins. Low quality toxicity.

◆ Picked up tools, fascinated by them.

**Day 4**

◆ Dream: My mother asked me for a remedy for herself and I realized the remedies I had given her had worked. Her suffering is old age and stoicism.

◆ One of my best friends while growing up was in mental hospital after taking mescaline in college. He suddenly called me and we had an interesting conversation. Days seemed to pass quickly.

**Day 5**

◆ Tutto sembra possible! I keep noticing this writing in the hallway.

◆ Salmon was not right for dinner.

◆ Time passes quickly.

**Day 6**

◆ Big a.m. hike, SOB on ascending.

Revelation: Stopped "trying;" new case taking stuff comes easily.

**Day 7**

◆ Got the instructions.

◆ Dream: D. was a shiny bug in a fly's armpit. (A parasite on a fly.)

**Day 8**

◆ Nose and ears itched in voluptuous way.

**Day 9**

◆ Bought salmon that was so beautiful. Rubbed oil on it for a long time. Into radishes. Kept walking to the fridge looking for something and it was not there. Did this hourly. Ate ice cream. Stuck head and hand into freezer and laughed and stayed there for a while. Wanting hot sauce less.

•Right kidney pain 5 on 1-10 scale, lasted 5-8 a.m.

**Day 10**

◆ Tried dark chocolate and really understood why people like it so much for the first time. The best I have had in my life.

◆ I keep meaning to get a haircut each day, but keep forgetting. Received a lot of overseas mail.

Left forehead sweat.
◆ Big party with drumming. Ecstasy.

**Day 11**
◆ Left forehead and right axilla perspiration.
◆ Had a key made for my car and keep forgetting to go pick it up.
◆ Overall feeling everyone else went through changes but not so much me. Big unfinished projects got finished and completed.

**Prover #4 · Male · 37 years old**

I don't think much happened but I had more dreams, intensely.

**Day 1**
◆ Dream: Two patients coming to me; a brother and sister, one with a goiter and the other with adrenal and kidney problems. Searching for a room to see them in and in one room my father was there sleeping. It was midday and odd that he should be there sleeping. I finally found a dusty, unfinished room, it felt like chaos and I could not properly take a case there. Male patient said he had pain in ears and neck when he urinated or ejaculated. Somehow were next to a pet store and I saw large turtles. Next I was studying Kali iodatum in books. Frustrated with the confusion.
◆ Next couple of nights could not recall dreams.
◆ Energy good overall.
◆ Went to a restaurant and while we were waiting a man was pushing his way through the line. I said, "You can get by me," and he answered rudely and smugly, "Are you confident about that?" I felt a very violent aggressiveness inside, like I wanted to hurt him, kick his ass. It surprised me. In the restaurant I got up to go to the bathroom and the light was strange and faces seemed to come out at me. The people in the restaurant seemed stranger than normal. Plates of meat and dead carcasses—strange, anguished, unconscious people—so ugly, broken, old, diseased. Like a low realm of life.

**Day 2**
◆ Dream I was looking into my dog's ear and it was 10x the normal size and there was green stuff in it.
◆ That day we were walking with my dog and there was blood from his eye dripping on his cheek.

**Day 3**
◆ Dream: a broken computer, the latch keeps breaking.
◆ Landlord asked if homeopathy could help her uterine fibroid.
◆ My son in bed with me and I get this timeless ancient feeling. Quiet—Deep state of timelessness, present ancient state, staring out the window at the mountains. Feel free

and a lot of space around me. No history, no self but self, only peace. It feels like my cured state but does not last.

**Day 4**

◆ Dream: of two teenage girls naked with a poodle. They seemed homeless, broken and yet surviving. One girl is emaciated and had large anus hole. The feeling is she had been abused, broken, tormented, no hope, doing what she had to do to live. She had an animal look in her eyes, no trust. Weary, hungry, frightened, jumping around like a primate.

**Day 5**

◆ Dream of someone I do not know but am friendly with and I am helping him with some task. I feel he is dangerous and should not be trusted and then he turns on me and we fight using our fists. He has so much hate. I am forced to protect myself and I hit him with a broomstick ruthlessly and he breaks his wrist and falls down. He is defeated. I think to give him Anacardium and wish someone would give it to him. The feeling is: "I do not want to fight but I have to or I will die." A friend who becomes a foe. A white trash male: scared, violent, fighting, bloody. I am scared but at the same time ruthless.

**Day 6**

◆ Dream: Of running away, of being pursued but getting away; scared but pleasurable. Dream: Vivid but could only remember a doorbell and the words Hura braz and Merc that brought me out of the dream. When I woke I kept hearing the doorbell. As though that was all I was allowed to know or needed to know.

◆ Pain in scapula and spine on left: mid rhomboidal spasm or pulled muscle.

◆ Strong desire for chocolate. Desire for yogurt and kefir.

**Day 7**

◆ Dream: Two old clients came and one is deeply depressed and suicidal. He is broken, from a low-class sick white family. The mother has been sick with cancer for 20 years and he was her caregiver and confidant since the father was detached from the family. Everyone in the house was suicidal. I woke and viewed the whole family a different way. Lots of suicidal feeling. Dark, sick unrecoverable. White broken Jehovah's witness suffering. Broken, white low-class impoverished: no way out, damaged feeling.

**Day 8**

◆ Dream: I was going down a fast river with four friends and we are going fast, on our bodies. I smash into a 16 y.o. kid and he bumps his head and is angry. He is red and spotted. I try to console him but it doesn't accomplish anything. He needs Belladonna. Then we are on a train and going fast and I want to take care of this boy and his companions. I feed them with food from my mother's kitchen, but they are greedy and grab it. White trash, broken, desperate, hungry, poor. We pass my stop but it is too late to get off. Pass my old landlord's house and there are picketers protesting against him. Lower class poor and downtrodden fighting for redemption.

**Prover #5 · Male · 50 years old**

**Day 1**

◆ Received the remedy on 2/2. On going to bed after taking the remedy, closed eyes and an image of a fine geometric pattern of wire with deep blue or purple pastel. Then another image delicate white wire pattern.

◆ Head: sharp pain in roof of right orbit.

◆ Stomach: queasy.

◆ Good quality sleep. Able to sleep in—usually get up early on Saturday morning.

◆ Dream: I was at a school or clinic searching for a creature and an object. Two pictures of Star Trek-like figures: one humanoid, one inanimate. Some kind of cover—up. An official blew off any evidence or clues I found. Went to get water and there were two glasses lying on their side in the water fountain. One was dirty, it was further proof that something had gone awry. I tell a person of something that is bothering me, but there is something else I do not tell him. Theme of secrecy and subterfuge.

◆ In another part of the dream, at a meeting at the school and there were two large red ellipsoid rocks. I was playing with the rocks and try to move them. I finally gave them a large shove and expected them to have a certain path when pushed because of their shape. It went with unusual speed against a wall. It bounced up and took an angled trajectory and struck an Indian sitting in the room. The rock was 4-5 feet x 1-2 feet. I was upset at this turn of events and I woke up. Feeling of perplexity. Surprised I could shove the rock across the room with so little effort.

**Day 2**

◆ Dream: We had to stay over another night in Berkeley because we had to take a later plane flight. Stayed at a condo-like place in a middle-class neighborhood. I got up early and went for jog before we have to leave for the airport. Not hurried.

◆ Dream: Intrigue and struggle. Low key feelings during the dreams and not anxious.

◆ I had lots to do and time went quickly, feel less time pressures.

◆ General energy level good, had restful nap in afternoon.

◆ Slight queasiness, frequent small eructations with offensive taste for about two hours after breakfast and lunch.

**Day 3**

◆ Dream: About practical issues in a group discussing where and how to practice, whether should buy a building for clinic.

**Day 4**

◆ Took another dose.

◆ Dream: Trees with square wooden frames holding water around base of trunk. Animal fetuses were attached to the roots. We had a special device and were supposed to suck out the fetuses. I did not want to. Looked like something in the rodent family. Wolves wandering around. We went to the store with something to repair (from an earlier part of the dream). Walked around afterwards. Lost shoes. Had three books to rebind. Also a segment with driving, trying to get into the right lane. I am struck by the lack of feeling in the dream.

**Day 5**

◆ Dream: My son borrowed the car and the hood was torn off with the engine exposed. There was some question as to who had done it but I found tortilla chips in the radiator and I knew he had done it. I did not have a strong reaction.
◆ Dream: Taking off my penis as though it was an attachment and put it back on. At some point I realized this does not make any sense. Wondered about the theme of detachment. I realize as I write this I am somewhat embarrassed to write about this dream.
◆ Decreased appetite.

**Day 6**

◆ Dream: Woke at 3:19 a.m., obsessing about two difficult patients. Realized it was not so hard, their problems are not that complex.
◆ Anxious feeling and burning in stomach while waking up.
◆ Decreased appetite

**Day 7**

◆ Dream: Driving down the streets to go home and police were there; I slow down. On the way home the streets were gridlocked due to bicyclists going through intersections when they should not. In another area, a video camera is posted, I know this is a speed trap. Lot of traffic and there was a playful feeling.
◆ Dream: Something about a test. I discuss the test with some people while others are retaking it. I am struck by how difficult it is to recall the details of my dreams. This suggests defensiveness to me.

**Day 8**

◆ Dream: Discussing homeopathy in the dream. About Tuberculinum. I was discussing with colleague whether it is dangerous to give it to someone who had TB in the past. I also recall a dream fragment of a window with a number of panes lying over a container of water. Eventually the panes became broken and one could see the water below.

**Day 9**

◆ Dream: Working on a group project. I was going to sea in an open boat. Some people walk to get off the boat willingly. A well-to-do passenger is afraid his friend is conspiring to kill him. The wealthy man kills his friend, but tries to make it look like an accident: He got stuck in the air duct and died. They were anxious to cover it up and buried his body quickly. Aside: I saw a TV program earlier in the day about how Mozart was buried quickly.
◆ Dream: The dishwasher broke because I turned it on too fast. I waited for the repairman who wanted to sell me a warranty. Again the theme of water and broken things.
◆ Energy level good. Better than usual.

**Day 10**

◆ Dream: Some sort of court proceedings involving a schoolteacher. Concerned with HIV transmission via underwear of adolescents.

**Day 11**

◆ Dream: Observing interactions of children. Later dogs. Conscious of dreaming and sure I'd remember dream but have poor recall later. Something about going to a gambling casino and sure I would win, confident of my ability; air of detachment.

**Day 12**

◆ Dream: Traveling and traffic. Eating takeout and there was not enough food. I was laid-back.

◆ More emotional and sentimental, grateful for my marriage. Taking things more personally, more vulnerable. Loving feeling.

**Day 13**

◆ Dream: Patient has weight loss 60 lb. unsure why. Perhaps wheat allergy?

◆ Dream: Traffic, wrong lane, but eventually parked the car and then could not find it. More perplexed than anxious about it. At one point drove to a restaurant with two other people for lunch break from class. While waiting for a friend who went to the bathroom, one of the waitresses began to fondle my hair and upper body. We take our food back to the classroom and there is a rustic fireplace there. I am disgusted by a cow or elk with two horns that is in the fire. Then it transforms to a human face. Theme of two again: two horns. I take some pretzel fish crackers in pita bread, but when I realize it is someone else's I return it to them. I realize they do not have enough food.

◆ Trouble recognizing humor in sarcastic remarks. I feel hurt rather than coming back with a snappy comeback.

**Day 14**

◆ Forgotten pens and pencils for the first time in the course. Yesterday had trouble finding an envelope.

◆ Dream: Frustrating experience. We are in meditation class and there was a substitute teacher and we were changing our seats around. Then it switched to stamps and letters and trouble getting the right stamps on. I licked stamps and had nothing to put them on.

◆ Dream: At an AA meeting, in order to check in must put your tie tack in a special rack. I could not get my tie pin stuck on in the right way. They were looking for a wanted man and he was trying to get out of the building. He befriended a bunch of homeless people and they were to transport him to prison but his family is in the car and we cannot drive away because the car is stuck in the building.

**Day 15**

◆ Dream: Trying to extricate a car that is parked in a blocked area. Huge pieces of puzzle and the car is stuck in them and trying to solve it still. At another level the puzzle represents political issues, but it seems as soon as I get up to write some details, they go

out of my head. While I am in bed I feel I can easily remember.
◆ Dream: Sort of a continuation of the first dream. At one level the puzzle became an authorization request for a patient. I am at a party and someone asks about a patient I am seeing. Someone reveals information inappropriately about a patient.
◆ Eyes more tired that usual.

**Prover #6 · Male · 41 years old**

◆ Dream: of chatting with someone in the hospital and he gave me tickets to the 49ers, great seats and surprised.
◆ Wept in the car hearing 35 primates died of smoke inhalation in zoo fire.

**Prover #7 · Male · 42 years old**

### Day 1
◆ After taking the remedy I argued with wife, highly unusual. The theme from her end is that I am too serious and I do not know how to play. My theme is that the pace is too fast and I want to slow down and not do it so fast.
◆ Calm and centered.

### Day 2
◆ Felt clear, calm and centered, almost floating, singing and cheerful.

### Day 4
◆ Working on writing a book and spend 14 hours typing on the computer. By the end of the day, feel excruciating restlessness, hyper as though had three cups of coffee, wiggling hands and jiggling feet, impatient, thinking very clearly. Need to get to destination with sense of urgency, to get to the movie in time. Some people called me and while I was talking to them, I was typing and working crossword puzzles and reading textbooks so only half of me was paying attention. It was unusual that no one noticed.
◆ I cursed one time that day, unusual.
◆ Marked, arthritic symptoms of hands, fingers and neck.

### Day 5
◆ Dream: Mechanical dream of putting brakes back on a woman's bike, no problem. Tiny screws, precisely managed.
◆ I wondered if the remedy was a mineral like a halogen.
◆ In a big hurry to get through my Sunday morning routine of working out the puzzles in the paper so I could get back to writing. Did not enjoy it but had to do it, I did not want to miss my crossword but rushed through it.

◆ Deep pain in M-P joint of middle finger. Left side in a.m.

**Day 6**

◆ Embarrassing dream: Me and my family are living on an island kingdom with a castle. I am the mother. My beloved son goes off to the crusades and he comes back half nuts, crazy on this wild stallion that is vital and beautiful and untamed. It comes running at me in this field and I have this stake and I plant it in the ground and the horse impales itself and dies. My son is very upset. He embraces me, his mother, and he kisses me and then it becomes sexual and I am willing and aroused. He says this is not moral and rejects me and I go to the beach to hide and find a place to sleep but all the huts are full. I sit on the shore and wait for whatever will come.

**Day 7**

◆ Dream: I have cancer in the spine, the neck and it is causing numbness of the arm and hand and am seeing a woman osteopath, and we are both concerned I am not doing enough for myself. In real life I got a call from a woman osteopath about a woman with breast cancer metastasized to spine.

**Day 8**

◆ Dream: I am cooking mushrooms. Feeling anxious I have become involved in a crime by cooking these mushrooms.

**Day 9**

◆ Dream: I am living in an old German city and we have been given a lease in a beautiful, old building. G. is making a separate floor—building a new level. I am inspecting the space.

◆ Dream: N. is offered the lead in an opera and it is a great honor for such a novice singer. I am taking her to meet the troupe and she is going to tour. As she is getting on the bus, she negotiates with the bus driver/stage manager for her salary. She asks for 2.5 million and he laughs and says: "$200,000 tops—take it or leave it." She keeps negotiating. He says it is only for one week. I am thinking: "Take it, take it." But I know enough to keep my mouth shut!

◆ Overall feeling: calm and heavy. Don't want to do too much and then forced to do too much and become hurried. Effort and heaviness and the conflict between these two. Feeling tired and earthbound.

**Prover #8 · Male · 43 years old**

**Day 2**

◆ Drawing tension in the stomach; in the epigastrum, a pulling upwards.

**Day 4**

◆ Erratic energy levels, stay up late with second wind and then tired the next day. More emotionally labile.

**Day 5**

◆ Tired aching left upper right ribs posteriorly; may be from recent exercises on new machines at gym.

◆ Discouraged from the rain, not able to go outside. Restless and unproductive feeling, revved up feeling, wasted much of the afternoon, feels unsettled.

**Day 6**

◆ Dream: A woman friend had an orifice in her abdomen and she passed a stone. (It was unclear if this was from the digestive, urinary or reproductive tracts.) I said that is curious and then more and more stones came out, gray in color and they filled a wheelbarrow. The sound was rhythmic and pleasant. This transitioned to a series of globular shapes, slightly furry like kiwis, the size of grapes. Then a tubular thing came out and it turned out to be a weasel. Shocking and disturbing. It got up and moved around. Feeling of fascination and disgust. Someone in the dream said it was a skunk but looked more like a weasel.

◆ Pressure and constriction in the chest and stuck a little forward, hard to sit up, inability to stand up fully or feel any opening in the chest area.

**Day 7**

◆ Woke with yellow discharge in the right eye that glued the eye shut. No pain or redness noted. It washed off easily without further trouble. (I wear contacts and have been wearing them long hours last few days.)

**Day 8**

◆ Beautiful sunny day. Went hiking in the mountains and felt ecstatic and out of my body, blissful and at peace. Good change of pace.

**Day 9**

◆ Dream: Nightmare of a military guy who was involved in nuclear war planning, and he sequentially murdered people whom he knew. I did not actually observe the murders, but they involved brutally bashing skulls in with a garden trowel. He was partially disabled and walked with a limp. He was nuts, diabolical, and there was a feeling of vengefulness in the murders. Someone else caught on to him and saw a bed filled with a pool of blood, so I have confidence he was about to be stopped. Not sure what I was doing there but felt endangered myself. He was crafty and completely ruthless. On waking I was not sure if I was a witness or actually in the story, but I was scared and was trying to figure out how to get him, not having any success.

◆ Felt trapped inside at my hospital job, waiting for a planned admission. I could not wait to get outside. Left the hospital early. Went running which was satisfying.

**Day 12**

◆ Dream: Nightmare that I had to go to naturopathic school after Hahnemann.

**Day 13**

◆ Yesterday went for a run and felt very peaceful and happy. Sat for a minute and it was very sweet a period of not having to do anything. Communal feeling of hearing birds, smelling flowers and trees.

◆ Walking across streets against the light without looking.

**Day 14**

◆ Very sensitive to alcohol; more than usual.

◆ Sleepy during a treatment at 3 p.m. and fell asleep.

# LAC LEONINUM

*Milk of the Lion*

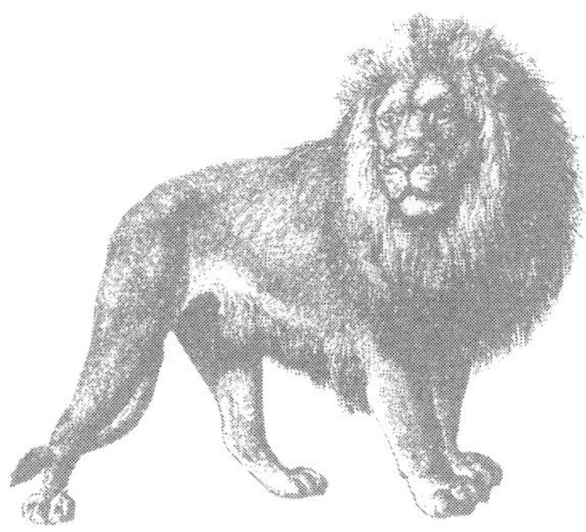

# LAC LEONINUM *Milk of the Lion*

The lion is a study in incongruity. He is both lazy and bold; he is a killer, yet he plays like a cub; he is the master of a large family, and he wanders the savanna alone. He is the archetypal "king of the beasts." In the children's fantasy film, *The Lion King*, all the animals face the great king and honor his new infant son by bowing to him. On the savanna, all the creatures face "the king" at the watering hole, but they do so in order to watch his every move and quickly leap away should he look hungry.

The lion has always been associated with power and prestige. Killing lions has been, throughout history, a symbol of manhood—reserved only for kings or for the very rich. Ramses II had a tame lion accompany him into battle. Ramses III said: "With my own hand I, the Pharaoh, killed from a chariot 102 wild-eyed lions." Endless myth and lore surround the lion. The Kalahari Bushmen believe the lion is a sorcerer and thus can hunt in complete darkness. They also believe he can cause a lunar eclipse by stretching his paw toward the moon and obscuring it. Other African tribesmen believe they can derive courage from eating the heart of the lion.

He is the stuff that legends are made of—magnificent beauty, pride, power, and majesty. In every culture, lions are symbols of courage and dignity. In Buddhism, we find Buddha on a throne upheld by two lions. One of the lions has a cub under her paw. This is an emblem of Buddha's universal compassion. Christ, also, is depicted with a lion, signifying Christ's role as the king of heaven. In medieval art, lions were pictured with halos, indicating that they are the symbol of Christ. In Hinduism, the lion is revered as the fourth Avatar whose form is half lion and half man. Another well-known half lion and half man symbol is the Sphinx, the guardian of the tombs of royalty in ancient Egypt. The lion and lioness together symbolize Shiva and Shakti, with the lion as the supreme lord and the lioness as the power of the uttered word. The Sumarian sun god, Marduk, uses the lion as a symbol of leadership, power, and strength. However, if we investigate a little further, we find that the lion has some areas of poignant vulnerability. In fact, we might say that the emperor (lion) has no clothes. (**NO CLOTHES**)

A large male lion is about eight feet long and weighs about 500 pounds. In contrast, the female is only about five feet long and weighs 300-400 pounds. The lion has a ravenous appetite and needs about twelve pounds of meat daily but is able to eat 70 pounds at one meal. A pride can eat an entire zebra down to bones in 30 minutes. Lions will eat anything from rats to hippos. The wild lion lives about eight to ten years. The female's gestation period is about 108 days, and the litter size is usually two or three cubs, although rarely, she will produce as many as six. Cubs are born every two years.

The lion's highly successful team approach to hunting is unique in the cat family. This has led to their living together as a family or pride, another characteristic that is unusual among cats, who are known for their independence. The pride consists of three to twelve females, two to four males, and the cubs. The females share the nursing of all the cubs, guiding them and protecting them daily from a series of dangers. Management of the pride is the responsibility of the females. Along with the all-important task of caring for the cubs, females move the pride when necessary to find water and food, lead all the hunting expeditions, and feed and care for the older members of the pride. Lions hunt mostly at night, especially during the waning moon. When the prey is caught, the males have the privilege of eating first.

The males' main task is to protect the pride from marauding nomad male lions who threaten to kill the cubs. Apart from this major responsibility, the males are content to eat, sleep, have sex, and to follow the female leadership in most other endeavors. Because vigilance and combat are the males' responsibility, they are freed from other tasks.

When we look at pictures of male lions lounging in the sun, what we are seeing is a head male, his brothers and his older male cubs. (**MEN RELATING TO OTHER MEN**) The cubs are tolerated as long as they do not spray urine or, in any other manner, assert themselves. The moment they start to "act like men," they are unceremoniously sent away forever, before their presence becomes too threatening to the sovereignty of their father. Life in exile is very difficult. They must struggle to find food on other lions' territories where they are distinctly unwelcome. Since all the land is claimed by one pride or another, there is nowhere for them to go. They slink and hide and take what meager game they can get. Eventually, as they grow bigger and more experienced, they will take on one of the established males in battle and either win their own pride or crawl away defeated—perhaps mortally wounded.

The hungry young males are constantly trying to dethrone the head males. (**PROBLEMS WITH AUTHORITY FIGURES**) Sometimes related males will form a team to try to unseat a head lion, or a brave single male will go at it alone. Ousting an established leader, though, is a very dangerous proposition and will often cost the young male his life. Should he win the battle and take over the pride as the new head lion, he immediately begins to kill the cubs of the previous leader. When it appears, during a fierce battle, that a new male will take over the pride, the female quickly goes into action. She attempts to move her cubs one by one to a safe location at the edge of the territory. Her intent is to hide them from the new male. (**CONCERN ABOUT PEOPLE AND DESIRE TO HELP THEM, ESPECIALLY CHILDREN**) This is usually futile because the male follows her scent, and when she returns to the pride for the next cub, he kills the one left at the new location. In this obsessive concern for lineage, lion behavior mirrors that of human kings. A usurping male lion will even kill large female cubs unless he can be persuaded to regard them as mates and not as the previous male leader's offspring. The situation is very dangerous for the female cub because she has no options; there is no place else to go. (**WOMEN AT ODDS WITH THEIR HUSBANDS**)

By killing the cubs immediately, the male forces the female to stop nursing and go into estrus quickly. Then he can mate with her and insure the continuation of his own bloodline. When the female comes into estrus, there is a bit of a frenzy for two or three days. She is motivated to mate aggressively every fifteen minutes. In one study, a male mated with two females 157 times in 55 hours. That means he mated every 21 minutes or so, without a breather, for two days.

When the new leader is established, older male cubs in the pride must leave quickly. They then become nomads and, in turn, spend their days wandering the perimeters of other lions' territories trying to establish their own pride. At best, when they do succeed, they can expect to be a leader for only two or three years before another male, or team of males, takes over their role. The defeated male then returns to the vulnerable fringes of pride society—the 20 percent of the lions who are nomads.

It seems, in one experience after another—as cubs, as adolescents, and as older defeated adults—that the life of the male lion is fraught with insecurity, danger and hardship. For most males, there is a brief period when they are on the kingly throne—with females, cubs of their own, and a territory. Even during this period of relative security, they must be constantly on the alert for interlopers. While for a time this emperor strides arrogantly, humiliation and defeat lurk around the corner. Lions are definitely thieves. (**THEFT**) Often the hyena, who is the lion's biggest rival, will make a kill, and then the lion, usually the male, will stroll in at the end and consume the meal. Lions scavenge up to 50 percent of their meat from the kills of other animals. Hyenas also steal from lions. Whichever animal group outnumbers the other takes the kill. The Masai, who are called the "people of the lion," are famous for their belief that all the cattle in the world belong to them. Wherever they wander, they assume ownership for cattle in that territory.

Lions are very aggressive. (**ANGER/RAGE**) A lion will stalk and kill a hyena for no reason. Often they walk away from a kill and do not even bother to eat a bite of the dead animal. The lion is particularly prone to making a surprise attack on a hyena clan, charging and killing the ruling female hyena.

### Analysis of the Proving

The real lion, as we have seen, is not quite as noble or dignified as the idealized image. The male lion, in particular, is not so much the leader as the follower, not so much compassionate as aggressive, and not so much the king as the thief and temporary stand-in. This proving brings out some of these dilemmas and issues. Particularly interesting was the issue of male-female relations. While it is believed that female lions are very attracted to their mates, the proving revealed that they can get frustrated from doing all the work and watching the males lounge under the local shade tree. The theme of stealing was a perplexing one to me during the proving analysis. I could not imagine how this would pertain to lions. Only after researching the lifestyle of the lion did I understand that stealing is a part of everyday life in the lion kingdom. Most striking was the amount of material related to cats—both dreams and experiences—though the provers did not know what substance they were taking.

I have used this remedy for individuals who project fierceness yet have a problem with behavior disorders; for those who love to play, too roughly, and yet are very dependent on and demanding of their mothers. In other words, it is useful for little boys. It may also be indicated for women who are strong and independent and who resent the laziness or playfulness of their mate. These women feel they carry "the lion's share" of responsibility while the man carries less of the burden. Intense sexuality seems to be a strong characteristic of those who need this remedy. They also project a striking feline image—they are graceful, slinky, very clean and beautiful. (**CATS/CATLIKE**) Other aspects are desire for exercise and a sense of playfulness. Left-sided headaches were strong in the proving, and this was a good confirmation because they were also strong in the old Lac felinum (milk of the cat) proving.

### The Substance

This remedy was obtained by a zoo keeper who is a friend of Rajan Sankaran, a world-renowned homeopath in Bombay. It was made from the milk of a nursing African lioness. (The Indian lion has been slaughtered into near extinction and is not kept in zoos. There are a mere 200 of them left, all individually named.) This African lioness is housed in a nature sanctuary just outside Bombay. She is allowed to roam the enclosed park during the day and is then put in a cage at night. At the time of the milk extraction, she was about six years old and had just delivered two healthy cubs. The milk was obtained by restraining the lioness in a cage, injecting her with a hormone to increase milk production, and manually milking her. It was exciting to receive this substance because it is extremely challenging to get milk from a healthy lioness. Our deepest gratitude goes to Dr. Sankaran as well as to the zoo keeper. Dr. Sankaran has also done a proving of this substance that we hope to see published soon.

*Lac Leoninum* **Themes**

*Milk of the Lion*

- *Anger/Rage*
- *Concern about People and Desire to Help Them, Especially Children*
- *Theft*
- *Problems with Authority Figures*
- *Women at Odds with Their Husbands*
- *Men Relating to Other Men*
- *No Clothes*
- *Playfulness*
- *Cats/Catlike*

# *Anger/Rage*

**#4** Anger, brooding; visit a patient who normally provokes a gentle loving feeling yet I feel anger towards him. I wonder if he is looking angry, but the mood continues after I leave. I feel this underlying arrogance—a sort of broody anger just generally towards almost anyone I think of.

**#1** On way to airport, realized left ticket behind. Taxi had to backtrack ten miles. Then once at school, I realized that I left bag at home, felt angry at self.

**#4** Irritable when speaking to sister on phone, but then I realize I feel really irritable with anyone and or any passing thought! It's a really new feeling to me.

**#1** Dream: The feeling of being unjustly accused or blamed for a bullshit crime evokes a feeling of rage and indignant feeling.

**#5** Dream: About to undergo unnecessary abdominal surgery as example for medical students. Slightly fearful of being out (due to general anesthetic), but more angry that I could not make them stop.

## Concern about People and Desire to Help Them, Especially Children

**#5** Dream: We needed to get home, no car available, so we borrowed a plane and my husband flew it; made children parachute out safely to places they needed to go. We arrived safely and landed on our street.

**#4** Anxious about daughter, who is unhappy in her new house, and her cat, who is finding it hard to settle down.

**#1** Sensitive to hearing or watching about bad news; unbearable to see sick children in hospital. Life is so brutal.

**#5** Dream: Trying to keep track of people. I was supporting mostly young adults with disabilities. People kept asking me to take in another one, and I could not remember all of them; felt worried I would forget one.

**#4** Dream: In a room in a house and it has two animals in it, and one of them is a huge tiger. Somehow I know the tiger is tame if treated carefully. My sister approaches the tiger to take it down off the shelf, where he is standing, but I am scared and I tell her we should leave him and run out of the room. Tiger starts swiping at her with his paw, and we run out quickly.

# *Theft*

**#6** I had a strong impulse to steal perfume while walking through a department store. I don't know why. I could pay for it if I wanted to. I have never had this impulse before.

**#3** Dream: Wife is accused of theft by another couple; I felt exasperated that my wife gave a statement to the police against my advice.

**#4** Dream: Kidnapper at large; while driving down street, I recognize a man as him through photos, wearing green patterned shorts and red shirt. He is taking a small child from a house. I tell other people but then realize I am in the house with the kidnapper and am in danger. Try to be friendly towards him, have a dialogue, but feel frightened. Begin to run in order to hide from him.

**#6** Dream: Someone was stealing a part of my sewing machine, and I couldn't finish my project. Amazed they would steal it because the part had no value, except to the machine.

## *Problems with Authority Figures*

**#1** Dream: Being pulled over by a police officer using radar. I was supposedly going 63 mph. I was very angry and indignant. Pleading with the cops. I noticed I was half-hour late and increasingly indignant and pissed. Cops had car towed. Went ballistic, then woke, and I felt immediately relieved but was still pissed about the way I was treated for an hour. The feeling of being unjustly accused or blamed for a bullshit crime evokes a feeling of rage and indignant feeling: "F— You! Don't control me! You have no right!"

**#3** Dream: In a car with spouse, taking turns driving. While wife was driving, she fell asleep and hit a house. Then it was me (who had hit the house). I did not want to get caught, so I ran up a hillside that became too steep to climb.

**#4** Dream: Walking with sister in green, grassy park. Met a veterinary surgeon. Sister is flirtatious with him, and I feel jealous and some anger. There are small battery operated police along the way.

**#5** Dream: About to undergo unnecessary abdominal surgery as example for medical students. It's taking place in large room like a kitchen. I needed to get dishes and laundry done before the surgery. Thought would be done under a local but then realized was going to sleep and shouted: "I have not signed a consent, you can't put me out!" Slightly fearful of being out but more angry could not make them stop. As soon as came to, I immediately jumped up and started folding laundry before the anesthetic wore off and the pain started.

## *Women at Odds with Their Husbands*

**#2** Irritable at husband who was late and kept family from attending a planned event on time. I was so irritable with him, I actually left home without him; but he caught up and made up later.

**#2** Unsympathetic towards my husband, who woke several times during the night with heartburn. Thought to self internally: "Why is he doing this? Why does he take up so much space?" But externally was considerate and helpful.

**#5** Very resentful of husband and demands of life. Actually told husband did not think I could go on with the relationship. Feeling of being overwhelmed.

**#5** Dream: I was lending money to a woman, but (the woman's) husband did not want me to. He said that she was unable to budget, and he wanted his wife to give the money back. I wanted her to have it but was unwilling to cause conflict between them. I was satisfied that I was not a spendthrift.

**#2** Details attended to of all the loose ends since I was gone for a week. Schoolwork, bills. Irritable with husband over how he is not keeping track of the checks since I do all the bookkeeping.

## *Men Relating to Other Men*

**#1** Dream: An old friend with whom I have mutual differences and unresolved problems in relationship. I have not, in reality, made an effort to complete or resolve our relationship problems. In the dream, there is a feeling of resolve, and we are accomplishing a task in the hospital. (It) felt relieving to be in harmony, with no discord, with him. (37 y.o. male)

**#1** Dream: friend from college have not seen for 15-16 years. Resolution feeling. (37 y.o. male)

**#3** Dream: In a house in the woods. I pee through a screen door. It is O.K.; it's only males present. A woman approaches, yells, "Stop," so she will not get peed on. She comes in, a Mexican whore with large, flabby breasts. She fondles me. Dream ends, unfortunately. (51 y.o. male)

## *No Clothes*

**#4** Dream: Lost clothes, looking for something to wear, so I wrapped self in rug.

**#5** Dream: Just out of the shower with no clothes on and started to walk to my room, when I notice a group of strange people in the house. I call to my husband to get me my clothes. He just laughed at me and didn't do it.

## *Playfulness*

**#1** Dream: Back at childhood home in backyard. People and children around, many are shooting off rockets.

**#3** Dream of sliding on a slide, feeling was fun.

**#3** Fleeting dreams of playing tennis, eating.

**#4** Sense of playfulness and stretching in the water when went swimming, freedom.

**#5** Dream: Riding a bike through the restaurant with a baby on the back doing headstands.

**#2** Big "date" with husband. Out to eat and to the movies. Fun, relaxing. Light.

# *Cats/Catlike*

**#4** Dream: An old boyfriend is sitting on ground, and he is very hairy. Sitting licking his leg and rubbing his face on it; sitting with a woman and tells her it is a magic way for him to be sure he will come back again. I feel interested and amazed at how hairy he has become.

**#4** Dream: A soft, milky-white skull; milky faces that are rather grotesque. Somewhere tigers and cats come into it.

**#4** Dream: Daughter calls in a panic saying that her cat has gone crazy being alone all night.

**#4** Dream: I've lost my new kitten. I go to a restaurant where my cat was served to me on a plate; it was skinned with its head intact like a bear rug. Felt very sad.

**#6** Dream: Cats, pleasant, warm feeling.

**#6** Dream: Cats again, this time feeling pursued.

## MIND

*ANGER, irascibility; tendency*
blamed, from being
contradiction, from
indignation, with
ANIMAL consciousness
ANXIETY; future, about
dreams, on waking from frightful
waking, on
ARROGANT
AWKWARDNESS
BUSY; evening
CARES, worries; full of; nature, for, animals, plants etc.
*COMPANY; aversion to, agg.*
solitude, fond of
alone; dreads being, yet lonely
desire for; to keep group together
CONCENTRATION; active
CONTEMPTUOUS
COQUETTISH; too much
DELUSIONS, imaginations; light, incorporeal, immaterial, he is (floating in air)
DESIRES; group together, to keep
DICTATORIAL, domineering, dogmatic, despotic
command, talking with air of
DREAMS
accusations
crime, wrongful of
adolescents
teaching French and piano to
amorous
anger, rage
indignant over event she is unable to stop
*animals, of*
*cats, felines*
pursuing him
kitten
gone crazy; being alone all night, from being
lost, missing
skinned and served; felt sad

DREAMS animals, of (cont.)
    pigeons
    pursued by
    snakes
    tigers
  anxious
  bicycling; difficult
  body, body parts; body hair; grooming and licking
    breasts
    head; skull, milky white
  boyfriend, of; old, amazed at how hairy he'd become
  bridges, building of
  capture; evading people's
  cares, full of
    about her children
    patients, for his
  caretaking
  child, children; about
    baby, on back of mother
    kidnapped, being
    something had happened to
  childbirth, of
    delivering baby by herself
  cleaning; spilled milk
  clothing; hidden her, someone has
  colored; purple
  curious
  drowning
  dying; teammates in a plane crash
  eating; at night
    unable to; because of another's dishonesty
  education
  feathers
  flirtation
  forgetfulness; streets, of well-known
  forsaken
  friendly, being; though frightened
  friends; mourning the departure of
    old, former
      relieved to have harmony with
  groups
    mourning departure of friend
  hiding from danger, of

- *house, houses*
    - *in the country*
- insults
- jealousy
- kidnappers
- licking body hair
- milk; cleaning spilled, of
- money; lending
- monsters
- *nakedness, about*
    - wraps self in rug
- overcharged by cashier
- planes
    - crashes and all killed
- planes; parachuting from
- playful
- playing
- police
    - pursued by, of being
- pursued, of being
    - man; kidnapper
- responsibility, of
    - towards disabled young adults
- restless
- school
    - of old; taking tour, with daughter
- schoolmate, meeting of old
- speech; giving
    - inspirational
- standing
    - not enough chairs at table
- stealing; impulse to
- surgery, of
    - returns to work before anesthetic wore off
    - undergoing unnecessary, as example for medical students
- sympathetic
- with those mourning a friend's departure
- teaching
    - adolescents
- theft, robbery
    - committed, of having
        - object of no value except to owner
- traveling
- urinating, of

DREAMS (cont.)
vehicles
war; space war
water
wedding
work
FEAR; bad news; hearing
FORGETFULNESS
possessions, of, leaves behind
FORSAKEN feeling
friends or group, by
FRUSTRATION
*HAUGHTY*
HELPLESSNESS, sensitivity to
IMPATIENCE
IMPULSE, morbid; shoplift, to
INDIGNATION
INDOLENCE; aversion to work
hot bathing ameliorates
INSIGHTFUL
INTUITIVE
INDUSTRIOUS, mania for work
evening
*IRRITABILITY*
JEALOUSY
LAUGHING; tendency; sad, when
LOVE; animals, for
LOVE; nature, for
MEDITATION
MOOD; changeable, variable
alternating
MUSIC; amel.
PATIENCE
PLAY; desire to, playful
QUIET; disposition
RAGE, fury
*RESENTMENT; husband, to*
SADNESS, despondency, depression, melancholy
SENSITIVE, oversensitive
cruelties, when hearing of
emotional
nature, to
people's inner nature's, to
surroundings, to

STRANGE; things, impulse to do; shoplift, to
SUSPICIOUSNESS, mistrustfulness
TALK, talking, talks; indisposed to, desire to be silent, taciturn
THOUGHTS; clearness of
TRANQUILLITY, serenity, calmness; morning, on waking
TRUTH; sensitive to people's truthfulness
*UNSYMPATHETIC, unscrupulous;*
  *friends and family, even towards closest; though acts as if she cares*
VIOLENCE, vehemence; helpless person, feelings toward
WEEPING, tearful mood; tendency
  morning
    waking, on
  sleep; because she could not
  amel. symptoms
WORK; desire for mental; evening
  aversion to mental

## HEAD PAIN

GENERAL; evening; agg.
  evening; agg.; six p.m.
  evening; agg.; six p.m.; four a.m., until
  lying, while; agg.
LOCALIZATION; Occiput
  evening; agg.
  extending; neck, to
    nape of neck, down
LOCALIZATION; Temples; left
LOCALIZATION; Forehead
  evening; agg.
    eight p.m.
PULSATING, throbbing
  evening
  Forehead

## EYE

SWELLING; lids
  upper
  right
  painless and red

## NOSE

SNEEZING
evening

## MOUTH

PAIN; sore; tongue; tip
DRYNESS

## THROAT

*PAIN; sore, bruised; morning; waking, on*

## EXTERNAL THROAT

CLOTHING agg.

## CHEST

PAIN; stitching; ribs
right
lower; right
aching; ribs; lower
pinching; heart

## BACK

ITCHING
scratching; amel.
PAIN; General; cervical region
lying, while; back, on
pressure amel.
PAIN; General; dorsal region; scapulae
right scapula
extending to; shoulder
PAIN; General; lumbar region, lumbago; right
turning
bending; agg.; backward
PAIN; aching; cervical region
bending head back amel.
supper, after, amel.
PAIN; drawing; cervical region
right
extending; shoulders, to
right shoulder while lying

- STIFFNESS; Cervical region
    - turning head, on; left, to
- TENSION
    - forenoon
    - Cervical region
    - Dorsal region
    - extending to; neck

## STOMACH

- APPETITE; diminished
- ERUCTATIONS; General; eating; agg.; after
- THIRST; large quantities, for
    - indistinct, knows not what for

## RECTUM

- CONSTIPATION
- PAIN; General
    - morning; seven a.m.
    - cramping
- FLATUS
    - offensive; spoiled eggs

## STOOL

- SLENDER
- COLOR; dark
- ODOR; sulphur, like

## KIDNEYS

- PAIN; General; left
    - General; evening
    - General; drinking water amel.
    - General; afternoon; five p.m.
        - five p.m.; seven p.m., until
- PAIN; pinching
    - twitching

## BLADDER

- PAIN; burning; urination; during
        - after

## EXTREMITIES

AWKWARDNESS
NUMBNESS, insensibility
  sleep, during
  Hand
    night; sleep, in

## EXTREMITY PAIN

PINCHING; Hip; walking, while; agg.
SORE, bruised; Foot
  walking, while; agg.
  sole; sitting
    walking, while; amel.
TENDONS
STIFFNESS; Joints
  motion ameliorates
TINGLING, prickling; Hand; night
  Forearm

## FEMALE

MENSES; frequent, too early, too soon
  two days too early
  seven days too early
MENSES; painful, dysmenorrhea
MENSES; short, too
MENSES; dark
  pitch, like
SEXUAL; desire; increased
  diminished

## SLEEP

REFRESHING
RESTLESS
SHORT; four thirty a.m. - six thirty a.m.
SLEEPINESS; afternoon; agg.
  one p.m.
  three p.m.; after
SLEEPLESSNESS
  night; first part of
    thoughts, from activity of
  restlessness, from
  thoughts, from
UNREFRESHING

- WAKING; midnight; after
  - two a.m.
    - pain in finger from
  - three a.m.
    - sore throat, with
- WAKING; dreams, from
  - frequent
  - pain, from; feet, in

## PERSPIRATION

- NIGHT; eleven p.m.
- ACRID
- HEAT; agg. during
- ODOR; acrid
  - strong

## CHILL

- EVENING

## SKIN

- ITCHING; scratching; amel.

## GENERALITIES

- AIR; seashore air; amel.
- FANNED; being; amel.
- FOOD and drinks; cold; drinks, water; desires
    - large quantities of cold water
  - cucumber; desires
  - fruit; desires; juicy
  - indistinct, knows not what to drink, desires
  - juicy things; desires
  - salt or salty food; desires
  - meat; desires
  - milk; desires
  - potatoes; desires
  - spinach; desires
  - vegetables; desires
    - green, fresh, raw
  - yoghurt, desire
- HEAT; sensation of
- UNDRESSING; amel.
- WARMTH; agg.; clothing

# JOURNALS ........ *Lac Leoninum*

EDITOR'S NOTE: *Punctuation, abbreviations, and individual stylistic nuances of the original journal entries have been preserved wherever possible.*

## Prover #1 · Male · 37 years old

### Day 1

◆ Son vomited within one minute of prover taking remedy. Child (4 y.o.) had never vomited before.

◆ Anxious feeling with a strong desire to take a deep breath.

◆ Chest: heart sensation of pinching, intermittent for 5-10 minutes.

◆ Sleep: Sleepiness 1 p.m.

◆ Dreams: An old friend with whom have mutual differences and unresolved problems in relationship. In the dream, a feeling of resolve and accomplishing a task in the hospital. A feeling of relief to be in harmony with him. No discord between us in the dream.
Mind: Awkward. Felt unusually socially awkward and did not know what to say.
Perspiration: body temp increased, sweating all over 11 p.m.

◆ Dream: Crossing a bridge over a river. Walk into fishing tackle store. Owner puts soft material in my mouth and wants me to chew it. I do but do not swallow it. I wanted to spit it out.

### Day 2

◆ Sensitive to hearing or watching about bad news; unbearable to see sick children in hospital. Life is so brutal.

◆ Chest: pain, aching bones and ribs, like going to have the flu.

◆ Musculoskeletal: Tension in shoulders, neck.

### Day 3

◆ Sensitive to music, could hear more deeply, enjoyable.

◆ Drawing neck pain extending to right shoulder. Dull aching deep, neuralgic quality.

◆ Extreme. < lying on back. > deep massage.

◆ Constipation.

### Day 4

◆ Head: pain severe 8-10 p.m. < standing up. Localized to occiput and left temple. Throbbing in frontal region. Neck at C-7 aggravated by touch. Massage ameliorates.

◆ Right shoulder and scapula painful.

### Day 5

◆ Head pain severe. < 6-10 p.m. Neck and occiput tension. Left temple. < lying. > massage.

◆ Dream of friends long past—old friends that I have not thought of. Enjoying the interaction.

**Day 6**
◆ Head pain severe 6-10 p.m., entire head, < left side.
◆ Dream: Old friends from past.
◆ Sexual energy high.

**Day 7**
◆ Head pain, 6:30 -10 a.m., tension in neck and shoulders.
◆ Sexual energy high.
◆ Kidney pain, left, 5 p.m. Pinching intermittently until 7 p.m. > after drinking water.
◆ Dream: Friend from college have not seen for 15-16 years. Resolution feeling.

**Day 8**
◆ Head pain 6-8 p.m.,mild tension type.
◆ Kidney pain, pinching, left, intermittent throughout day.
◆ Waking fatigued in morning, too lethargic to go to gym as usually does.

**Day 9**
◆ No headache.
◆ Kidney pain, twitching 6 p.m.
◆ Dream: At river to fish. Walk to river's edge. Start to slide down embankment, water deep.
◆ Sinking and drowning. Have fear at first, then surrender as moves into current of river, then awake.

**Day 10**
◆ Dream: With an old friend from high school, looking for house in the country. We cannot find it. Stop at a friendly person's house in area. He tries to direct us. We continue to search but fail to find it. I awoke with strange feeling of having been with this person I have not seen in over 20 years.
◆ Absent-minded. Left my lunch at office.
◆ Still slightly constipated.

**Day 11**
◆ Absent-minded, on way to airport realized left ticket behind. Taxi had to backtrack ten miles. Then once at school I realized that I left bag at home, felt angry at self. I'm surprised at my absent-mindedness.
◆ Dream: Of being pulled over by a police officer using radar. I was supposedly going 63 mph. I was very angry and indignant. Pleading with the cops. I noticed I was half hour late and increasingly indignant and pissed. Cops had car towed. Went ballistic, then woke, and I felt immediately relieved but was still pissed about the way I was treated for an hour. The feeling of being unjustly accused or blamed for a bullshit crime evokes a feeling of rage and indignant feeling like: "F— You! Don't control me. You have no right!"

**Day 12**

◆ Dream: Back at childhood home in backyard. People and children around, many are shooting off rockets in the air.

**Prover #2 · Female · 44 years old**

**Day 1**

◆ Woke at 2:30 a.m. with vague recollection of dream fragment—trying to get somewhere but prevented by an obstacle; familiar dream pattern, went back to sleep disappointed.

◆ Woke energetic.

◆ No urge for company.

◆ Irritable at spouse who was late and kept family from attending a planned event on time. I was so irritable with him, I actually left home without him; but he caught up and made up later. Conflict with spouse over relationship expectations; withdrew and cried, but overall good connection and sharing.

**Day 2**

◆ Disappointment with the proving process. What is wrong with me? If I was "cool," I would have symptoms or dreams or something. I really am boring!

◆ Irritable with spouse for waking me. Tired on waking, no energy for exercise > tea and watermelon breakfast.

◆ Anxiety over spouse and in-laws relations. We don't see the world the same and this is fine with him. It is harder for me. I withdrew some and cried some. But overall it was a good, open connection and sharing.

**Day 3**

◆ Took the remedy again.

◆ Details attended to of all the loose ends since I was gone for a week. Schoolwork, bills. Irritable with husband over how he is not keeping track of the checks since I do all the bookkeeping. Walked with a friend and listened to how he is depressed and wishing I could help more, but what to do?

**Day 4**

◆ Light sleep with frequent waking. Unsympathetic towards my husband who woke several times during the night with heartburn. Thought to self internally: "Why is he doing this? Why does he take up so much space?" But externally was considerate and helpful.

◆ Big "date" with husband. Out to eat and to the movies. Fun. Relaxing. Light. Appetite low.

**Day 6**

◆ Slept soundly. No dreams. I don't see any point in taking this any further since I'm not having any dreams or symptoms.

### Prover #3 · Male · 51 years old

**Day 1**

◆ While playing tennis, developed an acute pain in small spot in Achilles tendon five inches from ground; 95% better next day.

**Day 2**

◆ Dream: Sliding on a slide, feeling was fun. I rarely remember dreams.

**Day 3**

◆ Dream: Ordinary subjects and people; playing tennis, eating.

**Day 4**

◆ Dream: Spouse is accused of theft by another couple; I felt exasperated that my spouse gave a statement to the police against my advice.

**Day 6**

◆ Dream: Man giving dollar bills to pigeons. I saw him give them a dollar, a ten and a fifty. He left and I followed the flying pigeon with the fifty, hoping he'd drop the money. He did not.

**Day 7**

◆ Dream: In car with spouse taking turns driving. While wife was driving, she fell asleep and hit a house. Then it was me. I did not want to be caught, so I ran up the hillside that became too steep to climb.

**Day 8**

◆ Dream: In a house in the woods. I pee through a screen door. It is O.K.; it's only males present. A woman approaches, yells, "Stop," so she will not get peed on. She comes in, a Mexican whore with large, flabby breasts. She fondles me. Dream ends, unfortunately.

◆ Dream: Spectator in space war. Rocket ships, ray guns. Building is shaking so badly needs to hang on to the rafters. It is like a rock video, perhaps *Radio Days* by "Kiss."

◆ Woke with mild tenderness in right Achilles tendon. Same place as before. Didn't notice it during yesterday's tennis.

**Day 10**

◆ Dream: Met friend at airport, helped him with unloading the luggage.

### Prover #4 · Female · 46 years old

**Day 1**

◆ Dream: Walking with sister in green grassy park. Met a veterinary surgeon. Sister is flirtatious with him, and I feel jealous and some anger. There are small battery operated police along the way.

◆ Nasal passages feel clear suddenly. Breath feels easily flowing within minutes of taking first dose.

◆ Head pain 9 p.m. Frontal, pounding lasted one hour.

◆ Craved meat at lunch (I am a vegetarian).

◆ No appetite for dinner.

◆ Bladder: Burning during and after urination, like onset of cystitis but did not recur.
◆ Woke at 2 a.m. with sharp pain and stiffness in right index and middle finger for one minute.
◆ Lost in well-known streets; took several wrong turns going to a place she knows well; did not feel frustrated, but rather anxious for the other people she was driving there.

**Day 2**

◆ Dream: Kidnapper at large; while driving down street, recognized man as him through photos wearing green patterned shorts and red shirt. He is taking a small child from a house. Tells other people, but then realize I am in the house with the kidnapper and am in danger. Try to be friendly towards him, have a dialogue, but feel frightened. Begin to run in order to hide from him. There is a huge tank filled with water and dead fish, which are rotting. We change the water, but the fish remain brightly colored, stiff, and floating on the top.
◆ Woke feeling peaceful and full of well-being.
◆ Desire to meditate and be still in self. Sensation of being light in body and mind.
◆ Seaside ameliorates.
◆ Mind: Anger, brooding; visit a patient who normally provokes a gentle loving feeling yet feel anger towards him. I wonder if he is looking angry, but the mood continues after I leave. I feel this underlying arrogance—a sort of broody anger just generally towards almost anyone I think of. By the evening, it goes.
◆ Menses: Onset two days early. Very dark, tarry blood.
◆ Underarm perspiration smells strong and acrid.

**Day 3**

◆ Irritable when speaking to sister on phone but then I realize I feel really irritable with anyone and or any passing thought! It's a really new feeling to me. I try to work but just sit there, unable and unwilling to do anything. I take a hot bath and feel much better. I then work until late evening, back to normal, even better than usual. I feel a sort of deep sadness not far under the surface. I could cry quite easily but don't want to.
◆ Menses: dark flow almost black blood.
◆ External throat: intolerant to clothing around neck.
◆ Stool: long thin dark, smells sulfuric.
◆ Flatulence odor: sulfuric.
◆ Extremities: Sore soles of feet after sitting, > walking.
◆ Stomach: Craves green leafy veggies, spinach, and milk.
◆ Rectum: Pain spasmodic at 5 a.m. (return of old symptom)

**Day 4**

◆ Mind: I feel depressed, sadness, and lonely. Yet at the same time, I know it will change.
◆ Sleep: Sleepiness 3:30 p.m. eyes heavy, naps from 5:30 to 7 p.m. No energy to do anything.
◆ Increased energy at 7 p.m.
◆ Mind: Thoughts clean, efficient, clarity. Fear of the future. Feeling rootless.

◆ Nose: Sneezing repeatedly in the evening.
◆ Stomach: Thirst high for cold.
◆ Menses: Finished 1-2 days sooner than usual.
◆ Joints: wrists. elbows, knees, ankles, stiff. Better as soon as I started moving.
◆ Chilly in evening.

**Day 5**
◆ Woke in the morning, took a deep breath and started crying! Tears then fell as if from a deep pain, grief inside. Weeping throughout the morning. Weeping ameliorates.
◆ Fatigue at 3:30 p.m.; sleepiness; energy returns by 7 p.m.
◆ Crave salt, potatoes, vegetables.

**Day 6**
◆ Dream: Lost clothes, searching everywhere for something to wear, so I wrapped self in rug.
◆ Felt more rested and peaceful in my heart. Something resolved and healed from yesterday's tears. I feel more grounded than usual. A busy day with things that would normally irritate me, such as other people's slowness, but today I just accepted it and still kept to the things I had to do without feeling added pressure. Less scattered and more focused.
◆ Pain pinched right hip on walking.
◆ Connected and energized by trees and nature around me.
◆ Crave salt (3), raw vegetables, fresh food.

**Day 7**
◆ Dream: In a room in a house and it has two animals in it, and one of them is a huge tiger. Somehow I know the tiger is tame if treated carefully. My sister approaches the tiger to take it down off the shelf, where he is standing, but I am scared, and I tell her we should leave him and run out of the room. Tiger starts swiping her with his paw, and we run out quickly.
◆ Dream: Old boyfriend is sitting on ground, and he is very hairy. Sitting licking his leg and rubbing his face on it; sitting with a woman and tells her it is a magic way for him to be sure he will come back again. I feel interested and amazed at how hairy he has become.
◆ Dream: I am at a seminar, and it is in a room across the river. I get a sort of elevator that shoots across the water horizontally—but it misses the room and ends up a long way away. I crawl out and have to crawl along a precipice wall that winds around over the water to get back. J is with me and I am agitated as I am going to be three-quarters of an hour late. I had just arranged a seminar with a pianist, and I realized he hadn't known to play the right music. So I had to arrange another pianist. Eventually I got back to the room. Throughout all the dreams, there was this recurring feeling of the tiger lurking somewhere. Scary feeling.
◆ Woke unrested, anxious after these dreams. Sort of upset, sad, and worried as if something awful had happened.
◆ Pain of hip has moved to back, right lower < twisting, leaning sideways.

**Day 8**
◆ Feels focused and methodical. More patient in situations where I am usually impatient i.e. with slow people.
◆ Nose: Sneezing 5-6 times in row.
◆ Low appetite.

**Day 9**
◆ Sleeplessness on going to sleep, feels jumpy, many thoughts: plans for the next day, things have to do; body feels nervous and unrelaxed.

**Day 10**
◆ Dream: A soft, milky-white skull; milky faces, rather grotesque. Somewhere tigers and cats come into it.
◆ Thoughts seeing the connectedness and patterns in all things. Connected to animals, feeling their moods.
◆ Energy tiredish today—feels like not much sleep. Wired when I go to bed. Many thoughts and I can't get comfortable.
◆ Company aversion to, yet feeling lonely.
◆ Craving plain yogurt, cucumber, peaches. cold juicy things, marmite.

**Day 11**
◆ Dream: I've lost my new kitten. I go to a restaurant where the cat was served to me on a plate; it was skinned with its head intact like a bear rug. Felt so very sad.
Anxious about daughter, who is unhappy in her new house, and her cat, who is finding it hard to settle down.
◆ Anger alternating with sadness.
◆ Sense of playfulness and stretching in the water when went swimming, freedom.
◆ Neck stiffness turning head to left.
◆ Feels best walking among trees and the earth.

**Day 12**
◆ Dream: N is in kitchen wiping up spilled milk. She says her back is hurting her, and she starts chewing a piece of crispy ginseng. I suggest pain is due to anticipatory feelings over upcoming teaching. N denies, she says never gets that. Talk about the remedy Ginseng. Look at the other remedy in that rubric. N bakes a purple potato and eats it. She has a large flower and says the remedy she heard about is like this. It has large leaves which she folds into a braid like Comfrey, Stramonium, Delphinium.
◆ Dream: Daughter calls in a panic saying that her cat has gone crazy being alone all night and that her pen is leaking and sticky. I tell her to flush with water.
◆ Dream: Son is eating a bowl of corn flakes. Tells him it is O.K. to eat backwards when you work nights. (Cereal for dinner, dinner for breakfast.) He goes next door to restaurant with feathers on the window. There are singing gangsters there and an Oliver Twist-type boy putting up more feathers since it is Christmas.
◆ Sleep: Woke at 3 a.m. feeling hot with sore throat. Woke fine next a.m.

◆ Dream: At a wedding with man and woman presiding; have their feet on the lectern and are dressed in black, massaging their feet as they speak.
◆ Feels very good to be walking on the earth.
◆ Skin: Back itchy > skin brush in shower.
◆ Lost 6 pounds since starting proving.

**Day 13**
◆ Sadness, weeping thinking of past spiritual teacher who was hurtful to me. Sadness, gloomy for no reason.
◆ Aversion to speaking. Aversion to work, reading, concentration. Aversion to company.
◆ Thirsty but knows not what for.
◆ Laughing but only on the outside, surface, feels bleak, heavy sadness on the inside. Seeing deeper into others' natures in a very basic way; e.g. very sensitive to people's truthfulness, or lack thereof due to politeness. Felt uncomfortable about it. Felt very quiet and withdrawn.

**Day 14**
◆ Slept only one hour, felt peaceful, quiet, not agitated or anxious at not sleeping. Nothing bothering me.

**Day 15**
◆ Sex: low desire

### Prover #5 · Female · 48 years old

**Day 1**
◆ Dream: Frenetic activity.
◆ Sleep: restless.
◆ Throat: Pain, sore on waking, which faded early. Not severe.
◆ Face: Swelling eyelid, right with redness: no itching or pain.

**Day 2**
◆ Dream: Traveled to China with medical society; full of wonder at the many sights and the planned itinerary.
◆ Slept well but too short.

**Day 3**
◆ Dream: I was lending money to a woman, but (the woman's) husband did not want me to. He said that she was unable to budget, and he wanted his wife to give the money back. I wanted her to have it but was unwilling to cause conflict between them. I was satisfied that I was not a spendthrift.
◆ Dream: On a trip on a bus to see the Loch Ness Monster. I felt strange and out of place

but that people were depending on me for something.
◆ Felt chilled during sleep.
◆ Sadness. Frustrated. Resentful.

**Day 3**
◆ Extremities: Tingling, numbness hands, arms during sleep.
◆ Mouth: Dry.
◆ Sadness, do not want to do anything with husband in evening. Irresolution, underlying feeling of agitation.

**Day 4**
◆ Dream: We needed to get home, no car available so we borrowed a plane and my husband flew it; made children parachute out safely to places they needed to go. We arrived home safely and landed on our street.
◆ Dream: Trying to keep track of people I was supporting, mostly young adults with disabilities. People kept asking me to take in another one, and I could not remember all of them, felt worried I would forget one.
◆ Very resentful of husband and demands of life. Actually told husband did not think I could go on with the relationship. Feeling of being overwhelmed.

**Day 5**
◆ Dream: Going out for dinner with siblings. Everyone went ahead while I waited for last sister to arrive. I waited and waited until everyone else was finished with the meal. I had the feeling of being left out again. Riding a bike through the restaurant with a baby on the back doing headstands.
◆ Dream: Seeing patients in a building with a dome-shaped opening in the roof so the rain came in. I saw several adolescents who reminded me of my youngest son. I tried to teach one to speak French and play the piano.
◆ Still feeling agitated and anxious.
◆ Pain in left arch—hurts to walk.
◆ Mouth: dry.

**Day 6**
◆ Dream: Giving an inspirational talk to a group of women: "We can make a difference."
◆ Dream: Sister announcing bilingual education class, wonders if I should move my family so my children can take advantage of it.
◆ Dream: Just out of the shower with no clothes on and started to walk to my room, when I notice a group of strange people in the house. I call to my husband to get me my clothes. He just laughed at me and didn't do it.
◆ Dream: In line at hospital cafeteria, clerk overcharged and I could not resolve the situation so left tray behind and did not eat. Then at a talk in conference room. Lots of people seated around long table. I kept standing up because I felt so restless, then I lost my seat.
◆ Dream: Touring old high school with daughter, feeling curious and interested.

**Day 7**

◆ Dream: About to undergo unnecessary abdominal surgery as example for medical students. Taking place in large room like a kitchen, needed to get dishes and laundry done before the surgery. I thought it would be done under a local but then realized I was going to sleep and shouted: "I have not signed a consent, you can't put me out." Slightly fearful of being out, but more angry that I could not make them stop. As soon as came to, I immediately jumped up and started folding laundry before the anesthetic wore off and the pain started.

◆ Back: Dull ache in thoracic area.

**Day 8**

◆ Dream: Did sport physicals on ski team. Heard later they had all been killed in plane crash. Felt devastated.

**Day 9**

◆ Frequent waking, restless sleep.

◆ Dream: Sympathizing with group of people who were mourning a friend who was moving.

◆ Dream: Looking forward to daughter's return from living abroad.

◆ Dream: Of having a baby and delivering myself.

**Day 10**

◆ Sleep: Unable to sleep, feeling hyped up.

**Day 11**

◆ Mind: Crying from inability to sleep.

### Prover #6 · Female · 35 years old

**Day 1**

◆ Dream: Cats, pleasant, warm feeling. This is clearly different from my usual dreams.

**Day 5**

◆ Chest: Pain stitching ribs, right, lower, transient.

**Day 6**

◆ Sensitive emotionally.

**Day 7**

◆ Increased libido, increased sexual desire. Distracted.

◆ General: Warmth. More than usual.

◆ Female: Menses early one week. Cramping is less than usual.

◆ Emotionally labile. A 'wreck.' Suspicious. Jealous. Irritable.

◆ Awkward, broke a pot in a store. Clumsy, lost contact lens down the drain.

**Day 8**

◆ Moods: changeable, alternating. Frustrated, due to no outlet for increased sex drive. Still jealous and suspicious much more then my normal state.

**Day 9**

◆ Mouth: sore tongue tip.
◆ Mind: Frustrated.

**Day 10**

◆ I had a strong impulse to steal perfume while walking through a department store. I don't know why. I could pay for it if I wanted to. I have never had this impulse before.
◆ I couldn't help but talk to somebody about the state I'm in and the proving, even though I'm not supposed to. The person I spoke to is not in the proving group.

**Day 11**

◆ Dream: I dreamt of cats again. This time the feeling was of being pursued.
◆ Extremities Pain: Feet: soreness < walking.

**Day 12**

◆ Dream: Someone stealing a part of sewing machine and could not finish a project. Amazed they would steal it because the part had no value, except to the machine. It made me angry.
◆ Irritable and very tired.

## Prover #7 · Male · 52 years old

**Day 1**

◆ Irritability. Impatience.
◆ Warm < wool pants; > removing clothes, fan.
◆ Abdomen: Eructations after eating.

**Day 2**

◆ Dream: Building bridges and making progress.
◆ Dream: A woman training multicolored purple and green snakes. Cartoon-like.
◆ Throat: Sore on waking.

# LAC LUPINUM

*Milk of the Wolf*

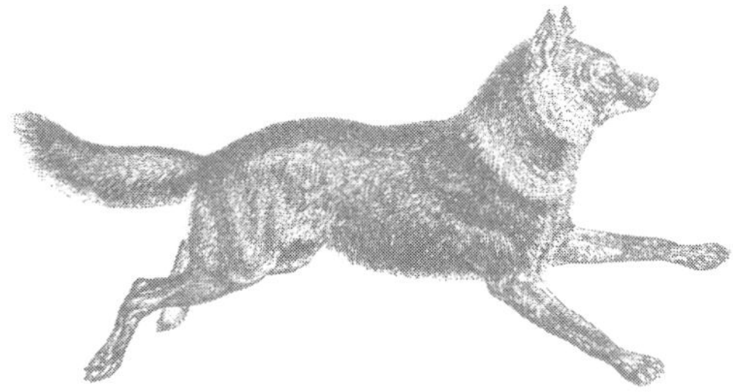

# LAC LUPINUM *Milk of the Wolf*

The gray wolf is a proud, intelligent, family-oriented, and highly socialized carnivore, but he has been despised and feared by most societies, with the notable exception of Native Americans. Wolves are powerful and robust creatures; the male grows to six and one-half feet in length and often weighs over 100 pounds. The female is somewhat smaller.

Wolves live in packs that range from three to 24 members or more. When sexual maturity is reached at about three years of age, rather than leave (as the lion does), wolves most often remain with the pack and mate with another member. The alpha, or superior, female produces from four to fourteen offspring in the spring. Unlike most mammals, all the members of the pack are deeply involved with the care, protection and feeding of the young. The adults play extensively with the pups—tossing and tumbling with them and enduring endless, sharp-toothed baby nips. The father wolf is an especially attentive playmate for his pups.(**PROTECTIVE OF CHILDREN**)

At birth, the pups are blind and have poor hearing but are equipped with an excellent sense of smell. From the very first shove toward the mother's teats, the individual pup shows its personality, and its dominance ranking quickly establishes itself. The leader, who is stronger and more determined than the rest, becomes the alpha pup and will probably be an alpha adult. The other pups fall into an order of descending rank.

Within the pack, this ranking is of great importance. Most of the time, there is an alpha pair who are mated for life, and these two are the leaders of the pack. Their responsibility is the safety and well-being of the other members. Usually one of the two is slightly more dominant than the other, and it is not unusual for it to be the female. Although smaller, she may be more aggressive and intelligent. The alphas engage in ritualistic altercations with their lower-ranked pack mates to demonstrate their dominance. These skirmishes often occur around food. The alpha always reserves the right to eat first and will snarl fiercely and put his or her incisors on the muzzle of the beta wolf who tries to steal food ahead of him or her. This is largely for show, and the bite is really quite gentle; yet it serves its purpose. The beta submits and rolls onto its back with tail between legs, all the while whining, smiling, and urinating on itself. This demonstration lasts just a few seconds, and immediately afterward, the pack will mob the alpha to show its support and submission. This mobbing, which consists of licking, kissing and jumping on the alpha, gives the entire pack a sense of unity and devotion to one another. It may seem anthropomorphic to interpret this behavior in this way, but doing these provings has made me understand the anthropomorphic conclusions animal behaviorists come to regarding their subjects. Man is, after all, an animal; animal is man.

Alpha wolves eat first; they must be strong and healthy at all times because to them falls the duty to counter threats to the pack's safety. They must be first to face danger and be the aggressor because the other wolves look to them for protection and leadership.

In the wolf world, there seems to be a great deal of excitement and enthusiasm. Wolves are extraordinarily fond of each other, and the bonds between them are so tight that the actions of each individual profoundly affect the entire pack. (**FRIENDS/LOVING**) Occasionally, an individual wolf will go off alone for a day or two. It then returns to a great hoopla of howling and joyous greetings, replete with play biting and chasing. This wayward traveler will also get a mild reprimand from the alphas. Once in a while a pack member is rejected and sent out to become a loner. When this happens, that wolf may seek another loner and team up to start a new pack. When an alpha is outranked in a battle for status, he or she may remain in the pack as a lower-ranked member or leave the pack as a loner.

Wolves are great hunters and will eat mice, rabbits, and birds. But their favorite meals are the large herbivores such as moose, deer, elk, and caribou. (**BROAD/WIDE/HUGE**) These creatures are large and well armed with horns and are a definite challenge to the hunting skills of the wolf. (**DANGER/DESIRE FOR DANGER**) First they stalk and chase their intended prey and, after the kill, gorge themselves until their stomachs hang down to the ground. Returning quickly to the den, the hunters go to the nursing moms and pups, and to any weak or sickly pack members, and amid much crying and whining and leaping, they regurgitate into the waiting mouths. The rest of the pack then feasts on the warm, dark, red meat. The pack takes care of an ill wolf until it gets better or dies. In fact, any adult will regurgitate for any other adult any time, on demand, if the other is unable to hunt on its own. Even alpha males have been seen doing this. (**TRYING TO HELP**)

The wolf is very useful in strengthening the herbivore populations because it hunts the most feeble members of the herbivore groups, thus ensuring the survival of the fittest. This is a symbiotic process that culls the herbivores while simultaneously strengthening the hunting abilities of the wolf pack. Of course, the wolf will do the same for cattle and sheep populations. This activity has been, unfortunately, the single most important factor in the wolf's demise. Although they do not significantly reduce livestock populations, wolves who poach give ranchers an excuse to kill. Wolves have been hunted, trapped, and poisoned wherever they come in contact with humans.

Wolves use all their senses intensely. Their sharp vision allows them to see and instantly memorize the height, weight, and shape of an oncoming intruder or friend. Wolves are particularly interested in colors that have red as a base, when these colors are perceived in a strong light. The wolf's senses of smell and hearing are highly acute. They use song extensively by howling in different tones and pitches to convey emotions and information. They signal their location, their excitement, their mournful sadness at the death of a pack member, and their tremendous joy in life through their singing. R.D. Lawrence best describes this in his book, *In Praise of Wolves:* "On the ground lying, sitting or standing, the wolves begin to howl. The throbbing, sweetly melancholy calls seem to fill the entire evergreen forest. To be in such a place at such a time....is an experience that awakens the primal emotions that each of us carries deep within his being."

Lawrence further discusses another special feature of wolf vocalizing, which involves the wolf's distinctive relationship with the raven. The raven's caw alerts the wolf that there is a herd or weak animal nearby. (**TRYING TO HELP**) The wolf then makes the kill, and the raven comes in for his share of the meat. In mutual celebration, both raven and wolf sing together in a song that Lawrence calls haunting, spiritual, and primitive.

Play is a big part of the life of the wolf. Making body contact, chasing, bumping, teasing, rolling, kissing, biting are everyday activities in a healthy wolf pack. The wolf burrows a chamber down a long, dark, twisted tunnel in the cool ground. (**CIRCLES/SPIRALS**) (**ENCLOSURES/CROWDED/TUNNELS**) There, in relative safety, the nursing mom and her pups are protected against intruders as well as the heat and bugs of the summer. Their coats are so warm and oily that they don't need protection from winter's cold.

### The Wolf Today

Schemes to kill wolves have been rampant throughout the world and throughout time. Some have been carried out by farmers banding together for the night to shoot local wolves. Others, in more ominous, well-planned and officially funded programs, have sought the total extinction of the wolf. (**MORTALITY/IMMORTALITY**) In Europe, the wolf had a reputation as a child killer, and thus all wolves were seen as a sinister menace to society. (**PROTECTIVE OF CHILDREN IN DANGER**)They have been completely decimated in most countries in Europe. Some still remain and continue to be hunted in remote regions of Spain.

In India, to the present day, the wolf is often scapegoated. In one scenario in the town of Banbirpur, villagers attributed the deaths of 33 children to wolves. An article in the *New York Times* stated: "It has been more than a century since India faced the threat of man-eating wolves on anything like the scale now terrorizing this region of the state of Uttar Pradesh." The article then went on to say that the villagers killed ten rampaging wolves and that even though men kept vigil all night, attacks continued. The article proceeded in this vein until finally, the truth was revealed: The villagers had been pressured into blaming wolves for the attacks, while the attacks were actually being conducted by men dressed as werewolves. Thus, for no particular reason, the wolf was blamed for something it didn't do.

In addition, we see that even a reporter from the *New York Times* was willing to prey on the prejudice against wolves and give readers the impression, at least in the first part of his report, that the wolf is a rampant child killer. The truth is, as David Mech, a Minnesota wildlife biologist and wolf specialist, is quoted as saying in an article by Aurelio Rojas in the *San Francisco Chronicle*: " 'There aren't any documented incidents of wolves attacking people.' " Just, it seems, people attacking wolves.

Another criticism of wolves is that they decimate herds of big game. However, a recent report from Idaho reveals that a fully recovered wolf population there would probably consume only 1,600 weakened or dead deer or elk a year while poachers illegally claim over 10,000 healthy deer and elk annually.

At various times in our history, licensed guides recruited hunters from Europe who paid large sums to shoot the wolf for sport. Other methods of slaughter by the government included the use of poisons, such as strychnine-treated baits and traps. (**DAMAGING LIQUID**) (**HOLES IN LEGS**) Finally, and perhaps most unfairly, airplanes were used, from which hunters shot the animals. (**VEHICLES**) (**PROTECTIVE OF CHILDREN IN DANGER**)

In the proving, many of the "feelings" of the wolf come out very clearly: **DETACHED, CONFUSED, CRITICAL, INTRUDER.** This proving was unusually rich in the number of strong themes. It had many more than any of the other provings I have done. The wolf, maybe because of its precarious position, which nears extinction, seems to elicit especially powerful dreams and sensations in the human prover. Particularly strong and poignant was, as one prover put it, "The feeling I was dying or I did not have the strength to go on living." The proving suggests that the wolf may feel that its end as a species is near.

### The Substance

The milk for this proving was obtained from a gray wolf bitch who lives in a large and forested enclosure in British Columbia. (**ENCLOSURES**) She and her pack receive humane treatment by the people who care for them. Melissa Assilem obtained the original substance and did the first proving on it. Melissa graciously assented to my request to do a second proving on the milk of this fascinating and complex creature. It will be interesting to compare the two provings once both are published.

### Further Observations

What is this unnamable fear that pervades humans whenever and wherever wolves are concerned? In 1977, President Jimmy Carter commissioned a report which stated that: "In no time in recorded history has the specter of species extinction loomed so ominously." The wolf seems to have been earmarked by humans for planned extinction. Many reasons have been set forth for this, such as the killing of children and mass slaughter of deer and elk, but as we have seen, these do not appear to be true.

When Jessica Jackson and I thought about the prejudice against and planned extermination of wolves, we made the correlation to one particular, large event in human history—the holocaust. Here, a group of people planned and methodically scheduled, on a large scale, the dissolution of several other groups of people. (**CONFUSED/ORGANIZED**) The victims of the holocaust included not only Jews but also Catholics and Gypsies. The story of the Gypsies has several close parallels to that of the wolves. Both wolves and Gypsies are inclined to roam freely in large territories, have a great love of music and song, possess mythic abilities to communicate over large distances (wolves by howling, Gypsies by broken twigs and signs in nature), and have extraordinarily strong family ties and rituals. Gypsies have a great love of beauty and flashy colors, especially the color red, and any wayward event in a town or village—any theft or murder—has often historically been attributed to Gypsies. This is also what has happened to the wolf, as we saw in the India news story. It seems that both Gypsies and wolves inspire exaggerated legends. The fairy tale, *Little Red Riding Hood*, comes from Europe and tells of the horrible, trickster, monster wolf who eats an innocent, little girl and her kind grandmother. Millions of children grew up being told that if they were "bad," the Gypsies would "come and get them." The reputation for killing, or stealing, small children has led to the persecution of both Gypsies and wolves.

While it is estimated that between 200,000 and half a million Gypsies were killed by the Nazis, the exact number will never be known because Gypsies were unregistered in their native lands. Many, many thousands of wolves were killed in the United States in the earlier part of this century. Once numbering in the hundreds of thousands in the U.S. alone, very few wolves remain in the wild around the world and only about 2,000 in the contiguous United States. Gypsies continue to be harassed severely wherever they go. In *Bury Me Standing*,

Isabel Fonseca says: "Since the revolution in Romania in 1989, there has been a sharp escalation of hatred and violence (toward the Gypsies). There have been more than 35 serious attacks.... Istvan Varga, for example, a three-year-old boy from Transylvania, was burned to death in a haystack." (**FIRE**)

Wolves can also be closely linked to Native Americans, especially the Nez-Perce tribe. Both wolves and Nez-Perce are hunters that travel in groups over wide territories, looking for game. Both were nearly destroyed to make room for settlers and their sheep. The Nez-Perce even used the cries of the wolf to find caribou and moose. Recently, the Nez-Perce received a small grant to study the behavior of wolves and opened the Wolf Education and Research Center in Idaho, where visitors are able to observe a pack of eleven wolves. According to Nez-Perce, Jaime Pinkham: "Today we see a reflection of our fate in the wolf. We were both displaced...and now, we are both trying to find our way home." (**LOST THINGS**)

One interesting fact that links two of the provings in this book is that researchers have discovered evidence that, at a certain point in history, wolves went into the sea. (**WATER**) Over millennia, they developed flippers and lost their legs. The dolphin is thought to have evolved from wolves or wolf-like animals. (**DANGER IN WATER**) (**FISH**) Given that three water-related themes came up in this proving, we can only speculate on the existence of a field of consciousness that still links the land and sea version of this mammal.

The wolf, whose family structure and devotion to its young is very similar to the best of human behavior, has a great deal to teach us, if only we will listen. The proving seems to tell us that we are not yet listening.

*Lac Lupinum*

# Themes

*Milk of the Wolf*

- *Mortality/Immortality*
- *Protective of Children in Danger*
- *Intruder/Outsider*
- *Danger/Desire for Danger*
- *Fire*
- *Damaging Liquid*
- *Danger in Water*

- *Detached*
- *Confused/Organized*
- *Critical*
- *Trying to Help*
- *Enclosures/Crowded/Tunnels*
- *Friends/Loving*

- *Broad/Wide/Huge*
- *Circles/Spirals*
- *Holes in Legs*

- *Fish*
- *Wallet/Purse/Lost Things*
- *Transportation/Vehicles*
- *Water*

# *Mortality/Immortality*

**#3** Dream: I walk into a cafeteria; sitting there is a friend of mine from grammar school who died when we were in college in Michigan. He had a heart attack on the basketball court at age 21. I never got to spend as much time with him as I wanted. "Hey I am surprised to see you," I said. "Your mom told me you had died." He looked embarrassed and said he wasn't well but he would be O.K. I told him I missed seeing him and having him as a friend all these years. Felt very sympathetic. I felt that I was getting in touch with the fact that we never really die; he really was there. I was talking to him and although he wasn't doing well, he candy-coated it for earth people. He wanted to be polite; I would not understand it. I thought, oh, well, that is what he needs to do, no judgment. Either way I knew inside I understood real life. His mother told me he died and it tore their family apart. His parents ended up getting a divorce.

**#4** Felt ethereal, disconnected from body but mind is very together and alert and conscious. Felt like my body not there, like I was dying, and I was leaving my body and didn't mind. I was too weak and disconnected.

**#4** I think I'm being really conscious of women's suffering, more so; feel like I see it in a new light. I feel ages of women, felt the pain of Othello's wife in the video, felt so sad and emotionally charged by her death, by all women's death by men.

**#5** Dream: At amusement park, a throw-up ride. We are leaving as a teenager arrives, he takes an elevator to the top of a building, jumps off screaming, and he kills himself. No one knows him or what's going on. Woke me up out of sleep.

**#6** Dream: ...Wondering if it is O.K. to let pigeons rest on you. We see pigeons flocked on a dead person. We think they are eating a homeless, dead person; but we get there and see he is O.K.

**#6** Had an actual experience with someone who wanted something (an emotional connection) from me. She has a tremendous need for something from me. I have nothing for her. I get a migraine headache from this experience. Up all night with it. That night I felt I was dying. No strength to go on living.

**#6** I wake up in the middle of the night having an intense anxiety attack. I am gong to go broke, bankruptcy, my business is going to fail. I am going to die. Sat for three hours trying to meditate the feeling away. Felt as if I was dying, too weak to go on.

**#7** Dream: My wife was being held forcibly by some men in the kitchen in our house. They were gagging her and she was terrified. I was walking toward her to save her. She was motioning to me to get away, and I was stabbed with swords, killed? He chopped me up with a sword. Do I want to die or do I want to go?

# *Protective of Children in Danger*

**#1** Dream: I was an early pioneer settler in the West. I was a child being attacked by Indians, and all children were hiding in one room. We could hear the attack outside. Could hear them outside yelling war cries, gunshots. Kids hiding huddled together in a room. I buried my head in my hands.

**#4** Another bad dream of men hurting, violating young girls.

**#5** Dream: Calling 911, "Man entering home. Mother has been knocked down." Two sons tell me a weird man outside is trying to get inside the house, we run around locking doors. As I'm locking the last door, the man bursts in and knocks me down, beats me. Terrified, protective of kids. Dream was powerful enough to wake me, fast, energetic, active, fearful.

**#10** Baby-sat a young child and felt unreasonably concerned about her safety. I kept looking down the hall and had a desire to run out.

**#5** Dream: Party at friend's, going water-skiing in the dark with ten year-old kids. Confusing because how can you water-ski in dark, how can you do this? I say I can't take my son into this situation. I come back from the bathroom, and they had left without me. I yell the hostess's name down the street. Fear, they left, there is danger and kids involved, they left without hearing what I had to say about it. Felt shocked, hurt, abandoned.

**#1** At 1 a.m. I heard tapping on the window that scared me to death. I heard my name whispered, drew curtains, and it was my mother. She had tried to call, but the phone was off the hook. She said she was worried about my three-year-old daughter and had a "premonition." She wanted to make sure she was O.K.

**#2** Dream: ...I insisted they leave. I struggled physically with the man, who became violent. He grabbed my daughter pulling her hair; she (was) arching her back. (His) pulling her hair (was) starting to hurt her. Felt violated—they pushed themselves in. I was trying to set a boundary, and they used my daughter.

**#4** Dreamt about a woman and her children being gassed and poisoned by a man in a car. A bad dream.

**#2** Dream: Intruders got daughter. Black magic, voodoo needles in her eyes; calling 911. My children are being hurt!

**#7** Dream: Walking around with father-in-law and daughter at Tilden Park in hilly area with steep path, large deep steps four to five feet high, leading down from the church. Lots of people around. Walked in front of daughter, carrying toy vehicle. Went back to get daughter, it was a long way back. Could not find her there in the church playground in the crowd of kids. Then found her lying on the ground; she had been hit on the head by some kid with a pipe. I felt upset, I had abandoned her.

**#9** A neighbor is riding on the front hood of his baby sitter's car while she is driving. An old man who looks demonic is speaking to him. I suspect the child is being abused. I talk to the mother. I'm concerned but not emotionally upset. "Who is your pediatrician? Can I be of help?"

**#9** There was this high structure, like a double cross, somehow involved with danger, somewhat similar to high-tension, electrical wires. A random, large group of people had been kidnapped and taken to a place that was deep underground where conditions were barely livable—horrible—incompatible with life. A young woman risks her life to escape and get help for the others (though it was known they were captured and not much was being done about it). A hopelessly threatening situation. I went with the young woman to her family. There were two young children, a man, and a woman. The children did not seem traumatized to have lost some family members. The situation seemed quite ordinary, not much emotion—maybe not enough food.

# *Intruder/Outsider*

**#1** I've been very sensitive. Had a disagreement over homeopathy and my beliefs with my family and got upset, almost starting crying. I had to leave the room. I felt like an outsider to my family, that I didn't belong. Also that they did not even care to hear my viewpoint. It made me feel unimportant and incidental.

**#2** Dream: A strange man and woman came dipping their fingers into our butter and dip, which was on the ground on leaves. I told them it was dirty, but they ate it anyway. They were very intrusive and pushed their way into the house, asking for more and more, and started stealing things throughout the house, hiding things in their clothes. I insisted they leave. I struggled physically with the man, who became violent.

**#3** ...I was more like a spirit watching—an outsider.

**#3** Dream: I was intruding on another man's place of residence, a large property fenced in, no buildings, living amongst junk. I needed something from him and was sneaking around. I didn't want his dogs to know I was there; they were sleeping. I came across an outside kitchen area with a refrigerator, and from the contents, I got a feeling the dogs got to eat meat and the man ate celery and carrots. But as I was leaving, I came across a dog and at first I was scared, but I gave it a carrot, which he ate, and he was fine. As I was leaving, it dawned on me. I was intruding on my own home. An intruder in my own world. Felt almost like a revelation.

**#3** Dream: I had a roommate who was moving out. Like a dorm room in college. He left some of his things, a few of which I was glad to have, like detergent, etcetera. I felt glad he was out of my space.

**#2** Dream: Intruders got (my) daughter....

# Danger/Desire for Danger

**#3** I need to be unprotected. Wanting to be raw, not hidden behind anything. I do not want to be sheltered, kept from anything harmful; wanted to be open to all experience with no boundaries i.e. drive without my seat belt. I sought out an unprotected place to come from. Neutral about the danger factor. Not seeking it, but if anything came along.... Wanting to be out there, at risk. When I am out there at risk, I feel relieved—an exposed state, enjoying the exposure.

**#2** Dream: I was outside a hotel in a large, concrete building in a round shape, like an amusement park ride.... A man was operating it and felt I was at his mercy. I was encouraging my daughter to jump on with me. It must have been fun.

**#3** Dream: Hiking with a guide and some others in the mountains, hanging by my right arm from a cliff.... I knocked a piton into a rock and was just hanging there. I was O.K. The feeling of, "How do you know I am O.K.?" It's feeling like I'm in a precarious position but O.K.

**#3** Dream: ...The stockbroker turns and says, "I hope that plane gets out of our way, and I asked if it wasn't far enough away. He flips the plane over, and we're flying upside down, ten feet above the water. He is turning into these sailboats. and we're having a great time. I am very calm about it, very matter-of-fact, and he is acting like he does this all the time. While weaving through the boats, he tries to communicate to me that this is the best way to be going....

**#3** Dream: I was driving around in a go-cart and was racing another boy. Big crowd of people were meandering over the track in a trance, like *Night of the Living Dead.* We can't race well because I didn't want to hit anyone; I was frustrated. I finally saw an opening between the guys, drove into it, and then the crowd dispersed and we could race. I was amazed that it was that easy to get the crowd away. That frustration gave way to wonder and surprise. Frustration gave way to success.

**#4** Dream: Before I was fully asleep, I had dreams of fireballs. Young boys, youths throwing or having huge balls like a meteorite, going past them like fireworks. I was just watching them with no real feeling.

**#4** Wanted to feel something, craving hot, spicy, chili peppers, can't get enough. Wanted to burn and be in pain, have a rush. Represented danger, but in a less destructive way.

**#4** Dream: I was whizzing around on the back of a firetruck with lots of women around. I felt safe.

**#7** Dream: New doctor wants to join clinic were I work. He did not want to buy disability insurance; says if he needed it, he would sue the clinic for his four dollars an hour. Another doctor there who is also a lawyer is sitting on this guy's lap, and when he hears this sue comment, he falls off the chair.

**#7** Dream: Camping deep in the woods with a large group of people. We arrive there by ice skating uphill on a new, concrete sidewalk. We cooked and ate without bear precaution, and as soon as we arrive, a grizzly bear enters our camp and starts eating our food. Then a polar bear arrives and chases us all through the tent a few times in circles and then leaves. The polar bear chased us walking like a human. Friends from my medical school residency are there. Scared all night about bears....

**#8** Dream: ...he went through the obstacle and on the closed road and around all kinds of dangerous stuff. He sped up the car so it would have momentum to fly over a huge gap in the road and land on the other side. I was annoyed and frustrated at being stuck in this situation, with a guy not very safe.

**#10** Dream: Pursued through old building.... Despair of being trapped with no way out.

## *Fire*

**#2** Dream: I'm keeping fires going in a huge store paying $130 a week for pallets....

**#2** Dream: Watching the sun or moon, a big fireball dropping into the sea; felt and sounded like a glass ball....

**#3** Dream: In a burning building, moving up there the floors in an attempt to escape the fire; not sure if it was out on lower floors, but it was chasing a group of us; feeling unsure about the danger; moving away from it but not sure if the fire was still a threat.

**#4** Dream: Before I was fully asleep, I had dreams of fireballs. Young boys, youths throwing or having huge balls like a meteorite, going past them like fireworks. I was just watching them with no real feeling.

**#4** Dream: I was whizzing around on the back of a firetruck with lots of women around. I felt safe.

**#7** Dream: Old house in woods, returning there with two people. I wanted to see if someone was O.K., but the two others were unconcerned. One had a bike and they went off. I went through double doors into a living room where everything was a mess, and looked around the doors to left and saw a toy ironing board, with a baby creature wrapped in swaddled blanket. It said, "Play with me," and I picked it up and realized it was this evil little thing called "Ichy," or whatever. I started to smash it with a toy iron, but it bit me on the finger. I became concerned about the safety of the little girl at home and went to the kitchen to find her. I took the evil creature and put it in the oven on "self clean" to destroy it; burned it to a cinder. All the appliances were on full blast, with oil all over them, making quite a fire hazard. There were pipes and burners everywhere. I turned them all off. When I yelled for help, no one was around. The kitchen was a maze of pipes, spooky. I felt this evil creature had done all this and was trying to burn the house down. Woke up.

**#10** Very hot. Sense of internal burning from the retreat. Feel like I am burning through the proving doses in 24 hours.

# *Damaging Liquid*

**#3** Dream: Two men had a damaging liquid that was damaging to humanity. One of the men was carrying it around in a pen like James Bond.

**#3** Dream: Sitting in an auditorium between two high school bullies. One of them started smacking me in the head. I was involved with some sort of ritual with oil. I got up and walked to the back of the room. At one point, I elbowed one of them in the face. I was disconnected; it did not matter, everyone was surprised I did not retaliate more.

**#4** Dream: ...Everyone shared rooms on the inside; children were playing in this purple liquid. I knew it was bad for them to be putting it in their mouths. I gave the children back to their mother, worried about the bad liquid a man gave them. They were sleepy, and I worried they were ill.

**#8** Dream: Person I know in waking time from school came to visit me with a test tube rack full of different types of chemical bottles and tubes of all colors and styles. Some look like perfume bottles more than test tubes. They are in disarray, haphazardly arranged in the rack, some close to spilling. We are inside a pink or salmon-colored bathroom, and this person is somehow holding this rack over me so that I look up at it. Some of the bottles/tubes were dripping their contents. I told him I did not want my face etched with acid. Later, I went back into the bathroom, and there were bubbles of creamy liquid on the floor, as if some of the chemicals from the test tubes had spilled there and were reacting. There was also something like sprinkles around that looked like cooked white rice kernels. The bubbles and puddles were creamy pink or yellow-colored, which I perceived as a disgusting, frustrating mess because I had to clean it up without getting anything on my hands.

**#7** All the appliances were on full blast, with oil all over them, making quite a fire hazard.

# *Danger in Water*

**#2** Friend swimming in water that became rough. He went under, I dove to bottom to get him; he wasn't breathing. The lady running the boat was very casual about the whole thing. Did not say to get help, nothing.

**#3** Dream: Two boys playing around in their motorboat, having fun. They came across something on the surface that indicated a problem, an older man trapped under the water. They pushed a pole down to him like a rescue pole and pulled him up. I was a bystander; I was not any of the people in the dream. I was glad because he didn't have much air left.

**#9** Dream: Boy is playing on edge of large, round precipice. He is not my responsibility, but I am watching him thinking, he may fall. He does fall very far down into the center—which is a body of water. I jump in right away, without a thought, to help him. I and another person struggle to pull him out of the water or he would have drowned. He was under for a little long. I wonder, Will he be okay? Will his mother be satisfied that we did our best?

# Detached

**#1** Who cares what others think anyway? I don't care about consequences of my actions or speech—only concerned with the here and now.

**#1** ...I'm a basket case. I feel like I'm in a daze. Feels like my head is separate from my body. It's like my body is doing one thing and my head is doing another.... ... Felt disassociated, not connected to my body. Disconnected from emotions, from things going on around me. Things were happening but I was apathetic: "Oh well too bad...."

**#2** Dream: A friend was swimming in water that became rough. He went under. I dove to the bottom to get him. He wasn't breathing. The lady running the boat was very casual about the whole thing. Did not say to get help, nothing.

**#3** Dream: My motorcycle is parked under a friend's house at the beach, and a big storm came through and trashed the underside of the house, including my bike. I saw all the water. He knew this but was hesitant to tell me. I was angry at myself because I knew not to leave it here. He was very detached from the whole thing, he was numb to it.

**#4** Realized I didn't want to pass through emotions. Didn't want to feel them.

**#5** Ahead of myself, a little panicky, short-tempered, out of body. External concerns. Felt off, felt not responding to what was happening in the moment.

**#10** Father has cancer; not very emotional with him—sense of detachment.

# *Confused/Organized*

**#1** Went to use microwave but put bowl of soup into cupboard next to the microwave and closed door as if to microwave.

**#1** Mind scattered, thoughts all over the place, difficult time focusing.
I felt anxious, like I need to get something done but not sure what.

**#2** Difficulty making decisions. Had to go back and forth, going somewhere and not sure what to wear. Went out the door with two different shoes on. (I) could not decide; forgot I was making the decision and realized I had two different shoes on. Normal, everyday, simple decisions were hard....

**#2** Got very energized at night and up late feeling very organized...or think I am, therefore feel calm.

**#3** Dream: I felt like I had a lot of work to do. Felt a little messy and confused. My place got screwed up, no shelter, a big piece of open property with junk lying around.

**#5** Dream: In a sitting room with other parents wondering if we should color-code a map. I start to explain why we should and then why we shouldn't, and I get totally messed up and upset because I don't know what I am talking about. We are being watched by someone sitting way up high.

**#5** Dream: Our assembly at school is getting ready to start. I find a room but have confusion about where to go. Someone thinks we have the wrong room. It is a huge auditorium with tiered seats, empty and vast.

**#3** Dream: I was hiking up a trail, which was very technical, with a woman who is wondering why I am leading her all over this mountain, wondering where we are going. I am obviously confused and don't know where we are going. I didn't even realize why I was in this confused state...poor planning, roaming around, unsure. Disorganized.

**#1** Dream: Organizing purse and then dumping out because not right and reorganizing it again.

# Critical

**#1** Dream: Planning my daughter's third birthday party. My mother came dressed as Minnie Mouse in a cardboard costume. I kept thinking she looks so stupid.

**#2** Strong inner critical voice. By letting it out, I felt better but did not want to do it. Felt bad being critical of things, even small things that normally would not bother me. But it was not a release because I did not like that I was being picky about things. It all seemed so trivial. The things that were making me uptight.

**#3** I am still feeling critical overall. I still want to fix things and contribute. Sort of critical and helpful at the same time. Seems to be coming through some of my dreams, more critical than anything.

**#5** Husband said I have been more critical, short-tempered, not myself, mentally depressed, looking for a way out or an excuse in my mind.

## *Trying to Help*

**#2** Dream: My daughter's teacher was going on vacation and wanted me to substitute. Looking at my calendar, each day was large and very detailed. I was free and could do it.

**#2** Dream: Had a dream of friend who would take my children and a lot of others from Friday to Wednesday until 7 p.m. I was surprised at how outrageous a babysitting offer this was....

**#3** Dream: I was teaching a friend how to deploy a parachute. He was going out for a flight with an older man in an airplane. I felt like I needed to offer him something, some sort of help, instruction or help somehow.

**#3** Dream: Hiking with a guide and some others in the mountains, hanging by my right arm from a cliff of some type. The guide on the other side of the ravine is dealing with other people who need more help, who are really struggling. They are afraid they are going to fall into the ravine. "Hey, what about me? I don't know what I'm doing!" The guide said to just do what he did. I knocked a piton into a rock and was just hanging there. I am O.K....in a precarious position but O.K. (In real life, I don't climb mountains.)

**#3** Dream: Learning and teaching a friend who had to deploy a parachute in case something went wrong on a flight with a father figure. I felt I had to offer him something to help with. I helped him deploy his parachute, yet I did not know what I was talking about, did not know if he needed to know it or not. I felt as though I had something to offer that might not be welcomed.

**#4** Feel like I have to help others less fortunate. I am so lucky, I have so much. I just want to help my friends and try and save their lives—help them have better, easier, healthier lives.

**#8** Dream: In a car with a repairmen who had been working on my house. I was not totally happy with him, but he needed help finding a parts store. I knew how to get to where the store was; showed him....

**#5** Dream: High school boyfriend was helping me with a math problem, getting ready for a test.

# Enclosures/Crowded/Tunnels

**#9** Dream: There was this high structure, like a double cross, somehow involved with danger, somewhat similar to high-tension, electrical wires. A random, large group of people had been kidnapped and taken to a place that was deep underground where conditions were barely livable—horrible—incompatible with life.

**#10** Dream: Moving silently through house at night. Very alert, not fearful. Trying to find someone in many rooms, like a maze. No fear but feeling of needing to avoid being trapped at all costs...kept looking down the hall; desire to run out.

**#4** Dreams of restrictions, in enclosure. Usually have open, airy dreams. This space was tunnel-like.

**#3** Dream: Intruding on another man's place of residence, a large property fenced in, no buildings, living amongst junk.

**#4** Dream: ...It was in this big building which reminded me of something Russian. Leaflets and posters were stuck on the outside, oppressed, negative, fearful feeling on the outside....

**#4** Dreams of hundreds of live chickens, all boxed in a room.

**#10** Dream: Pursued through old building: many rooms—maze-like.... Despair about being trapped with no way out.

**#5** Dream: ...Down a water tunnel. I am afraid to go down. I pull the rope back up and try to get at the sling-like hammock to sit on it, but it's all tangled. My breathing is short; I know it is fine, but I can't figure it out. I'm too hot, I can't breathe, I try to unbutton my shirt while I untangle the rope. I know I can do this if I can just.... Shallow breath, not claustrophobic. Sensations in the body woke me.

**#6** Dream of the far future: My family and I are waiting for a sea bus. There's total overpopulation, the beach is overcrowded with people and pigeons.

**#7** (I) had to crawl into crawl space to fix heating duct.

**#8** Dream: ...large building...made of cinder blocks...no windows or doors.

## *Friends/Loving*

**#2** Dream: Friend over, in the middle of the night, who had her son come under the covers to keep her warm. Somehow with her family in Spain, very old, another past lifetime. We were with them in Spain—her whole family traveling.

**#2** Dreams of familiar people. I feel aware and have deep knowing, recognition. Friend and her family were at their house; door was large, massive, with a large doorknob. Went to restaurant with group, left early....

**#2** Dream: ...seems close to reality. Friend, in dream at house with children, selling stickers, kids party. Sister backing up in old truck; told her to get out of here fast.

**#5** Dream: Party of teenagers, son off somewhere. I meet this guy I've met before, and we walk to the corner. I sit in a friend's convertible while he goes across the street. Son shows up from a friend's house, an old friend whom I haven't seen in awhile, and I realize it would be so good to see her.

**#6** Dream: Reconnecting and resolving things with old friends. We meet and...totally resolve everything. We agree to let everything go....

**#8** Dream at large party with many people, old friends from grade school and present.

**#4** I saw a man hugging a younger man, a genuine, loving fatherly hug. I felt a sense of appreciation and love for them and that I was missing some kind of male love and companionship. I wanted a fatherly hug or something, as if I saw male love for the first time, without it being tinged with embarrassment or sexuality or fear.

**#4** Feeling love and openness towards my friends. I am accepting myself more. I am enjoying life and what it brings, good and bad.

# *Broad/Wide/Huge*

**#1** Sensitive to criticism, Was shopping and sales lady asked my size and said, you're much broader than that. Normally, I brush it off but kept thinking about it. Bugged me that I was called "broad."

**#2** Actual event: Looking at the moon on Christmas Eve. Moon was very round, wide, but it had a black cloud in front of it with two white, radiant wings coming out from either side: white moon covered with black.

**#2** Dream: At an ocean bay seeing huge whale....

**#5** Dream: In old building, in an apartment with a man I know, seems to be my mate. I notice he is extremely big, with wide hips like three feet across—not fat, just massive. I look at myself and think how tiny I am in comparison, very strange.

**#6** Dream: Big neighbor (6 foot 10 inches) brings a baby raccoon over to our house.... He's a big, friendly, opinionated galoot with a big heart and a gruff exterior.

**#6** Dream: Big, fat man.

**#7** Dream: Walking with shoes that were very wide...quadruple E.... I actually have very narrow feet.

**#5** Dream: At wide crosswalk with many lanes of cars, afraid to walk across and in front of cars looming so big. Light says I can walk, but I'm sure I can't make it, so I don't move; felt fearful.

**#2** Dream: Of familiar people in dreams. I feel aware and have deep knowing, recognition. Friend and her family were at their house; door was large, massive, with a large doorknob. Went to restaurant with group, left early, driving around skateboard park, lots of water, at ocean.

# *Circles/Spirals*

**#2** Actual event: ...kayaking in bay...circled by seals, in the center, a moment of awe in this perfect circle, then they went back to their frolicking and playing. Felt a richness, a simple connection to the seals. Felt like a celebration.

**#2** Dream: I was outside a hotel in a large, concrete building that had a round shape like an amusement park ride. I was in an elevator, which was a chute or circle going up and down the outside of the building. The chute went in a circle, transporting me like an elevator. It would suck me into the spin to stay on. Feeling of rushing up and down, sucking me into a spin, suction. Wished for a belt or bar to hold onto, water swirling in it as part of the suction.

**#2** Actual event: ...looking at the moon on Christmas Eve. Moon was very round, but it had a wide, black cloud in front of it with two white, radiant wings coming out from either side: white moon covered with black.

**#2** Dream: Watching the sun or moon, a big fireball, dropping into the sea, felt and sounded like a glass ball....

**#3** I would almost be somewhere and then decide to go elsewhere and turn around, driving around in circles....

**#5** Dream: Happened in buildings or water. We go inside and open a secret door to find a slide like a spiral hamper chute. A woman who is my guide says this takes us down to her place. She pulls up a rope with a hammock on it and sits down on it and whoosh! Off she goes down the slide.

**#5** Dream: Children in class doing an Advent spiral, walking around a path usually made of pine boughs, but this one was weird, made from beanbags all pulsating up and down. All very nice feeling.

**#7** Then a polar bear arrives and chases us all through the tent a few times in circles, then leaves.

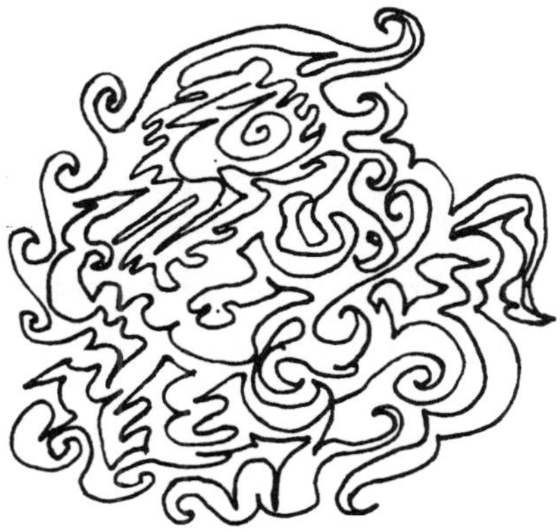

**Drawings/doodles that two different provers made in their notebooks during the proving.**

## Holes in Legs

**#1** Dream: Wearing holey leggings. Very vivid. The next day went to put on leggings, thought there should be holes; then recalled that was in my dream.

**#2** I put two different stockings on with holes in them. Had to keep changing them.

**#6** Dream: Two old high school friends—one kind of arrogant (and) has a hole in his leg, maybe cancer.... I am concerned and trying to...help him.

# *Fish*

**#2** Dream: Friend...transported them just to see the villa they lived in and left, though we were served dinner first, a lot of fish choices.

**#2** Craving fish

**#2** Dream: She had some Chinese takeout of real big containers, huge scallops. We could only serve so many....

**#7** My wife was cooking fish. I could not tolerate the smell; it nauseated me.

**#8** Dream: ...I'm looking at a still pool with an eddy, and my black cat suddenly can be seen swimming to the surface of the water from below, and then as she reaches the surface, she eats bugs that are floating there, like a trout would do....

**#8** Dream: I'm at a large party with many people, old friends from grade school and present. There's elaborately arranged seafood and vegetables on black plates given to us individually as we sit at an outdoor bar.

# *Wallet/Purse/Lost Things*

**#1** Dream: Organizing purse and then dumping out because not right and reorganizing it again. Sitting on bed doing this, with a mindless feeling. Not frustration.

**#3** Dream: Standing waist-high in clear water, with another man; my wallet had dropped to bottom of pool. I was freaked out that I lost my wallet—not sure if it was about the money or the loss of my identity—but then I found it and picked it up and started to dry it. Felt detached and didn't care that it was wet.

**#3** Dream: ...I could not find my wallet. Found it, not really lost, just next to the plane.

**#4** Kept losing wallet and keys, personal things, etcetera.

**#8** Left purse at restaurant; very unusual.

## *Transportation/Vehicles*

**#3** Car broken into and air bags, radio, glove box, whole dashboard stolen. Did not panic even though I then had no car and no mass transportation.

**#3** Dream: My motorcycle is parked under a friend's house at the beach....

**#2** Dream: Traveling in the countryside. Felt I was having a past life experience waiting for two friends on motorcycles....

**#2** Dream: My cousin and I in a dark dream, in the late night driving around a city in a rental red car. We got into an accident.

**#5** Dream: At wide crosswalk with many lanes of cars, afraid to walk across and fronts of cars looming so big.

**#7** Dream: ...walked in front of daughter, carrying toy vehicle....

**#3** Dream: I was driving around in a go-cart and was racing another boy....

**#2** Dream: ...driving around a skateboard park....

**#4** Dream: I was whizzing around on the back of a firetruck.

**#5** Dream: ...I sit in a friend's convertible while he goes across the street.

**#3** Dream: ...Then we were both in a plane, flying west from Alcatraz to the Golden Gate bridge, flying ten feet off the water....

**#8** Dream: ...buying a red, used boat, out on a huge lake....

**#6** Dream of the far future: My family and I are waiting for a sea bus....

**#3** Dream: Two boys playing around in their motorboat, having fun.

**#8** Dream: Bringing home a used car; dragging the car home by a string....

# Water

**#4** Dream: Lots of water, the ocean, and putting on a life jacket. Very realistic dream.

**#5** Dream: Water dream. An immense swimming pool, more like a slow-moving river with current, a strong current, but gentle. A lot of dreams with water. Feeling of soothing.

**#7** At a cabin in Minnesota, place I knew but it was all different, even the lake. JFK came to our cabin with secret service agents. Agents were in a small boat rowing on the lake, doing drills wearing life jackets. JFK was in a three-piece suit and wanted to go for a boat ride. I squatted down on the dock and dipped a soup bowl into the lake, and it was beef broth soup. The lake was all soup. Had it for lunch. They had to return to shore to pick me up. I was surprised to see all the secret service agents in swimming trunks and JFK in his suit.

**#8** Dream: ...Buying a red, used boat, out on a huge lake....

**#8** Dream: I'm near a stream or river bank, and it seems that I've been rafting or something like that. I'm looking at a still pool with an eddy, and my black cat suddenly can be seen swimming to the surface of the water from below....

## MIND

ANXIETY; control over senses is lost, with feeling that
ALERT
ANGER, irascibility; morning; waking, on
  irascibility; himself, with
ANXIETY;
  as if something needs to be done but knows not what
  business, about
  condition, about her
  sudden
ARGUMENTATIVE
AWARENESS; heightened; of body
    skin surface
BUSINESS; neglects his
CALMNESS;
  after car robbed and no transportation
  computer toppled off desk, when
  daughter cut herself on glass, when
CENSORIOUS, critical
CENSORIOUS, critical;
    blames others in her family
    find fault or is silent, disposed to, husband, of
    wants to blame others and make them responsible
    weather, the
CHEERFULNESS, gaiety, happiness; company, in
COMPANY; aversion to
COMPANY; aversion to; alone; amel. when
COMPANY; desire for
*CONFUSION*
  dazed
  *Disorganized, losing things, keys, wallets, purses*
    *planning, poor, roaming around, unsure*
*CONTENTED; himself, with*
DAYDREAMING
DELIRIUM; fever, during
  uncoordinated, in and out of consciousness
DELUSIONS; animals, of
    lions
  belong to her own family, does not

DELUSIONS (cont.)
body; erroneous ideas as to the state of his
lighter than air
separated, as if body or thoughts were
broad
broad, things are
burn, desires to
danger
enjoying the exposure, with a need to be unprotected, wanting to be raw, not hidden behind anything, did not want to be sheltered or kept from anything harmful, when at risk he feels relieved
depending, everything is depending on them
*dying; he is*
fortunate, he is
head, heads; separated from body, is
heavy, is
intruder, he is, and an outsider to his own family
light, incorporeal, he is
living
no strength to continue
looked down upon, that she is
murdered
women are by men
outside his body
roaming
separated; mind and body are
suffering women, conscious of, through the ages
victim, she is a ;
DESIRES;
danger
help, wants to, others less fortunate
pain
to run everywhere at a lope
to run down the hill
DESPAIR; life, of
*DETACHED*
DISCONTENTED, displeased, dissatisfied; everything, with
others, with
DISORIENTED with everything
DREAMS
accidents
car accidents
anger
at himself

  - *animals*
    - *bear*
      - polar
      - grizzly
  - black cat
  - deer
  - dogs
  - domestic animals, pets
  - fish
  - *insects*
  - lion
  - maggots
  - otter
  - *pigeons*
  - raccoons
  - rats
  - scorpions
  - seal
  - skunks
  - tiger
  - trout
  - whale
  - ball,
  - black magic voodoo
  - busy
  - children
  - attacked
  - baby-sitting, a
  - birthday party
  - child bullies
  - danger, in
  - doing advent spiral
  - dying from cold
  - gassed being
  - having hair pulled by violent man
  - murdered, being
  - *playing*
  - playing with dangerous liquid
  - teenager, jumping off building, screaming, dies
  - tortured, being
  - violated, being
  - weeping
- *choirs singing*
- circle

DREAMS (cont.)
competition
critical
danger
  children, to
  death
  drowning
  impending danger
  perils, of encountered
  dead, people, of
    *friends, long deceased*
    *talking with dead friends*
  despair
  dropping into the sea, with wings spread out of both sides of the ball
  falling, fear of,
    into a ravine, from a cliff

  fear of getting into trouble
  fights
  *fire*
  burn the house down, concerned someone is
  burning building
  danger from, chasing a group of people
  fireball
  firetruck, riding on the back of
  kept fires going
  evil little thing put in oven to self-clean and burns
  flipping over
  friends
  *childhood friends*
  meeting friends
  old friends
  seeing friends
  food
    dirty food, ate it anyway
  glass
  hanging from a cliff, by right arm
  *help*
    trying to
    yet he did not know what he was talking about
  helpless feeling
  hiding
    from danger
  holes

legs
stockings
home
childhood home
hose, garden, taking a plastic plug from a woman's faucet and putting it on his own
identity, lost
*Indians, he is among*
indifferent
intruder in his own world, felt like a revelation
intruders
*Journey*
liquid, damaging, danger to humanity, in an ink pen
lucid
music
*outsider, being an*
felt more like a spirit watching
*bystander, he was*
people
assembled
crowd,
family
his own family
cousin
daughter
father
mother
son
not seen for years
old
please, desire to, superiors
precarious position, feeling safe in a
purse, organizing
revelation, we never really die
he was an intruder in his own world
ridiculous
feeling
robbers
sneaking
social inferiority of
vivid, whom she sees and hears, as if awake
spinning
*stealing*
garden hose but he would return it when nearby again

DREAMS (cont.)

storms
        destroying, house, underside, and motorcycle
suction
swimming
teaching
*trapped, under water*
turning around
urgency, of
*vehicles*
    airplane
    beverage truck
    *cars*
    commercial airliner
    firetruck
    go-cart
    motorboats
        water-skis
    motorcycles
    parachute
    river raft
    snowmobiles
    toy vehicle
    used car
    victim, at the mercy of an amusement park ride operator
    *violence*
        *detached from it*
    vivid
    wallet lost
    watching me, two men
    *water*
        boat owner indifferent to man drowning
        *bottom of*
        danger from
        sea, of the
        swimming in,
            dove to get friend who went under rough water
    weeping
        music, with
    whale turning over and over like a skewer
    wild
DWELLS on past disagreeable occurrences
*ESCAPE, attempts to*
        angles of; looking for
        strategy, concern about

EXCITEMENT
desire for fun
FEAR; dreams, of; terrible
FEELING, loss of
HEEDLESS, careless
think, what others
HURRY, haste
IMPATIENCE
alternating with patience
*INDIFFERENCE, apathy*
INDOLENCE, aversion to work
INDUSTRIOUS,
efficient
IRRESOLUTE
*IRRESOLUTION, indecision; acts, in*
IRRITABILITY
everything causes
ISOLATION
JOY
giving out presents at Christmas
KILL, DESIRE TO,
beer bottle, a
LOOKED AT;
legs, aware her legs are looked at
LOVE
and openness, friends, for
appreciation for fatherly, between younger and older men
MOOD;
stuck and tight
OFFENDED easily
QUIET; disposition
calm, and
QUARRELSOMENESS, scolding; family, with his or her; husband, to
RELAXED feeling, letting go
SELF-CONTROL; loss of
*SENSITIVE, oversensitive; criticism, to*
noise, to
SENTIMENTAL
Christmas, at
SERIOUS
SIT; inclination to
observe world go by, and
SOCIABILITY
STRUGGLING

STUPEFACTION, as if intoxicated
*SUSPICIOUS, mistrustful*
    afternoon, feeling paranoid people are saying things she is not hearing, feeling righteous, something is going on without her, she did not know about, people do not talk to her straight
SYMPATHETIC
    daughter, with
TALK, talking, talks;
    expresses emotions
    indisposed to, desire to be silent, taciturn
THOUGHTS; clearness of
        night amel.
        reading amel.
    disordered
    distracted
    errors of perception
    excessive head chatter, mind whirling with picky things, tiring to listen to, hard to listen to
    hurried
    logical
    rush, flow of
    wandering
TRIFLES; agg.
    important, seem; evening
WEEPING, tearful mood; from; a story of father who poached a deer to
        feed his family and was imprisoned
        music; church music
        offense, from
        reading, while
        whimpering
            aches, everything
TOSSING about; sleep, during

## HEAD

CONSTRICTION
    Forehead
GENERAL; night
LOCALIZATION; Forhead, eyes; behind eyes; left
    *Sides; left; right, then*
PAIN; LOCALIZATION; Forehead
        extending; vertex, to
    PRESSING; Sides; both sides
    PRESSING; Temples
SWOLLEN, distended feeling
*TENSION*

## EYES

OPEN; sensation as if; wide
PAIN; burning
REDNESS
TIRED; sensation
WARMTH, sensation of

## VISION

VISION; ACUTE

## EAR

EAR; DISCOLORATION; redness; right

## FACE

CRACKED; lips
DISCOLORATION; red; heat, with
    red; cheeks
        mouth; around
            cold weather agg.
            eating agg.
DRYNESS; lips
*ERUPTIONS; pimples; lower jaw*
PROJECTS lower jaw

## MOUTH

DRYNESS
    evening
    night
    talking agg.
    thirst, with
MOUTH; SENSITIVE; GUMS; cold drinks agg.
SALIVA; copious

## THROAT

DRYNESS; painful
MUCUS; difficult to detach
PAIN; general; evening
    swallowing; on
SCRAPING

## EXTERNAL THROAT

EXTERNAL THROAT; PAIN; Sides; right
  SWELLING

## STOMACH

APPETITE; diminished
  increased, hunger in general
NAUSEA; odors, from; of fish
PAIN; General; evening
  lying; amel.
  nausea, during
  standing; while
  walking, while
PAIN; cramping, griping
  eating; after
RELAXATION
THIRST; desire to drink, without
  small quantities for; often
  unquenchable, constant
THIRSTLESSNESS

## ABDOMEN

ABDOMEN; PAIN; cramping, griping
  dragging, bearing down
  pressing

## RECTUM

RECTUM; URGING, desire; night

## STOOL

STOOL; TENACIOUS

## KIDNEYS

PAIN; aching; region of
PAIN; General; right
    afternoon; 2 p.m.

## FEMALE

- MENSES; copious
  - frequent, too early, too soon; five days
  - painful, dysmenorrhea
  - scanty
- PAIN; Ovaries
    - right
    - sharp
  - Uterus; menses, after
- SEXUAL desire; diminished

## CHEST

- PAIN; General; forenoon; 11 a.m.
  - cutting, sternum; like someone took a knife to my
  - inspiration, during
  - motion; agg.
  - pressure; amel.
- WEAKNESS

## BACK

- PAIN; general; Dorsal region; scapulae; right
    - spine
  - Lumbar region
    - night
    - right
    - extending to; abdomen
- STIFFNESS; Cervical region; right

## EXTREMITIES

- AWKWARDNESS
- COLDNESS; Hands; blue
  - Foot
- CRACKING; Shoulder; right
- HEAVINESS, tired limbs
- PAIN; UPPER LIMBS; left
    - Shoulder; right
      - extending to; chest
    - Fingers; first
  - LOWER LIMBS
    - right
    - Knee; right
      - left
  - CRAMP, like; Lower limbs, right
- TREMBLING; Upper Limbs
    - Hand

## FEVER

CHILL; with
CONTINUED fever, typhus, typhoid
RELAPSING

## CHILL

COLDNESS in general
NIGHT

## SLEEP

LIGHT
RESTLESS
SLEEPINESS; morning; waking; on
SLEEPLESSNESS; *night*
    thoughts, from
WAKING; 4 p.m.-5 p.m.
    dreams, from

## GENERALITIES

MORNING, 5 a.m.-9 a.m.
*NIGHT, 9 p.m.-5 a.m.; amel.*
BURNS; burning; sensation, internally
*ENDURANCE, increased*
FOOD and drinks; apples; agg.
        aversion
    chili, green or red, agg.
    creamy, desires
    fish; desires
    meat; desires
    spices, condiments, piquant, desires
    wine; desires
HEATED, becoming
HEAVINESS
STIFFNESS, rigidity; Muscles
TENSION; internally
WEAKNESS, enervation; daytime
        exertion, from; slight
WEARINESS; afternoon

EDITOR'S NOTE: *Punctuation, abbreviations, and individual stylistic nuances of the original journal entries have been preserved wherever possible.*

**Prover #1 · Female · 31 years old**

I held the remedy before taking it. Unable to hold bottle tightly, I felt a pulsating feeling that went up left arm.

**Day 1**

◆ I work the night shift, so I took the remedy and then up all night working.

◆ I felt confused and out of sorts; but happy, busy, going on with things and too bad if things didn't get done. Someone else will do them, that's what the next shift is for. (Very different from usual self.) I felt lazy and unmotivated.

◆ Twenty minutes after taking remedy, headache behind left eye, sore, felt like someone punched me. Pounding sore behind left eye. Lasted ten minutes. Then gone.

**Day 2**

◆ Unsociable, did not want to talk. When I do talk, I think I'm funny. Who cares what others think anyway? I don't care about consequences of my actions or speech, only concerned with the here and now. Hard time focusing, mind wandering, daydreaming about the upcoming holidays & upcoming events.

◆ Energy level good, considering I did not sleep. Felt weak physically when I went to push kids on swing, big effort to get it moving!

11:00 a.m. Tight sharp pains in chest, upper middle sternum, between and a little above breasts. Better pressure, worse inspiration, worse movement. Happened hourly at 11:00 a.m., 12:00 p.m., 1:00 p.m., each time lasted between ten and twenty minutes.

◆ Went to party alone. Usually would not have gone alone.

◆ Cheeks flushed, warm.

◆ Dry mouth, thirst for constant sips of water, went on for several days, mostly in evening.

◆ Hands and upper extremities tremulous.

**Day 3**

◆ Felt good, mellow: want to just sit and observe world go by.

◆ Went running, body did not want to move. I feel heavy, my legs are heavy. It's not that I'm tired, it's that I feel physically weak. Do not feel restless like I usually do. Usually it feels good to run, but today it was a definite effort. It took fifteen minutes longer to run usual course.

◆ Throat sore, worse swallowing, anything.

◆ Thirstless during day.
◆ Upper chest feels tight on inspiration.
◆ Dream: Organizing purse and then dumping out because not right and reorganizing it again. Sitting on bed doing this, with a mindless feeling. Not frustration.

**Day 4**
◆ Mellow, distracted, mind wandering.
◆ Klutzy, tripping over things, dropping things. Dropped baking soda into garlic, broke Christmas ornament.
◆ Eyes tired, burning and red.
◆ Sharp pain in upper right shoulder blade extending to right side of neck at 8:15 a.m. Lasted about ten minutes.
◆ Dream: In restaurant with another family, small boy starting to cry. Woman sitting at next table played her violin and the boy stopped crying when he heard the beautiful music. The woman stopped playing when she realized everyone was listening. We were all disappointed, enjoying the music.
◆ Dream: I was an early pioneer settler in the West. I was a child, being attacked by Indians and all children were hiding in one room. We could hear the attack outside. Could hear them outside yelling war cries, gunshots. Kids hiding huddled together in a room. I buried my head in my hands.
◆ It was a restless night. I had a lot of images of Native Americans through the night, quick flashes of Native American cultures, dress, ceremonial dance, tepee, flashes of different native cultures. Lots of brightly colored feathers. Feeling was of hopelessness and despair. Did not feel fear. But during the flashes, the images of Indian culture were comforting. Dream had a restless feeling, lots of movement, activity.
◆ Did not sleep well that night. At 1:00 a.m. I heard tapping on window that scared me to death. Heard my name whispered, drew curtains and it was my mother. She had tried to call, but the phone was off the hook. She said she was worried about my three-year-old daughter and had a 'premonition.' She wanted to make sure she was O.K. She had given me an old necklace and had premonition that my child would strangle to death if I had let her go to bed with it on. The necklace had a ribbon with a bunny and heart on it. Had belonged to me as a child. After that I didn't sleep very well.
◆ I'm having a difficult time going to sleep, actually not the sleeping part, but the just getting into bed. Then I'm very tired in the morning. My best sleep is after 4:00 a.m. or 5:00 a.m.

**Day 5**
◆ I'm a basket case. I feel like I'm in a daze. Feels like my head is separate from my body. It's like my body is doing one thing and my head is doing another. I'm losing things like important papers. Confused. Out of control.
◆ I was irritable and grouchy this morning after I couldn't find an important paper, but it didn't last long. I was frowning and scowling, I was mad at myself.
Energy level better, but the mornings are not so good. It takes me awhile to wake up. I feel sleepy until 10:00 a.m. and that's after I get up at 5:00 a.m.

◆ Klutzy.
Interview for new job went very well. While at interview oldest child cut herself on glass, the cut was not small. I reacted well, very calm.
◆ Went to use microwave, but put bowl of soup into cupboard next to the microwave and closed door as if to microwave.
◆ I think I am worse mentally before 10:00 a.m. and after 5:00-6:00 p.m., so that doesn't give me a lot of functioning time. Oh well, so much for taking any good cases right now!

**Day 6**
◆ Mind scattered, thoughts all over the place, difficult time focusing.
I feel anxious, like I need to get something done, but I am not sure what.
Tired during day, no energy, but much more alive at night, from 5:00 - 6:00 p.m. on. Had a lot of energy at night, wanting to be moving, had to think of things to do.
◆ Mouth dry, especially when talking, worse evening, night. Better drinking water, better not talking.
◆ I tried to sleep but was unable to because my mind was racing with scattered thoughts. I've had difficulty going to sleep at night, just going to bed to get to sleep is difficult.

**Day 7**
◆ I'm really klutzy, in fact, while running in the house to get the phone, I slipped, ran into wall and broke my little right toe. Felt disassociated, not connected to body.
◆ Disconnected from emotions, from things going on around me. Things were happening but I was apathetic, oh well too bad. Lost some important papers of client. Normally I would have been very upset about it but now, Oh well.

**Days 8, 9**
◆ Losing things, disorganized.
Tired, restless sleep. I am sleeping terribly. I have difficulty getting to bed, and then I toss and turn all night.

**Days 10, 11**
◆ I've been very sensitive. Had a disagreement over homeopathy and my beliefs with family and got upset, almost starting crying. Had to leave the room, felt like an outsider to my family, that I didn't belong. Also felt that they did not even care to hear my viewpoint. They made me feel unimportant and incidental.

**Days 12, 13**
◆ Poor sleep, restless, moving in bed. A lot on mind, thoughts racing, thoughts all over the place.

**Days 14, 15**
◆ Sensitive to criticism. Was shopping and sales lady asked my size and said, you're much broader than that. Normally I brush it off, but kept thinking about it. Bugged me that I was called broad.

◆ Dream: Planning daughter's third birthday party. My mother came dressed as Minnie Mouse in a cardboard costume. I kept thinking she looks so stupid.
◆ Dream: I was a runway model for Calvin Klein.
◆ Dream: Wearing holey leggings. Very vivid. The next day went to put on leggings, thought there should be holes, then recalled that was in my dream.
◆ Overall feeling was of losing things and not caring. Normally would have studied a lot for a case. Normally would have looked at homework right away, but kept putting it off. Only took one dose.

**Prover #2 · Female · 37 years old**

Note: Participated in the Proving for 14 days. Called Proving Master and said I wanted to quit. Often reminded me of horse's milk proving and felt I did not want to continue suffering.

**Day 1**
◆ Took at 12:00 p.m. Within a couple of hours I became energized. My eyes felt wide open, alert, clearheaded, vision crisp.
◆ Dream: Traveling in the countryside. Felt like I was having a past life experience waiting for two friends on motorcycles. Setting up an old couple in deli in isolated country. Kept emphasizing to friend don't kill the old man. Situation failed, we were trying to photograph something and the old man was disappointed. Thought I woke up to owner opening my front door talking to me about a play structure. Both dreams (this and one night before taking dose) felt very real, not dream state; felt like I was awake during dream. Very detail oriented. A lot of people from my past kept coming up.

**Day 2**
◆ Slight heart racing as if drank coffee. Mood labile, tight, stuck feeling.
Felt tight slight tension in head, stuck feeling. Tension, tightness in body.
◆ Conversation of partner being distant.
◆ Body lacked clarity, confusion. Hard to make decisions, feeling confused, what I wanted to do, where to be.
◆ Resentful of friend.
◆ Craving fish. Have not had any in long time, and went out and bought scallops and shrimp. Feeling this remedy is fish related, although spider came to me intuitively.
◆ Sleep was very light that evening, continued through proving, but restless sleep—physically thrashing at times. Not deep sleep.
◆ Got very energized at night, and up late feeling very organized.
◆ Dream: Friend over in the middle of the night, who had her son come under the covers to keep her warm. Somehow with her family in Spain very old, another past lifetime. We were with them in Spain—her whole family traveling. Somehow transported them just to see the villa they lived in and left, though we were served dinner first, a lot of fish choices.

◆ Dream: Daughter's teacher going on vacation and wanted me to substitute. Looking at my calendar, each day was large and very detailed. I was free and could do it.
Diving, swimming and competing in theater. I entered to help the children. Performing and being funny somehow had to do with children. Many different dreams, detailed vivid dreams, of people around me in life, so dream seemed real as if I were awake. Could not remember all the detail next morning.

**Day 3**
◆ Mood more stable. Felt clearer in head. Warm eyes in evening, felt warm and liquid, behind eyes.
◆ Dream: Cousin and I in a dark dream, in the late night driving around city in a red rental car. We got in an accident. I was scared, hiding in a bar/restaurant, renting a hotel room. Lots of chaos. Had to fix things, then blew it off and went to hotel room. Instead of dealing with it (the accident) went to a restaurant. Fast-paced, dark dream, wild, nonstop. Lots of action, movement, business, going from place to place, but delinquent about the accident—nonchalant about that.
◆ In real life out kayaking in bay and seals following us. Circled by seals, we in the center, a moment of awe in this perfect circle, then they went back to their frolicking and playing. Felt a richness, a simple connection to the seals. Felt like a celebration.

**Day 4**
◆ Dream: Had a dream of friend who would take my children and a lot of others from Friday to Wednesday until 7:00 p.m. I was surprised at how outrageous a baby-sitting offer this was. She had Chinese takeout of real big containers, huge scallops. We could only serve so many, I tried helping her sell them because they were going to spoil. Also huge trays of stuffed tomatoes. School event?

**Day 5**
◆ Feeling very organized or think I am, therefore feel calm.
◆ Sexual drive seems decreased in the last couple of days, affection and intimacy desired, though.
◆ Increased appetite, feeling more hungry at meals.
◆ Difficulty remembering dreams, awoke abruptly, had to struggle to get my dreams back.
◆ Got body work, felt stuck in my body, desperately needed release from this. Right neck, shoulder, upper back stuck; felt restricted, tense, tight. Ribs stuck; lung tissue on right stuck. Lasted throughout the whole proving.
◆ Also emotional.
◆ Strong inner critical voice.
◆ By letting it out, I felt better, but did not want to do it. Felt bad, being critical of things, even small things that normally would not bother me. But it was not a release because I did not like that I was being picky about things. It all seemed so trivial. The things that were making me uptight.
◆ Had conversation with my husband with "strong" words: "I don't want to torture her," regarding my daughter watching the horse lesson and not being able to ride. I was worried about her longing and suffering and contributing to her heartache by desires.

**Day 6**

◆ Lacking clarity, some tension.

◆ Dream: I was outside a hotel in a large concrete building that had a round shape like an amusement park ride. I was in an elevator which was a chute or circle going up and down the outside of the building. The chute went in a circle, transporting me like an elevator. It would suck me into the spin to stay on. Feeling of rushing up and down, sucking me into a spin, suction. Wished for a belt or bar to hold onto, water swirling in it as part of the suction. A man was operating it and felt I was at his mercy. I was encouraging my daughter to jump on with me. It must have been fun. This was the ordinary way to get from floor to floor, inside swirling water.

**Day 7**

◆ Period of tension in head continues.

◆ Afternoon fatigue with a boost in the evening. Down time is 4:00-5:00 p.m., pick up at 6:00 p.m. until really late, 12:00-2:00 a.m.

◆ Awoke abruptly.

**Day 8**

◆ Tension in head continues.

◆ Very sore throat, slightly dry with increased dryness in afternoon, nothing really bad.

◆ Woke up abruptly, knowing I had evening full of dreams but could not remember them.

**Day 9**

◆ Constriction in head, just there.

◆ Dream: Sitting at table eating artichokes dipping in butter and lemon, telling the truth to her, the secret I had been hiding. A strange man and woman came dipping their fingers in our butter and dip which was on the ground on leaves. I told them it was dirty but they ate it anyway. They were very intrusive, pushed their way into house, asking for more and more, started stealing things through out house, hiding things in their clothes. Insisted they leave, I struggled physically with the man, who became violent. He grabbed my daughter pulling her hair, she arching her back, pulling her hair, starting to hurt her. Felt violated, they pushed themselves in. I was trying to set a boundary, and they used my daughter.

**Day 10**

◆ Everything increased irresolution, annoyed, confusion. Ran over the curb with the car, very clumsy.

◆ Difficulty making decisions. Had to go back and forth, going somewhere and not sure what to wear. Went out the door with two different shoes on. Could not decide, forgot I was making the decision and realized I had two different shoes on. Normal, everyday, simple decisions were hard. I put two different stockings on with holes in them, had to keep changing them. Whole time had a sense of not flowing, increased effort, struggle.

◆ Not myself, out of balance. Numbness, not feeling like distant, but felt disconnected. A lot of excessive head chatter, mind whirling with picky things, tiring to listen to, hard to listen to.

◆ Occasional paranoid feelings, excessive worry but stronger than that.
◆ Dreams of familiar people in dreams, I feel aware and have deep knowing, recognition. Friend and her family at their house, door was large, massive with large doorknob. Went to restaurant with group, left early, driving around skateboard park, lots of water, at ocean.

**Day 11**
◆ More effort, less flow. Continued tension, lack of clarity.
◆ Tough to make decisions.
◆ Numbness to feelings.
◆ A lot of head chatter, mind getting in the way, paranoid feelings.
◆ Up late, little sleep. Went out to see neighborhood Christmas lights, taken by the details of everything, the details were important.

**Day 12**
◆ Dreams: Friends on journey, groups. Travel. Laundry, two machines, did not pay attention to which was mine.
◆ Dream: Friend swimming in water that became rough. He went under. I dove to bottom to get him, he wasn't breathing. The lady running the boat was very casual about the whole thing. Did not say to get help, nothing.

**Days 13, 14**
◆ Same symptoms next few days: same subtle tension, effort, lack of clarity.
◆ Slightly sore throat, dry.
◆ Woke up too fast, though I know I had many dreams.
◆ Dream: At the water again. Dream seems close to reality, friend, Rose, in dream at house with children selling stickers, kids party. Sister backing up in old truck, told her to get out of here fast. I was rebellious in group for not writing down or listening, and got called on it. Traveling the coast, I needed a taxi but chose to walk instead. Old, another time period, ancient but familiar.
◆ Real life looking at the moon on Christmas Eve. Moon was very round, wide, but it had a black cloud in front of it with two white, radiant wings coming out from either side: White moon covered with black.

**Day 15**
◆ Dream: I am keeping fires going in a huge store paying $130 a week for pallets. No one else in huge group was contributing. I announce this to group, but no one wanted to contribute. One felt empathetic. I threatened to stop it, some man said: "I hope you don't feel burdened." A man flirting with me, flipped me over upside down. I was hiding in bed under the covers, but had fun conversation with him later. I was working for him and afraid of getting into trouble. A choir of people singing.
◆ Dream: At ocean bay seeing huge whale turn over and over like a skewer. Watching the sun or moon a big fireball dropping into the sea, felt and sounded like a glass ball, the seas were crystal clear, something sharp. Wings spread out of both sides of it like the one

I saw in another dream, one I had that morning.
◆ Dream: Intruders got daughter. Black magic, voodoo needles in eyes, calling 911, my children are being hurt!

Note: Took Lac delphinum, which is my constitutional, to get off proving. Next day felt like I was in-between two stages—clear sensation of this happening. Then felt the new remedy came in and the proving left, I settled into a calmness.

### Prover #3 · Male · 36 years old

**Day 1**
◆ Have dull aching left arm at triceps about midnight.
◆ Slightly lightheaded, not present, not really there. Opened beer before supposed to leave. Took beer with me between my legs in car. Pulled out of driveway, foamed all over. I had just gotten dressed, I wanted to kill this beer bottle. Highly critical, confused at each other.
◆ Dream: Taking friend's car back to the shop after we both had cars fixed, I felt I had been approved of because my car was still fine.

**Days 2-3**
◆ Had extremely impatient, high energy level.

**Day 4** Took second dose
◆ Right shoulder crunchy feeling, got very intense. Crunchy feeling between shoulder blades: old symptom that was doing well.
◆ Going through stuff, doing martial arts, raining a lot, so not sure where symptom was coming from. Got locked up but crunched when moved it, sporadically tense, heard cracks and pops when moving.

**Day 5**
◆ Increased sensitivity to noise. Radio bothered me, preferred quiet. More impatient during the day but very patient and not caring in the dreams.
◆ Mellow, easy dreams. Can't remember context, but increased patience in dreams. No hint of confrontation, aggressiveness, in contrast to normal dreams of confrontation. Disconnected, unemotional in the dreams, opposite in waking life.
◆ Visions of lions during the day. They weren't doing anything, they were just present and close to me, and they were patient and non-confrontational.
I've been kind of quiet.

**Day 6**
◆ I need to be unprotected. Wanting to be raw, not hidden behind anything. I do not want to be sheltered kept from anything harmful, want to be open to all experience with no boundaries i.e. drive without my seat belt. I sought out an unprotected place to come

from. Neutral about the danger factor. Not seeking it, but if anything came along.... Wanting to be out there at risk. When I am out there at risk, I feel relieved—an exposed state, enjoying the exposure.
◆ Gums sensitive to cold, cold drinks only.
◆ In a hurry, rushed, continued for a week.

**Day 7**
◆ Dream: Stacking wood with superiors, wondering if I'm good enough, if stacking well enough, wondering if I was holding up my load with a desire to please. Guess I was because dad rewarded me with a large snowmobile. Was excited about it, got the snowmobile from my dad. Was getting changed to go out for a ride. Control issue—the snowmobile seemed too big and that it may be a challenge to control.
◆ Same dream, two men had a damaging liquid that was damaging to humanity. One of the men was carrying it around in a pen like James Bond. Their car crashed into ravine, two more men rush there to get the liquid before someone else got it. I was a bystander. Felt helpless like it was going on and I wasn't involved. I would have wanted to jump in and help get the stuff. I was more like a spirit watching—an outsider. Feelings of urgency and distrust.
◆ There is a hint towards polarities. The other day I started out feeling impatient and high energy, yesterday I felt the polar opposite—felt patience. That word, polar, comes to mind.

**Day 8**
◆ Dream: Driving around in a Volkswagen bus in the passenger seat with a long garden hose hanging out of van. I am supposed to keep the water inside from running out, but the hose is cut lengthwise like a gutter, so I have to keep it perfectly balanced, one end plugged, other not. I pulled over to take a plastic plug from a woman's faucet and put it on mine. I knew it was stealing, but I would return it when I was nearby again. Two men watching me. At times the hose is pluggable and other times not, a difficult situation. Feeling ridiculous, I had to control the uncontrollable, a menial thing. I was mad that it had to be important.
◆ Find myself eating less in past week, not clear on why.

**Day 9**
◆ Dream: Intruding on another man's place of residence, a large property fenced in, no buildings, living amongst junk. I needed something from him and was sneaking around. I didn't want his dogs to know I was there, they were sleeping. I came across an outside kitchen area with a refrigerator, and from the contents, I got a feeling the dogs got to eat meat and the man ate celery and carrots. But as I was leaving I came across dog and at first I was scared, but I gave it a carrot, which he ate, and he was fine. As I was leaving it dawned on me. I was intruding on my own home. An intruder in my own world. Felt almost like a revelation. I felt like I had a lot of work to do. Felt a little messy and confused. My place got screwed up, no shelter, a big piece of open property with junk lying around.

◆ Car broken into and air bags, radio, glove box, whole dashboard stolen. Did not panic even though I then had no car and no mass transportation. Another day the whole computer toppled off my desk and broke, and I did not panic at all.

**Day 10**

◆ Easily irritated, cloudy head and confused. A lot of confusion, had five errands to run and went up and down the freeway. I would almost be somewhere and then decide to go elsewhere and turn around, driving around in circles, getting nothing else done. Poor planning, roaming around, unsure. Disorganized.

**Day 11**

◆ Dream: Two boys playing around in their motorboat, having fun. They came across something on the surface that indicated a problem, an older man trapped under the water. They pushed a pole down to him like a rescue pole and pulled him up. I was a bystander, I was not any of the people in the dream. I was glad because he didn't have much air left.

◆ Dream: My motorcycle is parked under a friend's house at the beach, and a big storm came through and trashed the underside of the house, including my bike. I saw all the water. He knew this but was hesitant to tell me. I was angry at myself because I knew not to leave it here. He was very detached from the whole thing, he was numb to it.

◆ Dream: I walk into a cafeteria; sitting there is a friend of mine from grammar school, who had died when we were in college in Michigan. He had a heart attack on the basketball court at age 21. I never got to spend as much time with him as I wanted. Hey I am surprised to see you, I said, your mom told me you had died. He looked embarrassed and said he wasn't well but he would be O.K. I told him I missed seeing him and having him as a friend all these years. Felt very sympathetic. I felt that I was getting in touch with the fact we never really die, and he really was there. I was talking to him and although he wasn't doing well, he candy-coated it for earth people. He wanted to be polite, I would not understand it. I thought, oh, well, that is what he needs to do, no judgment. Either way I knew inside I understood real life. His mother told me he died and it tore their family apart. His parents ended up getting a divorce.

**Day 13**

◆ Dream: I was teaching a friend how to deploy a parachute. He was going out for a flight with an older man in an airplane. I felt like I needed to offer him something, some sort of help, instruction or help somehow.

◆ Dream: I had a roommate who was moving out from like a dorm room in college. He left some of his things, a few of which I was glad to have, like detergent, etc. I felt glad he was out of my space.

◆ I am still feeling critical overall. I still want to fix things and contribute. Sort of critical and helpful at the same time. Seems to be coming through some of my dreams, more critical than anything.

**Day 14**

◆ Dream: Sitting in an auditorium between two high school bullies. One of them started smacking me in the head. I was involved with some sort of ritual with oil. I got up and walked to the back of the room. At one point I elbowed one of them in the face. I was disconnected, it did not matter, everyone was surprised I did not retaliate more.

**Day 15**

◆ Dream: In a burning building moving up through the floors in an attempt to escape the fire; not sure if it was out on lower floors but it was chasing a group of us. We were feeling unsure about the danger, moving away from it, but not sure if the fire was still a threat.

◆ Dream: Hiking with guide and some others in mountains, hanging by my right arm from a cliff of some type. A guide is on other side of the ravine, dealing with other people who need more help, who are really struggling. They are afraid they are going to fall into the ravine. "Hey, what about me? I don't know what I'm doing!" Guide said to just do what he did. I knocked a piton into rock and was just hanging there. I was O.K., but was feeling how do you know I am O.K.? Feeling like I'm in a precarious position but O.K. (In real life I don't climb mountains.)

**Day 16**

◆ Dream: Standing waist-high in clear water, with another man, my wallet had dropped to bottom of pool. I was freaked out that I lost my wallet—not sure if it was about the loss of money or the loss of my identity—but then I found it and picked it up and started to dry it. Felt detached and didn't care that it was wet.

**Day 18**

◆ Dream: Learning and teaching a friend who had to deploy a parachute in case something went wrong on a flight with a father figure. I felt I had to offer him something to help with. I helped him deploy his parachute, yet I did not know what I was talking about, did not know if he needed to know it or not. I felt as though I had something to offer that might not be welcomed.

◆ Dream: College roommate moving stuff out, I was glad he was not in my space anymore. He left behind stuff and I was bummed, but as I started looking through it, I realized he left laundry detergent.

◆ Fairly critical, like no one can do anything right.

**Day 21**

◆ Dream: In an office where I used to work as a stockbroker in real life with seven other brokers. I was thirty years younger than the others. I was bringing money to my broker who was not working there anymore. The manager who offered to take my money was a rickety old guy who was vain: remodeled, working out, face lift. He said my broker was not in, and I was embarrassed to give him the money because it wasn't very much. Then we were both in a plane, flying west from Alcatraz to the Golden Gate bridge, flying ten feet off the water. Big huge commercial airliner was on the west side of the bridge up about 15,000 feet and ascending. The stockbroker turns and says, I hope that plane gets

out of our way, and I asked if it wasn't far enough away. He flips the plane over and we're flying upside down, ten feet above the water. He is turning into these sailboats, and we're having a great time. I am very calm about it, very matter-of-fact, and he is acting like he does this all the time. While weaving through the boats, he tries to communicate to me that this is the best way to be going. Then we pull into a dry storage dock and stop. I could not find my wallet. Found it not really lost, just next to the plane. (Note: second flying dream, second wallet dream.)
◆ In real life, left my wallet behind on the bed when I went out, never do it. Had awful feeling.

**Day 22**
◆ Dream: I was driving around in a go-cart and was racing another boy. Big crowd of people were meandering over the track, in a trance, like *Night of the Living Dead.* We can't race well because I didn't want to hit anyone, I was frustrated. I finally saw an opening between the guys, drove into it, and then the crowd dispersed and we could race. I was amazed that it was that easy to get the crowd away. That frustration gave way to wonder and surprise. Frustration gave way to success.
◆ Dream: I was hiking up a trail, which was very technical, with a woman who is wondering why I am leading her all over this mountain, wondering where we are going. I am obviously confused, and don't know where we are going. I didn't even realize why I was in this confused state. I went down this very steep hill in an open desert area and wondered if I could do it, and I looked over and saw another guy, a kid from grammar school for whom I don't have much respect. It was, if he can do it, so can I. He was making it down the hill so I got a little more confidence. Still didn't feel tremendously comfortable about it, but if he could, I could. Right then the other guy fell and caught his boot heel on a rock, and then he looks back to me as if to say, "What? No big deal, what are you worried about?"
◆ Very little hunger, decrease in appetite. Irregular bowels.

**Day 23**
◆ Dream: I am walking down a road at night and am avoiding skunks that are wondering around, but they turn out to be raccoons. Then I see a skunk that is about to spray a little puppy who is curious and ignorant. The skunk is conning the puppy and is about to take advantage of its good nature.

**Day 24**
◆ Dream: I'm wanting my mother to leave me alone as she is wanting too much attention. She is bugging me and I am feeling irritated. Trying to get to the course to teach (I teach in real life), and my car is broken down. It was snowing, so I cannot take my motorcycle. I went to mechanic's garage to find out why my car is not done, mechanic making excuses for not fixing it. Man drives a beverage truck into the garage and leaves, mechanic goes over and gets six Coors beer bottles—three old designs and three new designs. I am drinking Beck's beer. I was wondering if the truck driver would charge me for the Beck's beer, which was mine. He comes back and we are all talking about tennis. Then I'm at a wedding party for the marriage of a girl whom I used to date, but she was still attached to me, dialogue back and forth. She really wants to marry me, but is settling

for this other guy because I won't settle down and give her what she wants. Feeling was I was glad she was getting married because she was going to settle down and get what she wanted, white fence, etc.

**Day 27**

◆ Pain upper right neck.
◆ Calves sore and shifty feeling mobile.
◆ Intense pain behind right shoulder blade.

**Day 28**

◆ General weakness feeling and lightheaded and disconnected.
◆ Weakness in the chest.

**Prover #4 · Female · 28 years old**

*Note: Split with her boyfriend before taking the remedy so delayed taking the remedy because did not want that to affect her reaction to remedy.*

**Day 1**

(Took remedy at 8:00 a.m.)
Felt clear minded, efficient, mature and serious. Very logical.
Not hungry, nothing is appetizing.
Face seems to be red and hot.
Noon: Abdominal cramps—pressing, aching, dragging, pulling down even though mid-cycle.
2:00 p.m. pressing headache, temples and both sides of the head. More sharp on right side.

**Day 2**

◆ Wanted to feel something, craving hot spicy chili peppers, can't get enough. Wanted to burn and be in pain, have a rush. Represented danger, but in a less destructive way.
◆ Very meticulous and careful in my actions. Very centered mentally, very conservative with actions and emotions.
◆ Mucous in throat. Cannot get rid of it, cannot clear.

**Day 3**

◆ Took second dose very meticulously. Very centered in my actions.
◆ Painful stomach muscles deep aching cramps.
◆ Appetite increasing. Still crave chili hot pepper.
◆ Dream: Before I was fully asleep, I had dreams of fireballs. Young boys, youths throwing or heaving huge balls like a meteorite, going past them like fireworks. I was just watching them with no real feeling.
◆ Dream: Dreams of restrictions, in enclosure. Usually I have open airy dreams. This space was tunnel-like.

◆ I feel genuine—possibly because I felt ungenuine with boyfriend, towards others and friends.
◆ Had a really red face, hot & red all over with no explanation.
◆ Very extreme tight cramping in stomach as if hungry but I have eaten.
◆ Very painful lower back, worse than usual—pinching and continuous.
◆ Bunions hurt, cold aching, very painful (usually they only hurt if they have been squashed in tight shoes). Cold weather hurts them, too.

**Day 4**

◆ Dreams of arguing, discord, miscommunication. Fuzzy memory of dreams. Just woke up feeling a bit sad and frustrated, not an interesting, eventful or happy dream.
◆ Whole body very stiff, achy. Muscles hurt. Felt awful, shaky, very nervous.
Kidneys painful, like when I had kidney infection.
◆ Stomach nauseous and painful, worse walking and standing; much better sitting, lying down. Want to go to bed.
◆ Fever for 34 hours, almost hallucinating. Felt ethereal, disconnected from body, bumind is very together and alert and conscious. Felt like my body was not there, like I was dying and I was leaving my body and didn't mind. I was too weak and disconnected.
◆ Feel weak—like during menstruation. Cold, not much energy. Pain in ovaries.
Fever of 100-101 degrees Fahrenheit for 24 hours with huge painful back. Pain in lower back either side, worse on right, all through abdomen, and especially on surface, though not organic.
◆ Felt like whimpering and crying, everything aches.

(This all feels more to do with my finishing with my boyfriend, like I am finally relaxing, feeling free, getting rid of something that was making me unhappy. My body is reacting to the stress and relief of it. May not be the remedy because it feels so connected with finishing college and finishing with my boyfriend, who I still worry about.)

**Day 5**

◆ Emotionally felt fine.
◆ Little pain in back and kidneys. Stopped taking remedy. Realized I didn't want to pass through emotions. Didn't want to feel them.
◆ I saw a man hugging a younger man, a genuine, loving, fatherly hug. I felt a sense of appreciation and love for them and that I was missing some kind of male love and companionship. I wanted a fatherly hug or something, as if I saw male love for the first time, without it being tinged with embarrassment, or sexuality, or fear.
◆ I think my mental high has gone, not as astutely aware.
◆ Fear of feeling my emotions. I am admitting this to myself and recognizing it for the first time.
◆ Feeling extremely cold, especially at night. Hands go blue, purple.
◆ Whole right leg painful all day, bad circulation.
◆ Felt very thirsty.

**Day 6**

◆ Felt very tired and drained.

**Day 7**

◆ Not into Christmas spirit, blah.... Didn't care about Christmas, I usually love it, felt disillusioned this year. On Christmas I was bored and unsatisfied with my friends/acquaintances. Did not want to be there.

◆ Dreams of short, dark, very small pictures and feelings, not expressive or communicative.

◆ I woke feeling on edge, a little scared of what I just dreamt because I knew it wasn't very exciting or healthy or happy.

**Day 8**

◆ One week later, painful lower back, same abdominal pain, similar to menstrual cramps, but on the top muscle layer closest to skin.

◆ Tight stomach, worse as evening progresses.

◆ Tired, cold, with 104 fever. Went to doctor who told me I had a flu which lasted about 24 hours.

◆ Pain going around shoulder, over top & down back and front of chest.

◆ Headache left side, alternating right side.

◆ Kidney pain, lower back, but primarily localized in kidney.

◆ Thirsty for juice, water.

◆ Expressing emotions, talking.

◆ Feeling past emotions.

◆ Thinking logically and objectively of past.

◆ Dream: Dreamt about a woman and her children being gassed and poisoned by a man in a car, a bad dream. (Dream was during a nap at 5:30 p.m. because I've been up since 5:00 a.m.)

**Day 9**

◆ Went to party by myself which I normally would not do, very weird. Had fun at the party.

◆ Dream: I was whizzing around on the back of a firetruck with lots of women around. I felt safe. Was with my best friend who lives far away.

◆ Breasts painful, before menstruation. Menstruation seems early.

◆ Back still painful, sore after fever.

**Day 10**

◆ Had another fever, 104. Very painful back. Swollen head, neck. Legs painful. Lasted 48-58 hours, incapacitated. Centered in lower back, diagnosed with flu virus. Sore throat, worse evening.

◆ Very tired, sleepy most of the day.

◆ Sad weepy, strange dreams.

◆ In and out of consciousness, very delirious and uncoordinated.

**Day 12**

◆ Menstruation scanty, painful, very "unlike me," it didn't feel "right" somehow, almost unwilling to flow—I'm emotionally very happy to have my period, but my body seems to almost not "recognize" it. Hard to explain, it just doesn't feel normal—the flow, the pain, the whole ritual of it is unusual.

◆ Dream: Terrible dreams of sleeping on garbage riddled with ants, worms, maggots, bloated rats, smaller insects, smells of rotten things. I am lying down in it with my mother. Could not fall back to sleep after seeing we were in the garbage. I did not mind too much about the ants. Baby, embryonic mice & animals all dying from the cold and being hurt. A disturbing, horrible dream. I often dream of maggots and worms, having the maggots or worms inside of me. This was more about being immersed in them.
◆ Dream: Another bad dream of men hurting, violating young girls.
◆ I think I am being really conscious of women's suffering, more so. I feel like I see it in a new light. Feel ages of women, felt the pain of Othello's wife in the video, felt so sad and emotionally charged by her death, by all women's death by men.

**Day 13**
◆ Dream: Dreamt it felt pretty normal looking after two babies for a friend who lived in a large community with lots of strange people, men in leather and chains. Lots of old women and children, every different type of person you could imagine. It was in this big building which reminded me of something Russian, leaflets and posters were stuck on the outside, oppressed negative fearful feeling on the outside. Everyone shared rooms on the inside, children were playing in this purple liquid which I knew was bad for them to be putting it in their mouths. I gave the children back to their mother, worried about the bad liquid a man gave them. They were sleepy and I worried they were ill.

**Day 14**
◆ Period is painful, with very light flow. Sharp superficial pain. Usually have "unemotional" pain with my period—the pain is heavy, intense, and a "womanly," strong pain which I like. This feels altogether weak and "unwomanly!"
Sweat smells like onions, fear smell, smell of fear, when I get scared.

**Day 16**
◆ Dream: Dreams of hundreds of live chickens, all boxed in a room.
◆ Dream: Violent dreams.
◆ Feel like I have to help others less fortunate. I am so lucky, I have so much. I just want to help my friends and try and save their lives—help them have better, easier, healthier lives.
◆ Dry, cracked lips.
◆ Craving chili still.
◆ Calm and serious and quiet.
◆ Pains in ovaries. Worried about ectopic pregnancy, not that I could be pregnant! Pain is sharp, right side, very deep, pinching pain. Generally a scanty, "unflowing," sporadic period.
◆ Cold feet, always, tired and cold.

**Day 18**
◆ Particularly sensitive to noise, more so than usual.
◆ Feeling love and openness towards my friends. I am accepting myself more. I am enjoying life and what it brings, good and bad.
◆ Kept losing wallet and keys, personal things, etc.

**Days 19-21**

◆ Dream: Dreams unremembered, just memories of small, closed-in tunnels, slightly claustrophobic.

Angry at men's sexuality, especially when directed at me.

I am generally strong in my attitude and feel confident in decisions.

Sharp pains every day, especially a few days after my period, on right side of uterus. This worries me.

◆ Very thirsty, but never seem to quench it.

◆ I don't feel like eating chili anymore. It finally upset my stomach, and I had bad diarrhea, which also may have been caused because I ate a lot of beet roots, which seemed to cause cramping and irritate my stomach.

◆ Continuously painful lower back; it was only ever better when I did yoga, much worse when I am stressed, which I think I am because I don't have a secure, creative job, and I have not decided where I want to live or what it is I want to do. I would love to be innocent again and not worry so much, like when I was 17 and could have fun.

◆ Pimples around jaw line.

◆ Dislike apples for the first time in my life. They make me feel sick. This is weird. They have been a staple in my diet.

**Day 22**

◆ Dream: Teeth falling out, pulled them out. It was so real. I had braces on my teeth as well and I pulled them off. I just wobbled all my teeth and they were loose and rotten. I had a handful of molars, which someone had later stolen to sell.

◆ Dream: Lots of water, the ocean, and putting on a life jacket. Very realistic dream.

**Day 23**

◆ Pains in arms and legs like growing pains.

◆ Pain in mid spine 10:00 a.m. Very cold outside, therefore tense.

◆ Feeling self-pity because of..... Something? Men? Boyfriend? Because I am not "jolly," "happy-go-lucky?" Feel like I am not interesting, or clever or fun? Boo hoo!

**Day 24**

◆ Dream: Dream of tiger last night, very nice.

◆ Feel like eating meat—huge steak or hamburger—but I know it's wrong, bad.

Red around mouth like a rash, irritated by eating and by cold weather.

◆ Hot, red face.

**Prover #5 · Female · 45 years old**

**Day 1**

◆ Took remedy at 10:00 p.m. Immediately had vivid dreams.

◆ Sat bolt upright at night to go write down dreams.

◆ Dream: 4:00 a.m. looking for people with disease to come forward so we could do research.

◆ Dream: My husband, but it's not really him, says to me, "I've had it!"—meaning with our relationship. Woke up because I was so stunned and alarmed, panicked.

◆ Dream: At wide crosswalk with many lanes of cars, afraid to walk across and in front of cars looming so big. Light says I can walk but I'm sure I can't make it, so I don't move, felt fearful.

**Day 3**

◆ Vivid dreams, no other symptoms. Will take second dose tonight.

◆ Dream: Party at friend's, going water-skiing in the dark with ten-year-old kids. Confusing because how can you water-ski in dark, how can you do this? I say I cannot take my son into this situation. I come back from the bathroom and they had left without me. I yell the hostess's name down the street Fear, they left, there is danger and kids involved, they left without hearing what I had to say about it. Felt shocked, hurt, abandoned.

**Day 4**

◆ Dream: Calling 911, "Man entering home. Mother has been knocked down." Two sons tell me a weird man outside is trying to get inside the house, and we run around locking doors. As I am locking the last door, the man bursts in and knocks me down, beats me. Terrified, protective of kids. Dream was powerful enough to wake me, fast, energetic, active, fearful.

Fear did not linger but could recall as writing it down.

◆ 2:00 p.m. Aching in right kidney, dull, diffuse mid back on right side. Gone by 4:00 p.m.

◆ Increased urination.

◆ Bowel movement at night is unusual, stickier too.

**Day 5**

◆ Took another dose 11:00 a.m.

◆ Noon feeling paranoid, are people saying things I am not hearing? Feeling righteous. Something is going on without me, I did not know about it. People won't talk to me straight.

9:00 p.m. Ache in low back, right side. Used to have this sensation, but not for a long time.

**Day 6**

◆ Dream: In a bookstore. Teacher at school sculpted a beautiful clay hand, gorgeous. Son and I come in, I want him to read more, no talking on the phone till he reads more. I ask the teacher/sculptress if she had read *The Unfastened Heart*, a powerful book about women and relationships.

**Day 7**

◆ Before 4:00-5:00 a.m., woke up with dream: In a sitting room with other parents wondering if we should color-code a map. I start to explain why we should, and then why we shouldn't, and I get totally messed up and upset because I don't know what I am talking about. We are being watched by someone sitting way up high.
◆ Dream: Our assembly at school is getting ready to start. I find a room but have confusion about where to go. Someone thinks we have the wrong room. It is a huge auditorium with tiered seats, empty and vast.
◆ Feeling quite social, very joyous, giving out presents, talking, making things happen, unusual. A little ahead of myself, out of my body.
◆ Self-conscious a little. I wear a dress and teachers comment on seeing my legs. I am having an effect.

**Day 8**

◆ Dream: Happened in buildings or water. We go inside and open a secret door to find a slide like a spiral hamper chute. A woman who is my guide says this takes us down to her place. She pulls up a rope with a hammock on it and sits down on it and whoosh! off she goes down the slide. Down a water tunnel. I am afraid to go down. I pull the rope back up and try to get at the sling-like hammock to sit on, but it's all tangled. My breathing is short, I know it is fine but I can't figure it out. I'm too hot, I can't breathe, I try to unbutton my shirt while I untangle the rope. I know I can do this if I can just.... Shallow breath, not claustrophobic. Sensations in the body woke me.
◆ 3:00 p.m. Ahead of myself, a little panicky, short-tempered, out of body. External concerns. Felt off, felt not responding to what was happening in the moment.
◆ 10:00 p.m. left index finger painful and I have not done anything to it.

**Day 9**

◆ Dream: Scorpions lying in wait in people's shoes.
◆ Dream: Unknown man afraid of being touched. He is asked to pick me up so I am stretched lengthwise over his back, our bodies touching from shoulders down. He can do this and it is big deal since he is afraid of being touched.
◆ Constriction around top front half of skull, unpleasant, not hunger, lasted for a week.
◆ Feels like powers in the first dreams are dissipating.

**Day 10**

◆ Can't catch my dreams.
◆ Headache all day. Mild, diffuse, front of skull and over the top.
◆ Irritable. Started period five days early. In retrospect felt critical, short-tempered. Irritable due to the remedy, not premenstrual syndrome.

**Day 11**

◆ Dream: In old building, in an apartment with a man I know, seems to be my mate. I notice he is extremely big, with wide hips like three feet across, not fat, just massive. I look at myself and think how tiny I am in comparison, very strange.

**Day 13**

◆ Heavy day of period which started five days early. Premenstrual syndrome.

◆ On Christmas day having Christmas presents, husband opened pair of pants saying, "I can't believe you got me these!" I burst into tears, offended by his attitude, not that he did not like the pants. I was deeply stunned. He realized it was about his mother. Cut me to the quick very deeply. I was weepy for awhile.

**Day 14**

◆ Dream: Party of teenagers, son off somewhere. I meet his guy I've met before and we walk to the corner. I sit in a friend's convertible while he goes across the street. Son shows up from a friend's house, an old friend whom I haven't seen in awhile, and I realize it would be so good to see her.

◆ Heavy period continues.

◆ Not a huge appetite.

**Day 16**

◆ Dream: At amusement park. Throw-up ride. We are leaving as a teenager arrives, he takes an elevator to top of building and jumps off screaming and kills himself. No one knows him or what is going on. Woke me up out of sleep. Had other little mini dreams.

**Day 17**

◆ Ache inside skull

◆ Fighting over silly little things, being in the middle of it.

◆ Irritable but not able to stop it.

◆ Crying reaching my breaking point, little flexibility.

**Day 18**

◆ Dream: Children in class doing an Advent spiral, walking around a path usually made of pine boughs, but this one was weird, made from beanbags all pulsating up and down. All very nice feeling.

**Day 19**

◆ Husband said I have been more critical, short-tempered, not myself, mentally depressed, looking for a way out or an excuse in my mind.

◆ I feel like I'm waking up from being drugged. Only in retrospect am I aware of this altered state. I kept blaming it on other things. At first I thought it was premenstrual syndrome, but it didn't end. Then I thought it was my husband, then the kids were getting on my nerves. Then I thought maybe it's the weather. My dreams have lost that initial intensity, but the intensity is now in my emotional body. Depressed, looking for a way out. Very mental. Took a walk in the woods and found it very refreshing.

**Day 20**

◆ Dream: Water dream. Immense swimming pool, more like a slow-moving river with current, a strong current, but gentle. A lot of dreams with water. Feeling of soothing.

◆ Dream: High school boyfriend is helping me with a math problem, getting ready for a test. We have not finished studying yet, but are disturbed by our attraction for each other, so old, years ago, now we are both married. We kiss and then do more math problems. It's all a bit confusing and anxiety producing.

◆ I am liking staying up late at night. I feel better if I am quiet and by myself.

◆ Sleeping soundly till midmorning.

**Day 21**

◆ More thoughts on remedy: fear, doubt, violence, suicide.

◆ Felt like I am a victim.

◆ I am better when alone, more motivated, more in charge.

◆ When I am with others I want to blame them, make them responsible.

◆ I am better at night, late at night, reading a lot, which focuses my mind, constructive.

◆ Water is very soothing.

◆ Seeing a lot of movies, not exercising much.

**Day 26**

◆ Dream: Going to a baseball game with my son, walking in my old neighborhood, but I am the one who is going to play. I am putting my baseball uniform on but I am missing the shirt. Do I have time to run back? Can my son go by himself? No. Why didn't I take the car?

◆ Dream: Sailing and a big storm is coming up. How are we going to be O.K.?

◆ Husband and I are fighting over the silliest logistical things and totally misunderstanding each other. He feels I am undermining him, and I feel he is making a big deal out of nothing, being very oversensitive. It's better that we just don't talk and give each other space. Is this the proving? Hope so.

**Day 27**

◆ Seems better not to talk, keep my own space. Felt very antisocial. Better not to communicate but be on my own.

◆ Full pressing sensation, in pelvis only, for between one and two hours: heavy, dragging, very full sensation, like other prover mentioned.

◆ Kidney pain right side.

◆ Dream: About twins, everything was in twins.

### Prover #6 · Male · 47 years old

**Day 1**

◆ Dream: An acting company with a leading female who is a young vibrant poet, quite pregnant. She is in relationship with a poet/writer who is on the downhill: alcoholic, long nose like Cyrano. He negotiates contract with the managers to go with them, but he is being totally disrespected. He is asking for $325 a week, but they give him $80 a week as he is arguing under his breath.

**Day 2**

◆ Dream: Of the far future: My family and I waiting for a sea bus. Total overpopulation, the beach is overcrowded with people and pigeons. The pigeons cover everyone, if you sit down to rest, etc. Wondering if it is O.K. to let pigeons rest on you. We see pigeons flocked on a dead person. We think they are eating a homeless, dead person; but we get there and see he is O.K. Get on sea bus, seating is two-tiered and amazingly crowded, noticing a lot of pigeons.

◆ Real life: Several awarenesses of pigeons in last two days. Saw an injured pigeon, found it on a doorstep, it let me touch it. Almost took it to a vet but realized it was probably stupid. Saw a building flocking with them.

**Day 6**

◆ Got sick with malaise, aching, mild sore throat, upper respiratory infection.

◆ Anxiety that I will get much sicker, next day better.

◆ Left knee pain.

**Day 7**

◆ Right knee aching.

**Day 9**

◆ Dream: Big neighbor (6 foot 10 inches) brings a baby raccoon over to our house to give to me saying, "This is for the boy who was so good to my puppy." He is talking about me. I ask if I can keep him. "Yes!" he says. I go to thank him; he is a very friendly, connected kind of guy, discussing things with neighborhood boys. Everywhere he goes he creates community. He's a big friendly opinionated galoot with a big heart and a gruff exterior.

**Day 12**

◆ Got fluish again.

◆ Had an actual experience with someone who wanted something (an emotional connection) from me. She has a tremendous need for something from me. I have nothing for her. I get a migraine headache from this experience. Up all night with it. That night I felt I was dying. No strength to go on living.

**Day 14**

◆ Dream: Big fat man.

**Day 22**

◆ Took second dose.

**Day 25**

◆ Dream: I am with friends at a fancy hotel, considering going to eat at its restaurant, but we are mainly curious to see the interior. We are looking around trying to find a lost sweater. Also, I am hoping to connect with an old friend. People come and tell us we are not dressed properly, we do not belong there. Feeling of social inferiority.

**Day 27**

◆ Dream: Reconnecting and resolving things with old friends. We meet and we forget our differences, totally resolve everything. We agree to let everything go, not hold a grudge.
◆ Dream: Two old high school friends, one kind of arrogant, who has a hole in his leg, maybe cancer. Riding in a car or ride of some kind. I am concerned and trying to figure out what to do for him, how to help him.

**Day 29**

◆ Woke up in middle of night having an intense anxiety attack. I am going to go broke, bankruptcy, my business is going to fail. I am going to die. Sat for three hours trying to meditate the feeling away. Felt as if I was dying, as if too weak to go on.
◆ Tendency to jut my jaw forward for some reason.

## Prover #7 · Male · 36 years old

**Day 1**

◆ Took remedy 3:30 a.m.
◆ Dream: at high school reunion, trying to find bathroom in large home on wooded lot. Bathroom was a three-room suite. Put paper in old open suitcase, and almost had bowel movement in it. Thought, oh, how messy, and finally found the toilet. Girl, not a student of my high school, was at the party, not seen her for 23 years. Everyone wanted to get into the bathroom.
◆ Very sentimental, went to choral concert at church and got teary eyed at Christmas carols.

**Day 2**

◆ Very sentimental. Wept reading Christmas cards.
◆ Reading story to daughter about a poor family whose father had to poach a deer to feed the family and was imprisoned on Christmas. The girl, daughter, went to get father from town when he failed to return, and she was given gifts and got father out in time for Christmas. I could barely read the story, got so choked up could not finish the story. Teary eyed.
◆ Desire wine.

**Day 3**

◆ A lot of dreams but nothing there to write down.
◆ Clearing throat often.

**Day 4** (Repeated the remedy before bed, second dose.)

◆ Worked 8:30 a.m.-12:30, and 1:00-9:00 p.m. Busy, long day. Emotionally and mentally fine. Even-keeled.
◆ Dream: Walking with shoes that were very wide, like my brother's EEEE shoes when mine were AAA. I have very narrow feet.

**Day 5**

◆ Wife cooking fish, could not tolerate the smell. It nauseated me.

**Day 6**

◆ Dream: At childhood home in Illinois, very suburban neighborhood. Cops were outside chasing a crook in the driveway. Dog outside is growling at me. Went inside to check new addition, a long white corridor with a bedroom at the end. Turned on the lights and "Biff and Muffy" were in the room in the bed in street clothes. They weren't supposed to be there, so I took a doll and began to pummel Biff, using the doll as a butt. I was smashing the doll into his face as he was lying on the bed and as he was getting up. Absolutely no remorse, just beating the man.

**Day 7**

◆ Dream: At a cabin in Minnesota, a place I knew but it was all different, even the lake. JFK came to our cabin with secret service agents. Agents were in a small boat rowing on the lake doing drills wearing life jackets. JFK was in a three-piece suit and wanted to go for a boat ride. I squatted down on the dock and dipped a soup bowl into the lake and it was beef broth soup. The lake was all soup. Had it for lunch. They had to return to shore to pick me up. I was surprised to see all the secret service agents in swimming trunks and JFK in his suit.

**Day 8** (Took third dose at night)

**Day 9**

When doing errands, I got very frustrated/angry about our current money worries and was angry (again) that I was the sole breadwinner. Should we move, get a different job? Go to business school?

◆ Noticed pigeons going into building and had to shoo them out.

◆ Lower back pain. Not enough exercise or yoga.

◆ Had to crawl into crawl space to fix heating duct.

**Day 10**

◆ Developed cramping pain/soreness in right anterior/proximal thigh. Only physical symptom the whole month, felt like I'd been punched in the leg.

**Day 11**

◆ Very social with Christmas gatherings, events. Delightful day.

◆ Dream: New doctor wants to join clinic were I work. He did not want to buy disability insurance, says if he needed it he would sue the clinic for his four dollars an hour. Another doctor there who is also a lawyer is sitting on this guy's lap, and when he hears this sue comment he falls off the chair. I say, "He's not that slimy." None of these people looks familiar. One doctor has an old car in the clinic he wants us all to play with by filling a vessel with water and doing something with it. At the end of the dream, we are all standing behind curtains backstage, and I am trying to open the curtains for a final bow.

Cannot find opening, curtains are like blue sky above and rainbows stripes below. Turns out that we are in an auditorium at a Beatles concert, waiting for Beatles to come out. I go out for a bow—the stage is very high. The crowd doesn't clap as loud as I think they should until the Beatles come out. Then four ladders popped up for us to use to get off the stage. They all fall down, leaving us there.

**Day 12** Christmas day:
◆ Dream: About U.S. Senator Strom Thurmond. (Friend who hosted Christmas Eve party had told us she'd grown up in his hometown in South Carolina).

**Day 20**
◆ Dream: Walking around with father-in-law and daughter at Tilden Park in a hilly area with a steep path, large deep steps four-five feet high leading down from the church. Lots of people around. Walked in front of daughter, carrying toy vehicle. Went back to get daughter, it was a long way back. Could not find her there in the church playground in the crowd of kids. Then found her lying on the ground; she had been hit on the head by some kid with a pipe. I felt upset, I had abandoned her. I woke.

**Day 21**
◆ Dream: Camping deep in the woods with a large group of people. We arrive there by ice skating uphill on a new concrete sidewalk. We cooked and ate without bear precaution, and as soon as we arrive, a grizzly bear enters our camp and starts eating our food. Then a polar bear arrives and chases us all through the tent a few times in circles and then leaves. The polar bear chased us walking like a human. Friends from my medical school residency are there. Scared all night about bears. The tent is huge with partitions, and a colleague and I are asleep in one part of the tent separated from other areas. I dream while asleep in the tent about how would I get out if the bear attacked. Would the bear slash the tent open? Will the bear chase me? Should I roll down the hill in my sleeping bag, buried in the snow to escape? Why did we cook in the clothes we are sleeping in? Will the bear smell the food on us and come to eat us? I peer out at the fire area and the food is packed in steamer trunks in the clearing by the fire, some food is still on the ground, some poking out of the trunks. Why didn't we camp far from the food if worried about bears? If we did camp far away, would the bear come for the food and then smell us? Why no bear precautions? I am freaking out about this.

**Day 30**
◆ Dream: Old house in woods, returning there with two people. I wanted to see if someone was O.K., but the two others were unconcerned. One had a bike and they went off. I went through double doors into a living room, where everything was a mess, and looked around the doors to left and saw a toy ironing board, with a baby creature wrapped in swaddled blanket. It said "Play with me," and I picked it up and realized it was this evil little thing called "Ichy" or whatever. I started to smash it with a toy iron, but it bit me on the finger. I became concerned about the safety of the little girl at home and went to the kitchen to find her. I took the evil creature and put it in the oven on self clean to destroy

it, burned it to a cinder. All the appliances were on full blast, with oil all over them, making quite a fire hazard. There were pipes and burners everywhere. I turned them all off. When I yelled for help, no one was around. The kitchen was a maze of pipes, spooky. I felt this evil creature had done all this and was trying to burn the house down. Woke up.
◆ As I was waking up from the first dream this night, I was having another.
Dream: My wife was being held forcibly by some men in the kitchen in our house. They were gagging her and she was terrified. I was walking toward her to save her. She was motioning to me to get away, and I was stabbed with swords, killed? He chopped me up with a sword, do I want to die or do I want to go?

## Prover #8 · Female · 42 years old

Note: Only remedy I hesitated to take. When I got it, I did not want it with me, so I left it at mother's house. Felt apprehension about taking it. Took it evening January 3.

**Day 1**

◆ Dream: Slipped away from me very fast. Buying a red used boat, out on a huge lake with others in the boat, being just a speck.
◆ Dream: Bringing home a used car; dragging the car home by a string attached to it, also carrying large packages. It was difficult to manage the car and the packages. Walking near a large building that is a department store, made of cinder blocks. Seemed unnaturally large, square and plain, no windows or doors.
◆ Dream: Person I know in waking time from school came to visit me with a test tube rack full of different types of chemical bottles and tubes of all colors and styles. Some look like perfume bottles more than test tubes. They are in disarray, haphazardly arranged in the rack, some close to spilling. We are inside a pink or salmon-colored bathroom, and this person is somehow holding this rack over me so that I look up at it. Some of the bottles/tubes were dripping their contents. I told him I did not want my face etched with acid. Later, I went back into the bathroom and there were bubbles of creamy liquid on the floor, as if some of the chemicals from the test tubes had spilled there and were reacting. There was also something like sprinkles around that looked like cooked white rice kernels. The bubbles and puddles were creamy pink or yellow-colored, which I perceived as a disgusting, frustrating mess because I had to clean it up without getting anything on my hands. Then my black cat came into the bathroom, and suddenly a black dog came out of the cabinet and chased it away.
◆ Dream: In a car with a repairman who had been working on my house. I was not totally happy with him, but he needed help finding a parts store. I knew how to get to where the store was, showed him, but the road was closed so we needed to drive around to the other side to get here. Instead he drove through the obstacle and onto the closed road and steered around all kinds of dangerous stuff. He sped up the car so it would have momentum to fly over a huge gap in the road and land on the other side. I was annoyed and frustrated at being stuck in this situation, with a guy who was not very safe. Finally

we got into the shop and I wandered around in it.

◆ Dream: I'm near a stream or river bank and it seems that I've been rafting or something like that. I'm looking at a still pool with an eddy and my black cat suddenly can be seen swimming to the surface of the water from below, and then as she reaches the surface, she eats bugs that are floating there, like a trout would do or something. I was surprised at this, thought it was strange she was there at all, let alone be in the water and eating bugs. It was the same kind of context surprise that occurred in the pink bathroom dream. (I've never had my 'real' pets show up in my dreams before.)

◆ Had right-sided stiff neck or right-sided scapular pain.

**Day 3**

◆ Second dose.

◆ Quality of dreams has shifted; elusive on waking, cohesive while dreaming. Immediately on waking large sections of them slip away quite quickly, and I can't recall them. Even in other provings, this has not happened.

◆ This night's dreams are not as vivid or as real feeling as my normal dreams. They are less so than first dose dreams were as well. There is a softness or a dullness to them even though the actual content is not particularly soft.

◆ Dream: Domestic animals and pets.

◆ Dream: At large party with many people—old friends from grade school and more recent ones of the present. Elaborately arranged seafood and vegetables are on black plates, given to us individually as we sit at an outdoor bar. Inside the party is a large open room with wood floors & a dance band. Lots of large windows with a few people standing around in groups chatting. There is a lone white toilet in a conspicuous place in this open room. The people are talking about their bowel movements and how food affects them. I am sitting on the toilet totally at ease using it in public. I am constipated at the moment. Next, I am outdoors at the party, and it is dark now. There is a huge concrete raised slab with a fountain-type thing that makes a sheet of rain all around the perimeter of the slab. At first when you are standing near the slab you think it's raining because you feel the drops of moisture splashing on you. The people are lying around listening to the music. I passed through the water onto the slab to listen. The music was metallic, thready, synthesized music played on something like a sitar. I was thinking, "I've got a friend who would not like the unmelodic quality of the music."

◆ This dream had a sort of dull unemotional quality to it. In the dream I had gotten wet, figuring out how to get on the slab, which was unpleasant, but my reaction to it was dull. There was a certain subdued dullness to the whole party even though the food and surroundings were rather extravagant.

◆ Inside the dream, I was in a state of not being totally present myself, like I didn't really get into the food or the music or the people. I was there but sort of wandering and low-key, uninvolved, undirected, unmotivated about what I was doing, etc. This dream had a lackluster quality to it even though the potential was there for it to have been bright, shiny and extravagant, kind of like dirty or unpolished metal or gemstone or a dusty painting.

◆ In all the dreams both nights, there was a lack of intention or focus or clarity of purpose about what I was doing. This is unusual for my dreams.

◆ The domestic animals and pets were unusual for my dreams, although wild animals are common.
◆ Food is common in my dreams, but I always have an emotional response to it.
Left purse at restaurant, very unusual.

**Prover #9 · Female · 47 years old**

**Day 1**
◆ Dream: There was this high structure like a double cross somehow involved with danger, somewhat similar to high-tension electrical wires. A random, large group of people had been kidnapped and taken to a place that was deep underground where conditions were barely livable—horrible—incompatible with life. A young woman risks her life to escape and get help for the others (though it was known they were captured and not much was being done about it). A hopelessly threatening situation. I went with the young woman to her family. There were two young children, a man, and a woman. The children did not seem traumatized to have lost some family members. The situation seemed quite ordinary, not much emotion—maybe not enough food.
(I remember that the day before I heard a Czech playwright discuss his mom disappearing with the Nazis and his not being so affected by it.)

**Day 3**
◆ Dream: Boy is playing on edge of large round precipice. He is not my responsibility, but I am watching him thinking he may fall. He does fall very far down into the center, which is a body of water. I jump in right away, without a thought, to help him. I and another person struggle to pull him out of the water or he would have drowned. He was under for a little long—I wonder, will he be O.K.? Will his mother be satisfied we did our best?
◆ Detachment.
◆ Some issues of guilt.
◆ Sleep is a little better—sleeping through the night.
◆ Body temperature is warmer than usual.
◆ Sometimes I eat a lot, sometimes don't eat much.

**Day 4**
◆ Feeling wiped out, burnt out, everything is annoying me. I canceled Christmas Eve. Felt guilty. I don't attribute anything to the remedy.
◆ Dream: I am young. A neighbor is riding on the front hood of his baby sitter's car while she is driving. An old man who looks demonic is speaking to him. I suspect the child is being abused. I talk to the mother. I'm concerned but not emotionally upset. Who is your pediatrician? I am hers(?) Could I be of help?
◆ Dream: Talking about running with men and women. Supportive, friendly conversation. Talked about body odors. One not embarrassed. "Do you stink everywhere? Crotch?"
◆ Remedy repeated late at night.

**Day 5**

◆ Dream: Strong dream: Walking in unknown neighborhood trying to get to place I was staying—in the wee hours of the morning—knowing it was not a safe situation. A largely built man jumps out of the shadows and picks me up and carries me to his house. I say to him, "Please, just don't hurt me." He looks at me as if to say why would I do that. We are in his room in a large communal house. It is very friendly, a well-lit place, not like the dark street. We enjoy each other's company very much. I became very sexually attracted to him and aroused. We are putting up panels to make the room more private. I am the more assertive in the lovemaking. In the love dream the lovemaking is all foreplay—I wake up very sexually aroused.

◆ Dream: I am riding in a van with several people, listening to the baseball game on the radio. Then somehow I am watching the pitcher and catcher firing the ball with incredible speed back and forth, back and forth, multiple times. The comment is made, "That looks like good sex." The intensity of it, the working together, it is exciting, charged.

**Day 7**

◆ Dream: Being in Washington DC. I am trying to find my way back. I go to a large (government) building. People point out the window to give me directions from the main street I see. It takes me hours just to get to the street. I am not particularly emotional, or scared. It is just a long, convoluted experience. "I" in the dream may be a friend, a woman who is 94, very sharp, but just starting to lose her bright mind and ability to walk.

◆ Dream: Swimming in a clear pond with many different colored fish. I'm underwater with the fish, no trouble breathing, swimming around, no strong emotion.

◆ Dream: I am in a restaurant waiting to be served breakfast. We get a necklace free with the meal, a gold chain with 3 pearls on it. I order eight more when I go to pay the bill. (I saw a woman yesterday with a similar necklace and admired it—to myself).

◆ I wake up in the night, after one of these dreams. I am very alert and clearheaded and energized, but relaxed also and able to go back to sleep right away.

**Day 8**

◆ Dream: I am in an informal class situation with about ten people I have known for some time. I am covered only by a bright, large piece of cloth, bright orange or red. I keep adjusting it to cover my nakedness underneath. One man in the class seems to be aware of this, and is paying close attention. I keep shifting positions and becoming partially uncovered. I am somewhat embarrassed that my vulva keeps becoming uncovered. So I think I will turn it into parsley—then it can be eaten and will no longer embarrass me. The emotion is not so strong.

**Day 9**

◆ I have been all along—since the beginning of the proving—feeling quite thirsty, but no desire to drink. I have felt that in the past before the remedy, but it is much stronger and I note it several times a day. I make no effort to get a drink, though I am markedly thirsty.

**Day 10**

◆ I woke up early. It had been a restless sleep. I was full of anger. In my dream it had been anger in different situations, anger that was unexpressed. I was sitting on the anger.

◆ Dream: Sitting in a restaurant with three friends and my husband. They are discussing how to divide up the meat entree. I tell them someone doesn't eat meat. They cannot believe someone would not eat meat; I feel they are arrogant and insensitive.

◆ Dream: A group of little girls are playing in an area of three or four sandboxes. They keep getting into squabbles. Mothers come to break them up and send them back to their different sandboxes to play.

◆ Dream: I see an old friend from many years ago at the same restaurant as prior dream this night. I tart talking to her. She's already in a conversation with someone else. She pays no attention to me. I am upset about it, but I realize also that I just barged in and started talking. Frustration.

I repeat the remedy, third dose, in the evening.

**Day 12**

◆ Very relaxing day at home with my immediate family. Finally the season's rushing is over, and I feel deeply relaxed for the first time in weeks.

◆ I notice that my thirst - but no desire to drink (urge) isn't there today. Average thirst and am drinking to quench it. It feels good.

**Prover #10 · Female · 38 years old**

**Day 1**

◆ Holding remedy in hand. Power in pelvis; sense of legs and strength.

◆ More awareness while holding it. No fear, but very aware.

◆ More awareness of skin surface.

◆ Took remedy. More saliva for about two hours; then gone.

◆ Alertness persists.

◆ Some relaxation in stomach.

◆ Mind, thought processes more concerned about strategy than usual. Looking for angles of escape.

**Day 2**

◆ Still having sense of trepidation—not anxiety. Very aware of where exits are in room.

◆ Feeling slightly isolated and different from others.

◆ Energy level good; endurance good with activity.

◆ Appetite same—desire creamy foods.

◆ Dream: Moving silently through house at night. Very alert, not fearful. Trying to find someone in many rooms, like a maze. No fear but feeling of needing to avoid being trapped at all costs.

**Day 3**

◆ Another dose of remedy. Again heightened awareness and sense of suspicion. Interested in overhearing the conversation of others.

◆ Feel somewhat isolated although in the company of others.

◆ Go to airport to visit parents for the day. Flight delay. Sit on floor and watch people go by.

◆ Baby-sat a young child and felt unreasonable concern for her safety. Kept looking down the hall; desire to run out. Anxious about flying. Very unusual. Not wanting to be trapped in plane.

**Day 4**

◆ Energy level continues to show increased endurance.

◆ Frontal headache this morning.

◆ Somewhat constipated.

◆ Father has cancer: not very emotional with him—sense of detachment.

**Day 5**

◆ Start of retreat. Very hectic. Many people. Feeling much more claustrophobic than is usual for me.

◆ Feel like running everywhere at a lope.

◆ Very strong meditation with incredible opening. Sense of deep internal change.

◆ Very hot.

◆ Chest pain like someone took a knife down my sternum.

◆ Great difficulty sleeping.

**Day 6**

◆ Dream: Pursued through old building: many rooms—maze-like. Chased by three men. I realize their intention is rape but feel like I am going to be eaten. Despair about being trapped with no way out. Awoke with the feeling.

◆ Again very hot.

◆ Emotional turmoil that I keep putting down with my breath. Sense of incredible void inside myself. Very full. Realize that I cannot encompass the universe externally like I have been trying to do. Urge to go deeper inside.

**Day 7**

◆ No sleep again.

◆ Very hot. Sense of internal burning from the retreat. Feel like I am burning through the proving doses in 24 hours. Don't want to take another one.

# LAC DELPHINUM

*Milk of the Dolphin*

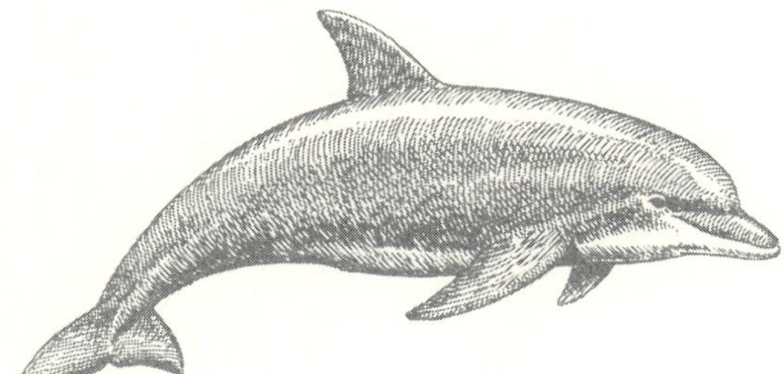

# LAC DELPHINUM *Milk of the Bottlenose Dolphin*

Humans and dolphins have an ancient connection. From stories such as those about the mystery temple at Delphi—Greek for "dolphin"—where the oracle gave people spiritual messages, to the mariner legends of the "singing mermaids"—thought to be dolphins—who lured and enchanted sailors, we continue to be intrigued by this winsome creature with the smiling face.

There are 43 species of dolphins and porpoises living in oceans and rivers throughout the world. The killer whale, who is not actually a whale but a dolphin, is 30 feet long, while the smallest dolphins are delicate, five-foot creatures. They can swim up to 70 miles daily and cruise at 20 miles per hour.

The dolphin, like the elephant, lives in a community with high levels of group cooperation. This is an important asset in the sea because it allows them to work together on tasks necessary for their survival. For example, they might herd a school of fish onto a rocky outcropping or trap them in a shallow cove. They might assist a mother dolphin by baby-sitting for her calf, or they can play group-type games. Teams of dolphins can be formed instantly to come to the rescue of a dolphin in distress and lift it near the surface of the water so it can breathe. They will then keep it there for weeks, carefully rotating places until the animal either dies or is healed. (**CALM**)

The dolphins' main social grouping is the pod, which, similar to the elephant, is comprised of adult females and their offspring in groups of two to fifteen. Within this group, mothers and calves swim in very close contact for up to five years. The calves are not fully weaned until 18 to 20 months of age. The mothers are ever alert to potential danger to the young. If the calf should stray near anything harmful or unusual, the mother will push him to safety immediately. When the daughters have their own offspring, they raise them with a lot of help from the senior females. Males join all-male groups and form very long-term friendships. Their daily activities include making the rounds of female pods, playing, and fishing.

Dolphins are legendary for their incredible vocalizing skills. They click, whistle, quack, bleat, and bark. Even when they are out of range from one another, they can locate and identify each other by each individual's unique whistle. When dolphins sing, they harmonize flawlessly in the same pitch, unlike wolves, who communicate by howling in various pitches.

In captivity as well as in the wild, dolphins love to play. (**PLAY**) They chase one another, race from a defined starting point, and use anything they can get their snouts on for a toy. A male will even use his erect penis to pull toys around the tank. They love to leap in and out of the water, soaring as high as possible for no practical purpose other than sheer pleasure. Groups of dolphins have been observed by underwater researchers performing complex, ballet-like dances in precise formation and rhythm.

In the wild, most of the aggressive behavior among dolphins is associated with sexuality. In captivity, if they are upset with another dolphin's behavior—such as parking himself in front of the trainer's fish pot—they may merely settle down on top of him until he moves away. Occasionally, there will be dominance skirmishes among the largest adults, including hostile acts such as ramming with the lower jaw or striking with a fluke.

Just like elephants and whales, dolphins love constant physical contact with one another. They rub their bodies together affectionately along their entire length while swimming and touch and pat each other throughout the day. They also engage in a curious maneuver where one dolphin will slowly push another dolphin around with its beak in the other's genital slit. Again, there seems to be no practical reason for this behavior. (**PLAY/PLEASURE**)

Dolphins are by far the most sexually exploratory and freewheeling creatures in the animal kingdom. To put it simply, they will have sex at any age, any time, anywhere, with anything: young and old, male and female, mother, father, daughter, son, toy or human—they are ready and willing. The female often lures the male. They chase and caress and nuzzle and rake each other with their teeth. They even knock their heads together. It is all done in a spirit of fun and play and lasts for hours. Most scars found on an adult dolphin are, in fact, created by the enthusiastic sexual activity of adolescence.

The biggest threat to dolphins are sharks, who find the calves delectable and manage to eat many of them despite the vigilance of the pod. Survival rate for the first year is less than 50 percent. This, for a creature who is very devoted to her calves, is a major trauma. Thus, the feeling among dolphins, especially the females, is that danger is all around. (**DANGER**) The threat is ever present and completely real, yet it does not mitigate the sheer joy and exuberance in the dolphins' daily life. Occasionally, the mother dolphins have a strong need to free themselves from the constant responsibility of caring for their calves. They will then go off on their own to play, explore, and fish. (**SEPARATION/DETACHED**) To do this safely, they leave the calves with the "aunties" (non-pregnant or nursing females) who, while baby-sitting, will form a circle and swim round and round the calves to protect them from danger. (**CIRCLES**) Thus, the feeling in the dolphin is that there is calm and safety in the center of the circle, even though there is danger outside. (**CALM DURING DANGER**)

Sleep is an interesting phenomenon in the dolphin's life. Consistent with the feeling in the proving of "danger all around," dolphins have evolved a sleep pattern whereby they rest only one-half of their brain at a time. The other half maintains vigilance by keeping one eye open to watch for predators. This became evident in the provers with symptoms such as: "restless sleep... in small, broken blocks...turning a lot, like a rotisserie, all night."

The Cetaceans have a remarkable lineage. Recent research has revealed that long ago a wolf-like, coastal mammal evolved to make the sea its home. Slowly, it lost its limbs and developed flippers and a sleek, hairless body. This may explain some of the similarities between wolves and dolphins, such as their haunting vocalization. While they look like large fish, the whale and dolphin are still typical mammals who give birth from a uterus, nurse with milk, and have internal heat regulation.

Perhaps due to subliminal fascination with a land mammal going into the sea, humans have always been especially drawn to dolphins. Aristotle studied them, and there are frescos of boys riding the backs of dolphins at the ancient palace of Knossos on the island of Crete. In 1975, John Lilly founded the Human/Dolphin Foundation to explore inter-species communication. In the present day, dolphins and whales have been found to be much more valuable as a tourist attraction than they ever were as a source of meat and blubber. People will now go to great efforts to save the life of even a single dolphin. When it was revealed that the tuna industry was killing dolphins as a byproduct of its fishing practices, there was a huge outpouring of sympathy and a boycott of tuna products, until the industry developed dolphin-safe nets. (They are still not completely effective, however.)

Anecdotes abound of dolphins interacting in surprising ways with humans. At Hahnemann Medical Clinic, we had a patient whose father had a heart attack while swimming in Hawaii. A dolphin magically appeared, swam under his unconscious form, lifted him up, and deposited him in shallow waters near the shore. (**CLAIRVOYANCE**) In western Australia, a group of bottlenose dolphins daily visits Monkey Mia beach, where visitors wade in the water to be with them. Here the dolphins are petted and loved by all. Many cultures around the world, from the northern Hebrides to Africa, have folk tales involving human-dolphin interactions.

Dolphins have a special affinity for the ill, especially children who are mentally or physically challenged. It has been reported that dolphins, when confronted with a group of children, will specifically identify and linger with the unhealthy ones. This is said to be particularly true when the children have emotional problems. There are, at present, over 150 dolphin-assisted therapy programs worldwide.

Progress has been reported in adults and children with disabilities ranging from Down's Syndrome, depression, attention deficit disorder, muscular dystrophy, spinal cord injuries, and mental retardation. Chris Harre of the Dolphin Research Center in Grassy Key, Florida says: "Mentally retarded children who swam with dolphins learned their lessons two to ten times faster than in a normal classroom setting."

Studies have shown that swimming with dolphins increases both the production of infection-fighting T cells as well as endorphins, the hormones that prompt a feeling of well-being and deep relaxation. (**CALM**) Some researchers believe this is due to the bombardment with sonar that the swimmer receives while in the water with the dolphins. David Cole, a dolphin researcher, states: "The dolphins produce an intense amount of echolocation energy. It resonates in your bones. You can feel it pass through you and travel up your spine." Dolphins' sonar is so powerful that it can echolocate a shark a half mile away in the ocean and be able to tell if its stomach is empty or full. A human being in the sea would be like an x-ray to the dolphin; the lungs and respiratory system especially would be completely transparent.

### Analysis of the Proving

This proving was done in a seminar setting on the island of Maui in Hawaii. It is the only one of the eight provings that was done in this manner, and it lasted for only eight days rather than the usual three weeks. The results were so clear and powerful that the core theme (calmness despite danger) became evident during the provers' meeting at the end of the seminar, unlike most provings, which require weeks of study before the themes are clear. Many synchronous events occurred during these eight days, but most striking was the sighting of a pod of dolphins swimming in the sea right outside the hotel while the final provers' meeting was taking place.

The feeling of calmness that comes through this remedy may be confusing. We see that sometimes the patient has the polarity or opposite of the state expressed by the substance. Thus, Sulphur may be either fastidious or extremely sloppy. Calmness may be the state that is desperately sought by our patient who needs Lac delphinum. They may be hysterical, with a constant fear that someone or something is going to get them at any moment. In the first long-term, cured case using this remedy, one of the patient's symptoms was an obsession about alarm systems and protection; she felt a constant, unnamed threat all around her. After Lac delphinum, she lost that feeling of fear and tension, and her life now is much happier.

I have observed in every Lac delphinum case so far (six) that the patient makes large gestures with his or her arms, often indicating a circle or a circular-type motion.

**The Substance**

The dolphin whose milk was donated was a *Tursiops Truncatus* species of Atlantic Bottlenose dolphin. She was a nine-year-old female named Shakta, and this was her first calf, Kolohi. Kolohi was born July 12, 1994. The researchers took some milk by breast pump from Shakta when Kolohi was only a few days old, in case of possible future need. The mother and calf were in captivity with six other dolphins in a large, sea-like enclosure next to a hotel where homeopath Melissa Fairbanks was staying. The dolphins were being studied by a group of researchers. Melissa convinced the caretakers to give her a very small vial (two drops) of frozen dolphin's milk. She immediately went to her room and, in sterilized containers, triturated it with granulated sugar to a potency of 3C. She sent it to Michael Quinn, at Hahnemann Pharmacy, who then potentized it to a 30C. I sent this same substance to Divya Chhabra in India, who had the original idea to prove dolphin's milk. She used it to produce an excellent proving in Bombay, India.

*Lac Delphinum* **Themes**

*Milk of the Bottlenose Dolphin*

- *Calm*
- *Calm During Danger*
- *Danger*
- *Play and Pleasure*
- *Circles*
- *Separation/Detached*
- *Clairvoyance*

# *Calm*

**#9** Wasn't bothered as much by little things. This has lasted to the present. Little things now don't bother me as much, like having everything where I like it so I can find it the next time I want to use it. I'm not as picky at my work bench, in the kitchen, or with my office staff. This shift was not gradual; it happened at the proving, and it has stayed. (This is a cured state.)

**#6** During infrequent visits with my parents, I have had a calmness and an acceptance of them not experienced in the past. Had an actual conversation about, "We need to listen to dad." It was a smooth visit, and I felt calm. Actually felt somewhat detached, and all the old stuff has not come up. Feel fully present with them. Now have better relationship to father.

**#5** General decrease in anxiety and worry. Everything is O.K. Very peaceful with my situation.

**#2** Felt as if I was a big rock in a harbor. Felt I was a strong influence. Solid. My friends would benefit from my strength by coming into my harbor. Overall feeling of solidity, very strong, stable. Usually just go through life without thinking about what I am, who I am, how I affect people.

**#3** Generally calmer, even in moments of emotional turmoil in her life. Positive, like this usually, but even more so.

## Calm During Danger

**#3** Driving and noticed a large jeep just behind me. He hit the back of my car on purpose. Never happened to me ever before. He backed up and hit the back of my car again and said: " You don't like this a—hole? You want to say something about this?" I pulled off to side of road; he pulled next to me. He shouted obscenities. He followed me cursing and flailing his arms. I was frightened but calm. This guy wasn't going to hurt me, but I wasn't going to be foolish either.

**#9** Dream: House flooded and had to use rowboat to get to friend's house. I was using a rowboat to get to and from classes and visit friends and go back and forth. Water was everywhere, and this was my mode of transportation. Calmness, no sense of danger.

**#2** Dream: All closest friends were dying in auto accidents. They were dying in groups. One accident had killed four people. When heard, not shocked—thought, that is interesting, that's the way we are going to leave the planet. Heard someone else had died in my little family. I was the only one left. When is my number up? Thought it was interesting, no fear. "An interesting way to leave, in batches like that."

**#4** Dozed off in class and had intense flashes of dreams which persisted on opening eyes. Like dream was carried over into waking state. One scene was of a wave crashing right over me. Normally I might have been startled, but wasn't.

**#16** Fearless on big waves. Plunged through giant waves.

**#10** Dream: A woman and I were walking in a circle clockwise, around the perimeter of a crowded mezzanine in a mall. I asked why was she walking in a circle, and she said enemies were coming to get her, and she has to keep going so enemies wouldn't catch up to her. Her walk was leisurely, but she kept looking over her shoulder as she was trying to avoid enemies. There was a languid swimming feeling as we were walking.

**#5** Less fear when snorkeling. Normally would worry in the water. Less fear, and less anxiety in general.

**#17** Fear of burglaries now gone. (This is a cured symptom.)

**#17** Fear of intrusion now gone. (This is a cured symptom.)

# *Danger*

**#15** I had a great fear of driving to that town in Maui where the Halloween parade was. I had the sense that something was going to happen and was very nervous about driving there with some companions. Nothing did happen, but I was worried about having an accident or something like that.

**#17** Delusion I wasn't safe (alarm system, dogs). (This is a cured symptom.)

**#2** Jerked eyes open with real panic feeling, as if was going to get run over. Like falling off mountain when you do this jerk.

**#14** Dream: I was in a house or building with other people, maybe women. Other people, maybe men, were making every effort to get into the building. The people in the house were moving from room to room, pursued by the outsiders. At times, the insiders could trap the outsiders in a place like a closet, but there was the sense of being pursued. When there was no place left to hide or move into, I remember turning on one of the outsiders and using my hand, pushed him back and away and over a piece of furniture and telling him I had had enough.

**#6** Dream: Saw this minister in a condo. I had to walk up steep steps to see him. Father said, "Don't go with him," but I went anyway and felt later that I had made a major mistake and was in danger. Something I shouldn't have done.

**#17** I was worried about my son all night. So I had some fear. I would wake up frequently and look over to make sure he was still in his bed and not still in the water. Several of my dreams, whenever I went back to sleep, we were in the slides or at the beach. I was looking for him in the water, as if I was distracted and I was being negligent and he was in danger.

## *Play and Pleasure*

**#5** Increase in joking, joviality, jesting, silliness, and an increase in laughing. A lot of playfulness during the week. This is not how I usually am. It's very different for me.

**#18** I had some moments of spontaneous joy; I laughed out loud, a deep hearty laugh. A real departure from my recent state.

**#9** Don't have as much self-control. Usually very disciplined, especially with diet. Chocolate, started eating it for first time in 17 years! Didn't care, not a big deal. The eating chocolate wasn't as much about chocolate as it was about an attitude: "This isn't part of my diet," lessening. I still eat it occasionally now, maybe a tiny craving for it. Ate it first at lunch. A chocolate chip cookie sounds pretty good right now! Also ate onion rings, which I would never have eaten before.

**#12** Dream: My usually celibate, female spiritual teacher wanted a male concubine. I auditioned for the job. I touched her, felt intense desire, and woke up with a wet dream.

**#17** The night was fun. Going from scene to scene to scene. Exciting. So many images, unusual images, without the element of surprise, just: "Wow, look at that." Fun. Playful. None of it made any sense, and none of it mattered. Element of surprise, it wasn't shocking, it was just fun, interesting. A curiosity. There was an excitement to it.

**#5** Desire to touch people, be near them, feel their presence, feel connection, to have fun with them, to laugh with them. Normally I want time to myself.

# *Circles*

**#16** Dream: Riding horses in an oval track area. I want to go fast. My horse was *perfectly* responsive, it ran full out and it was so smooth, completely satisfying and a thrill. Felt like being the wind.

**#6** I felt separated from the group during the proving. Like outside a window, looking in. Like standing outside a circle.

**#3** Dream: Heavyset man, big stomach, in yellow shirt being beaten up by three other young gentlemen. He was in the center of a circle.

**#10** Dream: On a merry-go-round, going clockwise.

**#2** Restless and turning at night. Like doing 360's. Laying on one side, then a few minutes later do a one-half turn, like on a rotisserie all night.

**#10** Dream: We were walking in a circle clockwise, around the perimeter of a crowed mezzanine in a mall. I asked why was she walking in a circle, and she said enemies were coming to get her, and she has to keep going so enemies wouldn't catch up to her.

**#10** Dream: Going to a horse racetrack. Again, the animals were racing clockwise. The main position was 6 and 9 on the dial.

## *Separation/Detached*

**#13** Dream: Large white rock passages. Solitary, lonely feeling. Me walking, looking for others but no one appears. I feel lost—not afraid but slightly sad.

**#6** Feeling of separation; I felt separated from the group during the proving. Feeling like an outsider, or outcast. Pervasive feelings lasted over three months. Wanted to be with people but felt shunned. Like outside a window, looking in. Like standing outside a circle. Very profound. Every time I talk about it, the feelings are very intense.

**#9** More detached, introverted yet still awareness of surroundings. Want to be in my own world, be inside myself. Preoccupied with myself.

**#18** Transient feeling of spaciness. I don't feel like I am really here. Its all just a movie and I am a detached observer.

**#1** Spacey, not spaced-out feeling, as much as if a fog is between you and the other person—like looking through a wet window or a pane of glass with rain on it. It was disfigured, disoriented.... ...disassociated feeling. Heard people talking, sounded like the hum of bees. Felt separate from this, not a part of it. Felt really like I wanted to isolate. Feeling like a loner.... Juststay on the beach and relax and not participate.

**#16** Felt a little separate, in my own thoughts.

# *Clairvoyance*

**#10** Dream: Researchers were working on a technique to literally transform substance, or to transmit thoughts.

**#17** Psychic ability and intuition heightened.

**#18** While in the midst of a conversation, I couldn't remember whether I had spoken some of my ideas or merely thought them. This never happens to me, and it felt very unusual and unnerving.

**#1** Dream: In house, front door with beveled glass, one of the pieces was broken. Was told it was too expensive to repair it. Told to cover it up. Refused to cover it up and wanted it fixed. Actual event several months later, my son was attacked, and the exact beveled glass door was broken by attacker.

**#2** Dream: Got a message in a dream, like it was a major revelation...All the mundane things in life will take on a significance and teach me about deeper things, like major learning. Felt this was so meaningful...felt this was a communication from my husband who had died one year ago. Felt good, he's still communicating to me. Felt like a blessing, a passing on of knowledge from the other side.

**MIND**

ACTIVITY; desire for
AFFECTIONATE
AILMENTS from; fright or fear
ALONE, feels he is
AMOROUS; disposition
AMUSEMENT; desire for
ANTICS, plays
ANXIETY; children; about his
family, about his
CALM
CLAIRVOYANT
COLORS; charmed by
desires bright
COMMUNICATIVE, expansive
COMPANY; desire for
wants to be watched constantly
CONSCIENTIOUS about trifles
CREATIVE
DANGER; surrounded by; yet calm
DELIRIUM; chill, during
DELUSIONS, imaginations
beautiful; things look
danger; impression of
yet remains calm
enemies, surrounded by
safe, she is not
separated
from the group, that he is
from the world that he is
visions, has, on closing the eyes
DESIRES; people
touch things
DETACHED
DOUBTFUL, of himself
inferior feels
DREAMS
attacked, son was
accidents, of

DREAMS (cont.)
  accusations
    denying
    having chemicals
  airplanes
    choosing comfortable seats
  amorous
    teacher, spiritual, celibate wants concubine; auditioned for job,
anxiety about
    with pollutions
  amusing
  anger
  animals, of
    dogs
      fur shaved off
    fishes
    horses
      racing
        clockwise
  anxious
  cars, automobiles, of
  child, children; about
    babies; nursing
      fulfillment in
    baby-sitting
    danger in water
    fondness for
    looking for
    loosing in water
    responsibility for
      does not want responsibility
    something has happened to
  circle; center of; he is in
      man is, violently beaten man is
    going clockwise toward a
    standing outside
    looking in
    walking in a
  clairvoyant, prophetic
  colored
    exaggerated colors and proportions
  cover up report card, son tried
  danger
    from seeing the minister

- desire, man has for her
- disoriented
- dispute legal, around poisoning by toxins
- distorting everything
- drown, fear son will
- dying
- encircled tightly, being
- enemies
  - pursued by
  - avoids
- enlarged, objects are
- exaggerated colors and proportions
- fearless
- flood
  - calm in
  - house is in a
- food
- friends, seeing, of
  - old
- glass, broken
  - covered up
- guilt
- hiding from danger, of
- houses, communal
  - rundown
  - wooden
- inadequate feels
  - as new paralegal resolving property disputes
- indecent behavior of men and women
- indignation at salesman
- large, all was
- laughing, people are, at him
- man putting hand on her crotch
- many
- meaningful
- mother, of
- murder
- music
- parties
- people, of; strange things, doing
- playmate since childhood
- purchase, making
- pursued by, of being
- quarrels

DREAMS (cont.)
  reproaches himself
  research on substance to transmit thoughts
  revelations from dead
  ridiculous, he is made to feel
  rocks, of large white
  rowboat
    is mode of transport
  secrets
  seminar, leading a
  shocking
  strangers, of
  surgery; grateful to have sperm and egg combined and put in uterus
  surreal
  swimming, languid feeling
  unremembered; morning, sleep, in
  violence
  water
  waves, washing over him
  woman, depressed, came to party
FEAR
  accidents, of
  crowd, in a
  danger; impending, of
  robbers, of
FEARLESSNESS
  big waves, plunged through
    danger menaced him, as if, but without fear
  water in the
INSECURITY, mental; sense of
INTROVERTED
IRRITABILITY
ISOLATION, sensation of
JESTING
JOVIAL
LAUGHING
  easily
LOVE; animals, for
OUTCAST
PLAY; desire to, playful
  water in the
PLEASURE
  in food, loss of self-control
RELAXED feeling, letting go

SELF-CONTROL; loss of
SENSITIVE, oversensitive; noise, to
        sleep, on going to
SENTIMENTAL
    music with
SPACED-out feeling
    as fog between self and others
TOUCH things, impelled to
TRANQUILLITY, serenity, calmness
    not bothered by little problems
    not caught up in pettiness
TRIFLES; important, seem

## VERTIGO

VERTIGO
CHILL; during
FLOATING, as if
LEANING; wanting to, towards the left
LEFT, swaying toward
SPACINESS with
TURNING; circle; he turns in a; right, to
VISION, with obscurity of

## HEAD PAIN

LOCALIZATION
    occiput
    temples
DULL
    Forehead
    Occiput
    Sides; right

## EYE

PAIN
    fever during
    burning
        reaction to perfume
PHOTOPHOBIA
REDNESS

**VISION**

ACUTE
    objects, for small
BLURRED, large objects seem
FOGGY

**EAR**

DISCOLORATION; redness
DRYNESS; sensation of
STOPPED sensation

**HEARING**

ACUTE
    evening; falling asleep

**NOSE**

CATARRH
    post-nasal; watery
CONGESTION to nose; agg. lying
CORYZA
    fever, with
FULLNESS, sense of
PAIN; pressing; posterior nares

**FACE**

PAIN
    pressing
    sinus, maxillary

**MOUTH**

APHTHAE
DISCOLORATION, tongue, red edges

**THROAT**

DRYNESS
    morning
    painful
    swallowing, on
INFLAMMATION

- PAIN
  - general; left
    - dry
  - burning
  - sore
    - left
    - lump

## STOMACH

- ANXIETY; eating, after
- APPETITE; diminished
  - enjoyment lost
  - increased, hunger in general; morning
- FLATULENCE
- HEARTBURN
  - coffee, after
  - eating; after
- NAUSEA
  - breakfast; first bite
  - morning
  - walking; while
- PAIN
  - burning
    - anxiety with
    - eating, after
    - eructations
    - hunger during
    - lying down on back
    - pressure amel.
    - warm applications amel.
  - gnawing
  - pressing
    - extending to; upward
- THIRST; cold drinks

## ABDOMEN

- FLATULENCE
  - eating, after

## RECTUM

- CONSTIPATION
  - bowels, action lost, as if with

DIARRHEA
FLATUS
    dinner, after
HEMORRHOIDS
    pain; burning, smarting

## STOOL

DARK
DRY
INFREQUENT
LOOSE
SMALL
WATERY

## BLADDER

PAIN
    burning
    sore
URGING to urinate, morbid desire; frequent

## URINE

ODOR
    offensive
    strong

## MALE

SEXUAL desire; increased

## LARYNX & TRACHEA

TICKLING in the air passages
    cough, with
    talking; on

## SPEECH & VOICE

VOICE; lost; excitement, from

## COUGH

DRY
SHORT

## EXPECTORATION

GRAYISH

## CHEST

GURGLING; breathing, when
INFLAMMATION; Lungs
    stages; congestive
PAIN; General; cough, during
    Heart; lying; sides, on; left; agg.
    Mammae; left
    ribs; right to left
    Sides; left, bubble like a

## BACK

MOVEMENTS, slow motion, as if
PAIN; dull; Dorsal region, lying

## EXTREMITIES

ERUPTION; Foot
ITCHING; Forearm; spots, in
  Hand; Palm
  Thigh
NUMBNESS; Leg; bed, in
    morning; bed, in
    motion, during; amel.
    rubbing amel.
    walking, while, amel.
  Upper Limbs; left, sleep during
PAIN
  Lower limbs; Toes; right
  cramp-like
    calf
    shins
      walking agg.
    toes
  throbbing
    toe; nails; touch agg.
      left, 10:30 p.m.-3:00 p.m. agg.
      sensation as if blister
      sheet agg.
PERSPIRATION; Foot

SWELLING; Ankle
Foot
Leg
Lower Limbs; heavy feeling

## SLEEP

ANXIOUS, Wake up on time, to
INTERRUPTED
restlessness, by
LIGHT
POSITION; changed frequently
turning 360 degrees all night
RESTLESS
bodily restlessness, from
turning left to right all night
SEMI-CONSCIOUS; hears everything
SLEEPINESS
SLEEPLESSNESS; night; latter part of night, in
UNREFRESHING

## FEVER

CHILL; with

## GENERALITIES

EATING, pleasure for instead of health
EXERTION; physical; aversion for
desires
FOOD and drinks; chocolate; desires
ice-cream; desires
onion rings; desires
PULSE; frequent, accelerated, elevated, exalted, fast, innumerable, rapid;
convulsions, during
SWIMMING; enjoys every opportunity
enjoys night diving
WEAKNESS, enervation
afternoon
3 p.m.-4 p.m.
exertion, from
heat, from
sun, of

EDITOR'S NOTE: *Punctuation, abbreviations, and individual stylistic nuances of the original journal entries have been preserved wherever possible.*

**Prover #1 · Female**

**Day 1**

◆ Took remedy Sunday night. Had a lot of dreams. Couldn't remember or get a real grasp on them. Disoriented dreams.

◆ Dream: In house, front door with beveled glass, one of the pieces was broken. Was told it was too expensive to repair it. Told to cover it up. Refused to cover it up and wanted it fixed. (Actual event several months later, my son was attacked and the exact beveled glass door was broken by attacker.)

◆ Dream: Son didn't want her to know how his report card was. He tried to cover it up, said he didn't get it.

◆ Dream: Dog running up the driveway with part of his fur shaved off.

Woke introspective. Sat up in bed, first morning, had spinal movement, like slow motion. Spacey, not spaced-out feeling, as much as if a fog is between me and the other person—like looking through a wet window or a pane of glass with rain on it. It was disfigured, disoriented. By the middle of the day, I could not stay awake.

◆ Wanted chocolate, or some kind of a stimulant about 3:30 p.m. Unusual for me.

◆ Desire to put ice on my feet.

◆ Took 2nd dose Monday night.

◆ Period had been two weeks late, kind of wondering about that. Period started that night.

**Day 2**

◆ Again disassociated feeling. Heard people talking, sounded like the hum of bees. Felt separate from this, not a part of it. Felt really like I wanted to isolate. Feeling like a loner. Spacey floating feeling, and again next day. Just stay on the beach and relax and not participate. Sleepy and hard to stay awake

◆ Chest: Night: Pain under rib cage. Moved from right side, then it went to left side.

**Day 3**

◆ a.m. Feeling as if the top of thighs sunburned. Hard time focusing. Tried to read something.

Vision not clear. Bad headache, chilly. Delirious with chills this afternoon.

◆ Couldn't come out of it. Sleepy and hard to stay awake. By 4:15 p.m. bad headache, headache temple occiput and eyeballs with fever, sore throat, eyes sensitive to light, still are. Itching thighs, throat painful.

◆ Woke in middle of night unable to swallow. Dry pain.

**Day 4**

◆ Dream: In galley of ship. Mother walking down hallway. Homeopath took my mother's case, she had incontinence problems. Excited my mother was getting better. Someone told me that my father had many other children from many other wives. Real shock. Woke feeling disoriented again.

◆ a.m. Throat still very sore, felt like head cold. >> after breakfast. Throat, dryness, like a ball in my throat, in center. Dry, hard to swallow. Fever—clammy feeling came up and down.

◆ Slept for three and one-half hours in middle of day. Fitful with many dreams. As if delirious. Unable to wake, to come out of sleep.

◆ After waking took short little walk while feverish, spacey, chills, no appetite.

◆ Ache. Felt like a full-on head cold << movement. Nasal obstruction. Spaciness. Kept saying to myself this cannot be the proving.

**Day 5**

◆ Everything came and left quickly.

◆ Sentimental with this music, for past Hawaii experiences. Took acute remedy.

**Day 6**

◆ Glad it's over.

◆ Feet sweating today, red stripes on edge of tongue, like red serrations.

◆ Chancre sore.

**Generals during the acute:**

Pulse is quickened.
< exertion or movement.
Achy. Wiped out.
Thirsty for ice cold drinks. Not real thirsty or hungry.
Desires ice cream, Hawaiian shaved ice.

**One year later, this prover reported:**

Sinus problems ever since remedy.
Pressure, congestion in frontal sinuses.
>>water i.e. swimming, showering.
<<a.m., after lying.
Creates headaches.
No discharge.

**Prover #2 · Female**

**Day 1**

◆ Took remedy at 4:15 (Sunday). On going to sleep 8:30 p.m., closed eyes. Saw vehicle coming at me in the wrong lane. As I closed my eyes, I saw this. Not even going to sleep. Jerked eyes open with real panic feeling, as if was going to get run over. Like falling off mountain when you do this jerk.

◆ Dream: Someone trying to get into my house. I was afraid of them, but it wasn't someone to do me harm but someone coming for a specific purpose to do a survey, but I didn't want them to notice that I was there, so I was sneaking around in my house trying to avoid being seen. Didn't want to be noticed. Peeking through the window to see if he was there. Actually had eye contact with the man. A feeling of being exposed and wondering if I was, feeling like a two-way mirror where you can see out. Had eye contact with a man, bushy hair, sleepy-looking like a private detective. Feelings of nervousness, worry about exposing myself, since pretending not to be there, mystery.

◆ In morning nausea when walking. Came in 2-3 waves.

◆ Blister on left big toe which I already had. Physical symptoms started here. Felt throbbing as if it was bright red and needed lancing, as if it would explode with all this pus, but when looked at it, didn't look like that at all. Objectively blister was white and calm, a little swollen. Throughout day, got worse and worse, even considered a wheelchair. I am not going to be able to walk very much. Felt like a major injury, but couldn't see physical evidence of all the pain I was in.

**Day 2**

◆ Couldn't sleep that night. Went to bed at 9:00 p.m., up at 10:30 till 3:00 a.m. with throbbing toe. Even pain from sheet hurt it, had to stick foot out. Whole consciousness on this throbbing toe. Nothing helped for two days. By third morning was just like normal blister.

◆ Began menses on second day. Menses very early, one week or so early.

◆ Restless and turning at night. Like doing 360's. Laying on one side, then a few minutes later do a 1/2 turn, like on a rotisserie all night.

**Day 3**

◆ Took 2nd dose.

◆ Dream: All my closest friends were dying in auto accidents. They were dying in groups. One accident had killed four people. When heard, I was not shocked, thought that is interesting, that's the way we are going to leave the planet. Heard someone else had died in my little family. I am the only one left. When is my number up. Thought it was interesting, no fear. "An interesting way to leave, in batches like that."

◆ Dream: Got a message in a dream, like it was a major revelation. On waking, it didn't make much sense. The message was take something mundane and attach some significant thing to it, to remember, and that way I will use all the mundane simple things in life to learn something really important. All the mundane things in life will take on a significance and teach me about deeper things, like major learning. Felt this was so

meaningful. Wanted to wake up and tell everyone, but then realized this means nothing. Felt this was a communication from my husband who died one year ago. Felt good; he's still communicating to me. Felt like a blessing, a passing on of knowledge from the other side.
◆ Enjoyed effort and sweating of exercise and the power of it. Felt I could keep going and going and going. This is unusual for me.
◆ Overall sense during the week, felt as if I was a big rock in a harbor. Felt I am a strong influence. Solid. My friends would benefit from my strength by coming into my harbor. Overall feeling of solidity, very strong, stable. Usually just goes through life without thinking about what I am, who I am, how I affect people. I usually just am in the present.

## Prover #3 · Female

### Day 1

◆ Dream: In a friend's office with a friend, with whom I used to work, and the three of us laid down on the couch. Male kept putting hand on my crotch, I kept moving it away. In life, I am a lesbian and know him and am not at all attracted to him sexually, although we are friends. I tell him that I am dreaming of him. He has assumption that I will be his lover. He says no, he cannot do that, he has to be sure of me. I introduced him to my lover, a woman who is lying on couch next to us.
◆ Dream: My brother in new apartment and his girlfriend, who was my play sister from childhood. We walked through the hallways and saw yellow stick-ums everywhere in the hallway, with my mother's handwriting on all of them. Told mother that I planned to move to a larger apartment, she said she would move in with me.
◆ Dream: Brother and I are running from the same man who had repeatedly put his hand on my crotch. Ran into a barbershop where brother would get a haircut. Stopped at a phone booth and used the phone to call my mother and partner. My brother said mom was going to call right back. Waited but no call.
◆ Dream: Heavyset man, big stomach, in yellow shirt being beaten up by three other young gentlemen. He was in center of a circle. Woke after that.

### Day 2

◆ Dream: Professionally dressed, leading a seminar; to group of young women.
◆ Dream: Another sexual dream which is unusual for me. Man desiring me. Someone I know. No contact, just desire. Sex and violence kept coming up.
◆ Actual event: Driving and noticed a large jeep just behind me. He hit the back of my car on purpose. Never happened to me ever before. He backed up and hit the back of my car again and said: "You don't like this a—hole? You want to say something about this?" I pulled off to side of road, he pulled next to me. He shouted obscenities. He followed me cursing and flailing his arms. I was frightened but calm. This guy wasn't going to hurt me, but I wasn't going to be foolish either.
◆ Generally calmer, even in moments of emotional turmoil in my life. Positive, like this,

usually, but even more so.
◆ Sleep is not good, but energy is very good, considering the sleep I am getting. Wanted very much to go into the whirlpool daily.
◆ I had diarrhea, which is unusual.
(As an aside, I thought of this after I knew the remedy. I was in a helicopter over Maui for the first time, but I was scared to death. Then I settled down to enjoy the clouds and felt calm and very serene.)

## Prover #4 · Male

Before remedy. Hay fever getting worse from the time arrived on this island.

**Day 1**

◆ Some hours after remedy, increased obstruction left nose and left-sided sore throat with mild euphoria.
◆ Increased thirst.
◆ Acrid post nasal drip.
◆ Flatulence. Stool more dry, less mass, less frequent. Still persists.
◆ Sleepy in the lectures.
◆ Dozed off in class and had intense flashes of dreams which persisted on opening eyes. Like dream was carried over into waking state. One scene was of a wave crashing right over me. Normally might have been startled, but wasn't. Other mundane scenes. When opened eyes, the dream images were superimposed on the scene in the room.
◆ Head: marked tenderness left temple, better with pressure, although no headache.
◆ Throat: symptoms mild ameliorated by cognac, but not by any other beverage hot or cold, nor by food. Dry and mild burning character of throat. Disturbing acridity in throat like post nasal catarrh.
◆ Small tasteless belches just before sunset.

## Prover #5 · Female

**Day 1**

◆ On going to sleep lying down: aware of sensation pressure behind my eyes pushing outward to temples, and feeling as if brow furrowed. Constriction in throat, sense of suffocating, as if I could not breathe. Hands feel heavy and swollen. Restless sleep, turning a lot, from left to right, from left to right.
◆ Dream: Didn't make sense. Parents in dream bought two more white cars, in addition to the one they let me borrow, so had three cars. Two had been in accident and were in garage one on top of the other. Felt guilt about this happening and that they were spending money on me and my brother. Woke with guilt.

◆ Strong, offensive odor to urine.

◆ Stools darker and softer, 2 -3 x a day. Usually I tend to constipation. A real increase in gas and bloating. Always a bloated feeling lasting 3-4 days.

◆ Body feels very ,very heavy and very tired with deep lethargy throughout my whole body, definitely aggravated by heat. Lost all desire to run and exercise as I usually do. Did not feel the need to move my body as I usually do.

◆ General decrease in anxiety and worry. Decrease in brooding. No thinking. Everything is O.K. Very peaceful with my situation.

◆ Increase in joking, joviality, jesting, silliness and an increase in laughing and a real desire to be around people, which is unusual for me. Usually prefer to be alone. Found it easier to open myself up to people. Wanted to be close to people and to touch them.

◆ Decreased interest and enjoyment in food. Unusual, as this is typically a big sensual experience for me. Had no taste for it. Did not enjoy it.

◆ Averse spicy and increase in thirst for cold drinks.

◆ Woke in the a.m. ravenous. Really, really hungry.

**Day 2**

◆ Increased sensitivity to noise at night. Will be completely aware of a noise, and it will annoy me that I could not go to sleep.

◆ Dream: Had a baby a year old. Responsibility in taking care of it. Felt very guilty as I ate tomatoes and child is allergic to tomatoes. Felt guilty for not having taken responsibility.

◆ Headache, right occiput, as dull ache extending to temple. Dull constant ache. Took aspirin as had the feeling it would get really bad.

◆ Sharp localized pains in body here and there. Worse in heat and aversion to sun.

◆ Less fear when snorkeling. Normally would worry in the water. Less fear, and less anxiety in general.

**Day 3**

◆ Dream: Pregnant, but not sure if I was, and feeling of responsibility, and not wanting to take on that responsibility.

◆ Lying in a hammock, all anxiety left me. I felt connected and deep relaxation.
Decreased desire to exercise and move my body and desire for company the most pronounced, unusual for me. Desire to touch people, be near them, feel their presence, feel connection, to have fun with them, to laugh with them. Normally want time to myself. Guilt dreams not common to me, although there is a situation in my current life to make me feel guilty. Guilty to be here, it was a fluke that I got to be here. Three nights of guilt in dreams.

◆ Playfulness during week. Not how I am. Very different for me.

◆ Vivid dreams and feelings around them.

◆ Dreams: Same, two nights in a row during proving, none like this before or since: Strong feeling of having and nursing a baby. Strong feeling of my breast. Strong feeling of fulfillment.

**Prover #6 · Female**

**Day 1**

◆ Took Remedy Sunday 4:00 p.m. Within half hour noticed that burning stomach pains, which I had been having for one month, pains like acid congestion, went away and have stayed away. (CURE) Immediate amelioration of six months of hiatal hernia reflux pain. Completely cured, never came back again.

| | | |
|---|---|---|
| Location: | center of solar plexus extending to mid chest | |
| Type of pain: | periodical, ~ daily; | |
| | | pressing from down upward |
| | | burning, acid |
| | | pain with eructations |
| Pain extensions: | upward moving from center of solar plexus | |
| | | extending to mid chest. |
| Modalities: | >> | warmth; |
| | | eating; |
| | | pressure, laying on stomach |
| | << | food |
| | | coffee |
| | | hunger |
| | | laying down on back |
| | | anxiety, generalized |

◆ Toenails so sensitive that I could hardly stand to have my feet touched by pedicurists. Very sensitive around the cuticles.

◆ Bladder: pain. Burning sensation and fullness in bladder with desire to urinate frequently.

◆ Gas and burping the evening is unusual for me.

**Day 2**

◆ Took 2nd dose.

◆ Strong reaction to smell of perfume, had to move outside after 45 minutes so that I could breathe the fresh air. Eyes burning, eyeballs burning, red at lower, outer sclera. Stopped nose, dizzy. Stayed with me a few days.

◆ Head: dull headache in forehead.

◆ Pain in bladder.

◆ Colic in abdomen also.

**Day 4**

◆ Dull headache and eyes burn.

◆ Sinuses burn and are full.

◆ Bladder seems sore when full.

◆ Extremities: legs, ankles and feet are very swollen, hands, too.

◆ Dream: Husband and I on airplane looking for comfortable seats. Seats very unusual, big, comfortable, lots of walking space around. We could choose back or front, front seats were down really steep stairs, like stadium stairs, and it was dark down there so we chose seats in the back. When my husband and I turned to go back to our seats, I saw someone I haven't seen for four years. I was surprised to see her on the plane, didn't take the stairs. Funny, interesting, amusing to see her on the plane.

**Day 5**

◆ Legs ankles and feet and hands still swollen.
◆ GI: flatulence after dinner.
◆ Extremities: very uncomfortable with swelling in legs and feet.
◆ Dull headache.

**Day 6**

◆ p.m. Stomach symptoms coming back. Lots of burping.
◆ Swelling in legs and feet is a little better today.

**Day 7**

◆ Feel calm and a little sad.
◆ Right-sided dull headache.
◆ Eyes feel blurry. Hard to focus without squinting. Eyes, especially right, burning. Redness on eyeballs. Feels irritated.
◆ Mucous in sinuses and can cough up some gray mucous.
◆ GI: stomach heartburn. Acid condition is back.
◆ By break time in the morning, headache is gone. Right eye still burns.
◆ Right ear feels stuffed.
◆ Dreams: Each morning at five a.m. or so has dreams not remembered well enough to relate, but themes had to do with people I do not really know well, but have seen regularly. Dreams also of cars, houses, and airplanes.
◆Dream: Saw a minister in condo. Had to walk up steep steps to see him. Father said don't go with him, but I went anyway and felt later that I had made a major mistake and was in danger. Something I shouldn't have done.
◆ During infrequent visits with my parents, I have had a calmness and an acceptance of them not experienced in the past. An actual conversation about: "We need to listen to dad." It has a smooth visit, and I felt calm. Actually felt somewhat detached, and all the old stuff has not come up. Feel fully present with them. Now have better relationship to father.
◆ Cure: Complete amelioration of acid reflux stomach problem. Never came back.
◆ Rug pulled out from under my feet regarding my emotional stability:

Doubting Self
Insecurity in all social situations
Unsure of self
Took three months to go away.

◆ Every time I talk about this, the feelings come back. Pretty profound, not real pleasant. Not to degree of old feeling. This was a serious amplification. Really unsure of myself. Like in Jr. High—kids making fun of you. You know deep down that you're a

good person, but the teasing still gets to you. Juvenile, adolescent awkwardness: the stuff you're so glad you got through. The proving was, "Oh no, not this again!!"
◆ Circular theme: ruminating thoughts regarding insecurity.
◆ Feeling of separation: separated from group during proving. Feeling like an outsider, or outcast. Pervasive in feelings over three months. Wanted to be with people, but felt shunned. Like outside a window, looking in. Like standing OUTSIDE a circle. Very profound. Every time I talk about it, the feelings are very intense.
◆ Unsuccessful attempts to communicate at seminars. Wrote a letter to communicate the experience, but it didn't convey what I wanted, so I didn't send it. By the end of the weekend, I had lost my voice!! I felt so unable to communicate I lost my voice!!! I didn't want to grab her and say, "You *have* to hear this!!" I couldn't do it. Low self esteem? Insecurity?
◆ By end of January, '95 on solid (emotional) ground again

## Prover #7 · Female Child

*(This is mother speaking about daughter)*

**Day 1**

◆ My daughter took the remedy Sunday 5:00 p.m. One hour later, she became very awkward. Fell three times in 15 minutes for no reason. Stumbles. She was dropping things that she picked up, and stumbling.
◆ Stomach: pain in belly after dinner, short-lived.
Slept well, all night which is unusual for her, and didn't have to urinate all night. Usually wakes at 11:30 p.m.

**Day 2**

◆ Flushed at 12:30 p.m., lunch time, very red. Gone by the evening.
◆ 5:30 p.m. in the car, in evening complained too warm, even though air conditioning was on and skin not warm to touch, and then too cold. Nothing O.K., weeping which is unusual for her.
◆ Again pain in the belly after 15 minutes of feeling too warm or too cold. Episode did not last long.
◆ That night woke 4:30 asked me to read her a story. She is very insistent, "Read it now. I want it now." We had an argument. Then demanding all kinds of things. Curtains open, another pillow, another sheet, drink water. Wanted to get dressed. Wanted this shirt, that shirt. Persistent, pulling at me. Weeping when put back to bed. Cried for a long time, Could not calm her down.

**Day 3**

◆ At breakfast very little appetite. Very unusual. Ate only bread.
◆ During the day, very impatient, much more than usual. Could not wait for anything, and everything had to be done now. Usually she can wait if talked to. Demanding,

despite explanation as to why she couldn't have things a certain way, she just asked again immediately, repeatedly, 4-5 times. I had the feeling she didn't understand what she was saying. She wasn't as bright as usual, understanding things not as quickly.

◆ Demanded constant attention from me. Could not be alone at all. She always loves attention, but now it is much stronger. Had to have my attention.

◆ Playing on the beach, she gets stung by a bee. I pull out the stinger. No swelling no reaction. She's not even extra careful when playing afterward, and she doesn't mention it anymore the rest of the day.

◆ Respiratory: dry, intermittent painless short cough.

◆Nose: left nostril red and swollen but no coryza.

◆ Mind: Still impatient. When I am talking to others, she starts talking loud to get my attention and pulling my hand and or clothes and wants to go. Very hard to deal with her as she could not accept, understand my explanations.

Sleep: waking at night, once saying she wanted to go to beach.

◆ Two nights waking and crying for 15-20 minutes, could not calm her, then goes back to sleep.

◆ Stomach: doesn't have an appetite. Does not want to eat. Fussy.

◆ Our daughter didn't want to be looked at. We couldn't stand it, so we gave her two teaspoons of decaffeinated coffee.

**Day 5**

◆ Impatience is much less. She can wait again, not fussy. Appetite is back.

## Prover #8 · Male

**Day 1**

◆ I hurt my left shoulder at the beach.

◆ Dreams of waves.

◆ Waking at 3:30-4:30 a.m.

Other days: dreaming of day's events. Nothing unusual.

## Prover #9 · Male

**Day 1**

◆ Don't have as much self-control. Usually very disciplined especially with diet. Chocolate, started eating it for first time in 17 yrs. Didn't care, not a big deal. The eating chocolate wasn't as much about chocolate as it was about an attitude: 'This isn't part of my diet,' lessening. I still eat it occasionally now, maybe a tiny craving for it. Ate it first at lunch. A chocolate chip cookie sounds pretty good right now! Also ate onion rings, which I would never have eaten before.

◆ Mentals got better and stayed that way.
◆ Digestion got worse and stayed that way.
◆ Seconds after took remedy felt immediate change as if all energy came into a vertical line inside me. More detached, introverted yet still awareness of surroundings. After this, felt a little weak and trembly.
◆ First evening wanted to be in my own world, be inside myself. Preoccupied with myself. Wife said I was touchy, irritable, more than usual. I felt I was less irritable than usual.
◆ Wasn't bothered as much by little things. This has lasted to the present.
Little things now don't bother me as much, like having everything where I like it so I can find it the next time I want to use it. I'm not as picky at my work bench, in the kitchen, or with my office staff. This shift was not gradual, it happened at the proving, and it has stayed.
◆ Took one dose the first day and a second dose 3rd day since I didn't think anything was happening. Hard to tell I was proving the substance, till during the extraction meeting, I realized I had been all week.
◆ After 2nd dose Wed., felt slightly sad, sense of wanting to cry.
◆ Gnawing pain in stomach.
◆ Felt rage, but it was different. I was inside myself, but the rage was outside of myself. Thought, this is strange, where did all this rage come from? Not something I manifested, just felt.
◆ Dream: Second in charge of things in two or three dreams.
◆ Dream: House flooded and had to use rowboat to get to friend's house. I was using a rowboat to get to and from classes and visit friends and go back and forth. Water was everywhere and this was my mode of transportation. Calmness, no sense of danger.
◆ Two dreams of rowboats, being in them, on the ocean.
◆ Dream: Stereo store to pick out stylus for stereo, which in life I had not listened to for many years. Picked one by mistake which was the wrong one. It was the most expensive one. The salesman objected as it really was the wrong one. He said you have to hook this up to your computer to use it. I felt very indignant, thought, who is this guy to tell me what I don't want. Wanted to purchase it just to show him that he couldn't do this.
◆ Vertigo, slight, intermittent; wanting to lean to the left.
◆ Left-sided headache.
◆ Ears: plugged, pressure sensation, < left.
◆ Mouth: more canker sores, stinging pain, little ulcerations. Old intermittent symptom that came up during proving day three. Had bit the side of my cheek before proving, and sore seemed to heal a bit more quickly.
◆ Throat: Left-sided sore throat, right after taking remedy. Very sore throat in the week with post nasal catarrh aggravation in morning. Soreness unrelieved by anything. << a.m. on getting up. Would be << if woke at night. Lasted until I got a very bad cold two weeks after proving.
◆ Neck pain, dull, constant, >> lying down, >> massage.
◆ Back pain, upper thoracic, dull, constant, >> lying down, >> massage.
◆ Left inguinal pain, << rotating left hip.
◆ Abdomen: chronic digestive problems got worse and lasted indefinitely.

◆ Bloating <, flatulence <, both associated with eating in general, nothing specific.
◆ No stomach symptoms.
◆ Left knee aggravated.
◆ Sleep: didn't sleep well during whole proving. Restless sleep. Woke few times each night, deep sleep in small, broken blocks, not continuous. Woke feeling unrested.

## Prover #10 · Male

**Day 1**

◆ Dream: I woke from a dream that a woman needs to take the remedy Crotalus Cascavella. Was quite sure of this. We were walking in a circle clockwise, around the perimeter of a crowded mezzanine in a mall. I asked why was she walking in a circle, and she said enemies were coming to get her, and she has to keep going so enemies wouldn't catch up to her. Her walk was leisurely, but she kept looking over her shoulder as she was trying to avoid enemies. There was a languid swimming feeling as we were walking.
◆ Heart: As woke, had an oppression or a cramp in my heart, very strong, causing me to turn to my right side. Normally prefer to sleep on left.
◆ Sleep: insomnia. Woke early and couldn't sleep.
◆ Energy: overwhelmingly sleepy in the afternoon.

**Day 2**

◆ Dream: Going to a horse racetrack. Again, the animals were racing clockwise. The main position was 6 and 9 on the dial. (Same as in the first dream.)

**Day 3**

◆ Dream: On a merry-go-round, going clockwise.
◆ Throat: Woke each a.m. with dry sore throat. Each evening for three in a row, if tried to speak, had a tickle in throat that made me cough, aggravated by deep breath. Tenacious mucous, throat and lungs.
◆ Watery diarrhea.
◆ Dream: Man in the dream has a dream of a bird in a cage, which he feels is significant. He thrills to reveal the dream to the waiting world. As soon as he tells the dream, he is made to feel ridiculous. Everyone Is laughing and telling him this dream is not significant. In the dream, researchers were working on a technique to literally transform substance, or to transmit thoughts.

### Prover #11 · Female

**Day 1**

◆ Dream: I was in a communal house, a big house, with lots of rooms and bathrooms. There were a lot of different people around. We had to try to figure out where to put everybody. A tawny-faced, thin woman came to a party with us—she was really depressed, a former patient. She was really uplifted after the party, felt a lot better afterwards. A Latin American man also wanted me to help them. Then, some other women were outside next door in a garden. They were stuffy. They accused us of having some kind of chemical product. I said I was a well-educated professional and didn't appreciate their accusing me of that and that we didn't have any such chemical.

◆ Comments: Before I took the remedy, I stubbed my left big toe and the nail came off. It was very sensitive for the next few days.

### Prover #12 · Male

**Day 1**

◆ Dream: My usually celibate female spiritual teacher wanted a male concubine. I auditioned for the job. I touched her, felt intense desire, and woke up with a wet dream. Felt some issue of performance anxiety.

**Day 3**

◆ Dream: I was a new paralegal who had to prepare briefs to resolve a property dispute between two families. I didn't know how to prepare the papers, but I tried to help them resolve the dispute anyway. I felt somewhat inadequate to a difficult task, and unprepared.

**Day 4**

◆ Rectum: burning. Hemorrhoid appeared. Lots of gas and bloating, flatulence.

◆ Fatigue. Loose stool. Waking 4:30 a.m.

◆ Emotional: more irritable for no reason. Passed quickly. Felt inferior to other homeopaths who had thought a lot more deeply than I had.

### Prover #13 · Female

**Day 1**

◆ Strange whirring sounds in ear as going to sleep.

◆ Dream: Large white rock passages. Solitary, lonely feeling. Me walking, looking for others but no one appears. I feel lost—not afraid, but slightly sad.

**Day 2**

◆ Sensation of loss of balance, to the right. < night. Mild exhaustion, irritability, 3-5 p.m.

**Day 3**

◆ Sore throat begins on left. > warm drinks.

◆ Energy better.

**Day 4**

◆ Tickling sensation leads to cough. Throat. Very sore. Now < left.

◆ Tired weak, nasal congestion. Feels like an upper respiratory infection.

## Prover #14 · Female

**Day 1**

◆ 8 p.m. slight sharp fleeting pain in left chest wall. Superficial, like a bubble moving up and gently dissipating.

**Day 2**

◆ Poor sleep last night, restless. May be due to loud ocean waves.

◆ Sore wrist on right dorsal surface, may be due to being bashed in the surf.

**Day 3**

◆ 9-10:30 a.m. Slight headache in forehead, like a dull pressure. It went away without eating or drinking.

◆ Slight pressure headache in forehead after eating dinner.

◆ Late afternoon one vesicle on left foot, below the ankle, but above the instep, not red or itchy.

◆ I met an old friend, someone I haven't seen for 28 years.

◆ I notice air conditioning is very cold.

**Day 4**

◆ Woke 12:30 a.m. with dry sore throat and slightly dry eustachian tube. Could feel the pressure in the tube.

◆ Slight post-nasal drip. Watery, thin, bland. Sneezing three times during the night.

**Day 5**

◆ Woke in morning with all the above symptoms, plus stuffed nose on left side, the side lain on.

◆ Skin vesicle gone in 24 hours.

**Day 6**

◆ Some itching in palate.

◆ Tightness in left calf.

**Day 7**

◆ Low-grade cold all day, slight pressure headache in forehead.
◆ Slight congestion of nose both sides.
◆ Slight runny nose, mostly right-sided.

**Day 8**

◆ Woke 2 a.m.
◆ Dream: A bit hazy but, I was in a house or building with other people, maybe women. Other people, maybe men, were making every effort to get into the building. The people in house were moving from room to room, pursued by the outsiders. At times the insiders could trap the outsiders in a place like a closet, but there was the sense of being pursued. When there was no place left to hide or move into, I remember turning on one of the outsiders and using my hand, pushed him back and away and over a piece of furniture and telling him I had had enough. I was now angry instead of anxious or fearful. It seemed then that the whole group stopped their aggressive behavior and went to a football game or planned to go to a game.

**Day 9**

◆ Slight cold symptoms. Frontal pressure, headache, sniffles, congestion.

## Prover #15 · Male

**Day 1**

◆ Dream: Dreams busy.

**Day 2**

◆ Felt like I had a hangover in the morning. Very dull congested feeling. This is not uncommon for me when I take any remedy; however, I also had one glass of wine the night before, but I usually don't feel quite that bad from one glass of wine.

**Day 3**

◆ Unpleasant gnawing sensation in the pit of my stomach.
◆ The fogginess and general feeling of congestion left after about noon.

**Day 4**

◆ Busy dreams.
◆ Overall, my digestion has been poorer than usual, tendency to constipation, almost like a great inactivity of the bowels. At the same time, great appetite. That is most unusual.

**Day 5** *( Information gleaned in prover follow-up one year later)*
◆ On Oct. 31, 1994, I had a great fear of driving to that town in Maui where the Halloween parade was. I had the sense that something was going to happen and was very nervous about driving there with some companions. Nothing did happen, but I was worried about having an accident or something like that—similar to what other provers reported.

## Prover #16 · Female

**Day 1**
◆ Took remedy in water at 11:20 p.m. Sunday night and fell right asleep. Felt excited to take it; usually I'm a little apprehensive.
◆ Dreams of rooms, and of Sunday comics, didn't get to see them.
Having dreams one after another, trying to keep them in my mind.
◆ Bit surprised by wake-up call, felt sleepy. Can't remember dreams very well, but a sense of being enclosed.
◆ Very briefly queasy at first bite of breakfast—Unusual.
◆ Warm, itching rash on face along lower jawline up to ears. Around 10:30 a.m. On right cheek first, then both.
◆ Ate chocolate after lunch, delicious. Seemed especially good.
◆ Very drowsy after lunch, ~ 2 p.m. Annoyed and embarrassed to be drowsy.
Somewhat bored and intolerant of others.
◆ Brief darting pain in left breast.

**Day 2**
◆ Fell asleep fast Monday night.
◆ Extremities: Woke once with left arm stretched above head and the limb *completely* asleep—no sensation whatsoever. Lifted it with my right hand to place it parallel with my body, was briefly amazed at the numbness and fell back asleep.
◆ Dream: All dreams remembered were in same location—a sort of run-down wooden building on the slope of a hill, you had to walk up a path to get to it, a sort of rambling very loose communal household. First I went there for an operation to take eggs from my ovary (seemed left side) and put sperm with them and place in uterus (although in dream it seemed they were placed back in ovary). This was done quite informally with me lying on my back in one of the rooms, wide awake and not looking at my abdomen but watching, attentive to the whole procedure. No pain. Some sense of an anesthetic being used, but no detail of that. The person doing this procedure was a man, competent but informal. No one I know, but in the dream he was an old friend, and I was very grateful to him for doing this, and in fact, during and after the procedure, I feel so warm towards him and very grateful and turned on. Partly because he was so kind and skilled but low-key about it. I was grateful and awed with the immensity of what he had done for me, and I hugged him.

◆ Dream: Walked into this same house and heard a fairly serious dispute about one member of the household being poisoned by toxin in paint used to outline a drawing. It was vaguely the lips of a clown and was a light lavender, although people in the dream kept referring to it as magenta; then I realized what color they called magenta. The person who had used the paint could be in some legal jeopardy, and the people in the household were talking over how seriously to pursue this. It seemed difficult. He had meant well.
◆ Dream: At this house and also my house. My next door neighbor asked me to take care of the little baby she is being a foster parent for. She wanted me to watch him for three hours but didn't ask directly. I was mildly annoyed at the imposition, but agreed. Once she brought him over, I was very solicitous of him and found him very cute. I really felt fond of the little boy (about five mos. old—a twin whose brother is being cared for elsewhere and whose mom has postpartum depression). (In waking life, I see him but don't actually participate in his care.)
◆ Before breakfast, when getting dressed, very briefly saw bright gold flecks in front of my eyes after had bent my head slightly then looked up, relaxed, very mundane moment. These were flecks I saw (with my vision) not in my eyes, and unaccompanied by any other sensation.
◆ Some more itching in the face, late morning and later in day 1:30 p.m.
◆ Day went fairly routinely. Felt a little separate, in my own thoughts.
◆ A bit impatient on walk. I would say: "Lets go in the water, now, let's get out."
◆ Left palm, below thumb itches a little. Evening tingling, burning sensation in left palm, sort of stinging, biting.

**Day 3**
◆ A bit grumpy. How can I be grumpy in paradise?
◆ Didn't get enough sleep—anxious to wake up on time.
◆ Dream: Riding horses in an oval track area. I want to go fast. My horse was perfectly responsive, it ran full out and it was so smooth, completely satisfying and a thrill. Felt like being the wind.
◆ Enjoyed swimming and imagined being a sea creature. Fish amiable. Have been swimming at every opportunity.

**Day 4**
◆ Went on a night dive. Hadn't done a night dive before or used scuba for 10 years.
◆ After proving group meeting, these are things I'd add:
Concurred with others on restless sleep, drowsiness, especially afternoon after lunch.
◆ Sensitivity to noise.
◆ Several nights of strings of dreams that didn't stay with me.
◆ Less stool even though I've been eating more than usual.
◆ Back stiff, less stiff on Friday a.m. after dive.
◆ Slight cramps in the toes while on dive.
◆ Partner's observations:

Fearless on big waves.
Plunged through giant waves.

Felt definite about next day's snorkel trip.
Disgruntled. Conference over at 10 p.m. and was cold all evening.
Unenthusiastic. Didn't sleep well. Complained outside noise kept her up.
Generous. Helped me with snorkel stuff a lot. Later she said I was courageous. Thrilled. Snorkeled with unusual glee.

## Prover #17 · Female

**Day 1**

◆ Increased appetite. In two days ate more than previous 3 or 4 days.

◆ Full night of dreaming.

◆ Dreams: All images exaggerated: Like viewing the movie Fantasia. Vignettes. Distortions, exaggerations, not necessarily a theme running though.

◆ Dream: Clearest one: In a hotel room, female friend is with me, kids are sleeping in other bed, my husband woke up since he couldn't sleep, he went outside. Friend woke up, she couldn't sleep, so went to talk to husband outside. Friend told him she was uncomfortable about a man that was in the room. I woke up in the dream with this man standing next to the bed, and where his penis would be, there is this huge log attached. Here is where the images start getting really big. It was exactly like a log with the bark attached and everything. He was an older man, and he had this gray wavy hair, not just wavy hair, but really wavy (gestures big) exaggerated hair. I asked: "Who are you?" and he said he was her son's big brother, and he started laughing hysterically. He fell back on the floor laughing. Even his laughter was loud and filled the room. Taking it all in. Felt in wonderment. Not surprised or shocked, but in awe. Started laughing, thinking my son is four, and here is this gray, old gentleman, kind of like a wise old wizard, with everything on him exaggerated, which was comical, because it was an impossible thing.

◆ Dream: Was in upcountry, very rural setting. Flying though the air on huge horses, going from horse to horse, and they were really big (gestures with arms in a circle). Some sort of celebration or wedding occurring, so there were a lot of people doing things. At one point, there was a line of traffic, which was impossible on this little rural country road, going up the hillside, but it was packed with these cars. And they were racing, zooming. At one point, I turned the car I was in around and was in this car with them zooming up the hill and me zooming down the hill, between them, which could not have happened. Then I was taking metal nails hammering them into sand. And the nails had huge heads on them because I was going to do headstands, which you can't do headstands on a nail, but I was hammering those nails in, into sand, so the sand was even expansive, and the grains of sand were really big. I could get the nail in, but I couldn't do a handstand since the texture of the sand made the nail not very stable. But the head of the nail was really big. Laughing though all this because it was very comical. Sand was in this rural country area. Then left that scene to go into an airport, which didn't look like an airport at all. It was just another little glass cubicle, but it was supposed to be an airport. I was meeting an old friend, and when I arrived, the old friend wasn't who he was. He was more like a native of this island, with another person—a native—and when I went to shake hands, his hand was huge, again. Another exaggerated image. It had all these bumps in it. Again, I wasn't surprised, I just shook it. He said, didn't you know , and we started laughing, shaking this huge hand. At this point, I almost expected it, there was this pattern. It wasn't frightening, or scary, it was just, oh yeah, almost normal.

◆ Dream: It was this dark environment. There seemed to be people I knew, work related. Someone was preparing food and handed me this plastic bag full of pasta and sauce, and it was really huge. The plastic bag was huge, and the pasta was really big, but they were trying to hand to me, which was again really exaggerated. Another scene, back in the country, where someone had made a cake for someone, so big you couldn't carry it, rectangular shape, with frosting all designed around edges, huge designs, pouring over the edges, but it didn't fall off, it was supposed to be there. Enormous. The thing that's different from my normal dreams is the proportions. Normal is going from vignette to vignette, scenes will switch, and I'll frequently dream all night, and I'll remember them. They may have more of a theme, they may go together more. These were like viewing the movie Fantasia, in the colors and the brightness, and the exaggerations, and the proportions not making sense. The lyrical, almost_musical quality to it, the sound.

◆ Sleep: The quality of my sleep was different in that when I (usually) dream, I go into a deep, deep sleep. But this was as if I wasn't sleeping at all. It was a very shallow sleep. I was aware of the ocean sounds, the waves, movement in the room. Whereas when I usually sleep, its very sound. I woke up as if I hadn't slept. Not that I was exhausted, I felt O.K., but the sleep felt shallow. Felt like when I was in my 20's, and I had partied all night and had experiences that were a little bit crazy. It was that quality. The night was fun. Going from scene to scene to scene. Exciting. So many images, unusual images, without the element of surprise, just "Wow, look at that." Fun. Playful. None of it made any sense, and none of it mattered. Element of surprise, it wasn't shocking, it was just fun, interesting. A curiosity. There was an excitement to it. It was a really fun evening, like I was at the movies all night. Which I feel often anyway because I dream that way often. My dreaming can have the detail, intriguing quality, but not the surreal quality that this (night of dreaming) did.

Woke up, was a little dizzy. Unusual.

◆ My ribs were really sore.

**Day 2**

◆ Appetite seemed increased.

◆ That evening I had a series of dreams, more practical dreams, back to my regular dreams.

**Day 3**

◆ Repeated the remedy 6 p.m.

◆ Went to sleep. It was agitated sleep. Didn't sleep very well. Dreamt like usual dreams, with interruptions, I woke up a lot. Partly I was thinking about this morning and wanting to be awake, not wanting to sleep through coming here this morning and doing this.

◆ Some of my dreams were about my son, how he had done the slides. I was worried. I was worried about my son all night. So I had some fear. Not sure if this was related to the remedy or not. I would wake up frequently and look over to make sure he was still in his bed and not still in the water. I had had a sense of losing him in the water during the day, and that kept coming up in my dreams. I'd wake up with a start, look over to make sure he was still with us. Several of my dreams, whenever I went back to sleep, we were in the slides or at the beach. I was looking for him in the water, as if I was distracted and I was being negligent, and he was in danger. So I'd wake up and make sure he was still with us in bed, even though the scenes were the danger in the water. So I don't know if it is remedy related. Just that I was agitated. Frequently. And every time I woke up, I was looking for my son.

**Follow up of prover one year later:**
History of right-sided headaches CURED
Leg numbness CURED
Fear of burglaries CURED
Fear of intrusion CURED
Delusion I wasn't safe (alarm system, dogs). CURED
Fears. Have two huge dogs, pets as protectors, alarm system, on when at home, neighbors. Left there, moved to more rural place, all doors unlocked and open. No security measures. Therefore, after the remedy, internal world secure and safe. Aware of danger but not affected by it.
Couldn't get "into my legs" till Rx helped me transition to being on the earth. I am ocean-born NOW.
Leg numbness, below both knees CURED
Numbness was uncomfortable, >> moving, rub, rub, get up, walk
>> pressure, >> rubbing, >> walking. >> getting out of bed and walking.
My body worker had said, get into my legs and be on earth.
Slight right-sided Headache. Things "off" CURED.
Pain annoying, up neck, back side of head, up over to eyeball.
>> pressure, on bone, over eyeball on skull. (Retook Rx later and symptoms disappeared.)
Face: Hot red ear with right sided headache.
Exaggerations: Gestures, dreams, big breasts, depths, diving. Every detail exaggerated. Food on huge plate.
Son had right toe pain days after remedy during the proving.
Son and mother had same dream of spiders recently.

**Further curative responses from prover #17:**
◆ Psychic ability and intuition heightened. Much more valued and used now than before. Life changed directions: On path of Truth.. Layers are gone. Only the core. Others around me are living more authentically. Synchronicity in life is stronger. Information coming to me.
◆ Validating truth, validating authenticity. Living in higher self. Daily life realities have

shifted. Not caught up in pettiness. If we leave the house with the kitchen still dirty, it'll get cleaned later. Things don't have to be in their place. It can get cleaned later. Heart is most important. How we're feeling is what matters, not pettiness. Cure. Life is of abundance. Joy, heart, love.

◆ Intense vertigo since March '93. CURED (Tail end of poison oak, dizzy state, unclear state in life.) Lost vision, Temperature hot to freezing cold. Dizziness episodes, I'd have to lie down immediately. Rx: *Lac delphinum* straightened things up.

◆ Huge boost in immune system. Kicked into high gear. Last year everyone sick around me, I was untouched by it. Have history of pneumonia in self, family. Lungs, chest cold problems. Cured. Took that susceptibility away.

> Past deep bronchial infections CURED
> Pre-onset, tightening of chest.
> Symptoms were: chest gurgley not dry: painful, deep, junky, loose, yellow, green, brown expectoration.
> Chest hurt, I had to grab it when coughing.

◆ Eye: Acute clarity. World is clear, crystallized, like with new glasses. Saw clearer, sharper, details bigger. In some ways this continues.

Nose: Participated in another proving, got sinus problems. After proving, retook Lac delfinum and the effect was immediate, all things settling in on a healthy level.

Sleep: Deep quickly.

Respiration: Respiratory system better

Extremities: Leg numbness >> with remedy. Solidified my sturdiness

Sex: I'm more heightened that way (after the remedy), longing always to rub, stroke.... Stroking, beautiful, graceful motion.

## Prover #18 · Male

### Day 1

◆ Afternoon. I had some moments of spontaneous joy, I laughed out loud, a deep hearty laugh. A real departure from my recent state.

◆ Late evening head: a dull ache in right parietal occipital region. Mild, lasting less than 30 minutes. Headaches in that area are a very unusual occurrence for me.

### Day 2

◆ Morning. First noticed itching circinate red lesion one cm diameter with smaller satellite lesions on anterior left forearm. Target appearance, paler in center. Itches a lot.

◆ Midday. Transient feeling of spaciness. I don't feel like I am really here. Its all just a movie and I am a detached observer.

### Day 3

◆ Relaxed, perhaps tired.

**Day 4**

◆ Late morning. While in the midst of a conversation, I couldn't remember whether I had spoken some of my ideas or merely thought them. This never happens to me, and it felt very unusual and unnerving.

◆ 9 p.m. Extremely tired, exhausted. Need to sleep.

**Day 5**

◆ Second dose. Very difficult to wake up. I've been sleeping deeply and not keeping late hours these past few nights, yet during the day, I am constantly sleepy and fatigued.

◆ Dream: Had a disturbing dream last night. My spouse and I were visiting a big city like Portland and had a big disagreement. She was gathering things together to leave me and go off with other people. I became enraged and woke screaming and sputtering. This woke up the whole family.

◆ Noon. I notice the rash on my left forearm has settled down a bit. Still itchy, not as bad. Lesions aren't as dramatic. < scratching.

◆ 1 p.m. return to hotel room during lunch break to find the rest of my family, wife and three kids, still sprawled around on the beds, glum, low energy. They all said they'd had a bad morning. This was four hours after we ate breakfast. Our youngest, age seven, had spent an hour crying this morning, he almost never cries, everyone was feeling down, low energy, unhappy. Snorkeling during lunch break snapped us out of it.

◆ Sitting by the ocean, I had a strong feeling of despair about the passing of time. Everything is fleeting. change happens so fast. We cannot hold onto anything. Even the finest experiences are immediately lost, similar to a feeling I've had after orgasm.

◆ Lip: noticed a canker sore on left lower lip.

**Day 6**

◆ Dream: I was climbing around on a lava flow. My wife and kids were there, we are on vacation. She's reading book, I'm throwing a Frisbee, the kids are digging in the dirt. I keep calling my family to watch the magnificent thing my Frisbee is doing. They make half-hearted attempts to humor me. I can tell they are not interested. I hurl the Frisbee, and halfway through its course, it changes into a large black bird. The bird soars around. I am calling to my family, but they don't even look up. As the bird glides down a lava flow below me, I notice there is a man sprawled over the rocks—face down, as if exhausted; he's medium large build, black, in his middle years. As my bird swoops by, the man suddenly grabs for it and jumps onto its back. He glides on down the lava flow to the bottom, then hops off and walks away. All this time, I am yelling until I'm hoarse—trying to get my wife to look. She never sees it. I know later I'll be charged with hallucinating.

**Prover #19 · Male**

◆ Busy complicated dreams.

◆ Confusing, with lots of people in them.

# MAIASAURA LAPIDEA

*Fossilized Bone of the Dinosaur*

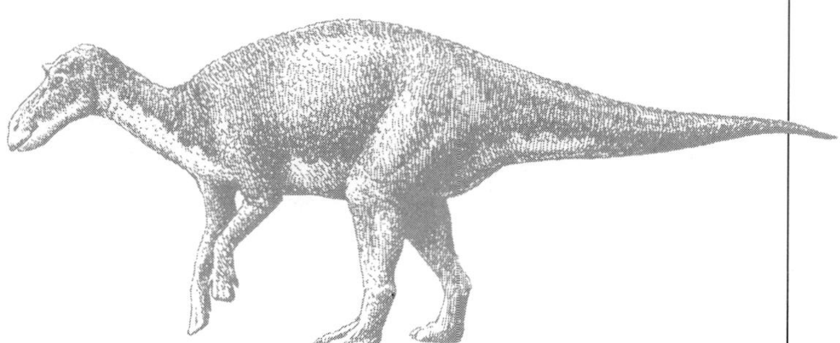

# MAIASAURA LAPIDEA

## *The Fossilized Bone of the Dinosaur*

Maiasaura dinosaur was unique in the world of prehistoric, reptilian creatures. It lived in the late Cretaceous period, approximately 80 to 65 million years ago, toward the end of the dinosaurs' time on earth. Its native habitat was what is now Montana, between the Rocky mountains and a prehistoric interior sea. It was in the family of hadrosaurus.

Anthropologists found the first remains of egg nests next to adult females bones. The nests were scooped-out holes, six feet across, filled with vegetation and mud. They would hold up to 20 sausage-shaped eggs. As they baked in the sun, the vegetation rotted and produced heat, which helped the hatching process. These same nests also contained the bones of older juveniles. The juveniles had worn teeth and unformed limb bones and were about three feet in length. From this, it is apparent that the mother must have kept the young in the nest until they were quite well-developed. She brought food and nurtured and protected the young for a long period of time, until they were able to forage for themselves. (**HELPING/NO ONE HELPING**) This is unusual in the dinosaur or lizard realm, where the eggs are usually abandoned after they are laid. Thus, paleontologists named her the "good mother lizard." In Greek the name, "maia," means "mother" and "saurus" means "lizard." This is the only dinosaur to receive a feminine name using an "a" at the end instead of a "us," such as in "Albertosaurus."

Using fossilized skeletons, paleontologists have constructed what they believe to be a fairly accurate model of the Maiasaura. She was approximately 30 feet long, had a long, snout-like face, a duck-like bill, and big, gentle eyes. She also had a solid, horn-like crest above her eyes, which was probably used in combat and in courtship rituals. She had five fingers on her hands and three toes on her feet and could stand and move on two or four limbs. She had wide feet and a wide stance, which gave her a reasonable turning radius. However, the forelimbs were only two-thirds the length of the hind limbs, so she could walk on them but not run on all fours to avoid enemies. The juveniles had large heads, short snouts, and huge, helpless eyes. Scientists conjecture that the helpless appearance of the young produced a maternal response in the mothers.

The males were probably larger and had more dramatic coloring and cresting to attract the females. They also had an inflatable sack near the nose for display during combat or courtship. It is also speculated that this sack was in some way related to a "hooting" sound all hadrosaurus made to maintain contact and to identify each other sexually. Not much else is known about the sexual behavior of Maiasaura, but the proving may give us further insight. (**DECADENT SEXUALITY**) (Dream: "Then there was some sexy sex in a sleeping bag; quick and rough sex...." "I ended up seducing my wife's sister. I'd just told my wife how much I loved her." "He complained about having four homes. I said it must be a lot to keep up. He said it's good for his liaisons, looking matter-of-fact and decadent.")

Possibly to escape their neighbors' carnivorous appetites, as well as to satisfy their own vegetarian appetites, Maiasaura was forced to travel frequently and in immense herds. This would offer her and her young a modicum of protection—especially if they could place themselves near the center of the large group. They traveled from the western United States to the Arctic where, due to nearly constant summer sunlight, there was an enormous amount of vegetation for them to eat. Maiasaura was large and bulky and would eat approximately 200 pounds of plants per day (the word, "hadrosaur," means "thick" and "strong"). We know from fossilized feces that her diet consisted of ferns, palms, cycads, and woody conifer stems.

Even though she had a bill like that of a duck, Maiasaura had no webbing on her toes. Recent evidence has contradicted earlier theories that Maiasaura was an aquatic creature and thus able to swim away from danger. While many dinosaurs had armor-like scales, which served to protect them from vicious, meat-eating teeth, Maiasaura had only wrinkled and thick skin with bony knobs on it.

Although it is all scientific speculation, the manner in which the Maiasaura is discussed by paleontologists is unusual. Researchers use words like "maternal," "loving," "kind," and "protective." The assumption, based on fossilized remains in the nesting colonies, is that this dinosaur cared for her young in a tender manner. Remains also indicate that Maiasaura lived in huge colonies, 10,000 strong, and might, therefore, have been sociable. We do know for certain that Maiasaura was a herbivore and had huge and violent carnivorous neighbors, such as the infamous Tyrannosaurus Rex.

Should all these suppositions be true, it would seem that Maiasaura was indeed a very vulnerable creature in a harsh and cruel world. She was large and bulky; she stayed with twenty eggs as they hatched and then fed her young until they were quite large; she couldn't swim or run well; and she was a mild-mannered herbivore without an armored skin. It is not surprising then that the main feeling that came out in the proving was an intense state of apprehension and a feeling of danger. (**APPREHENSION**) The following quotations from provers reveal this fear: "Something really bad is going to happen; I got a huge sense of fear, just a tremendous feeling of fear. It first came like a free-floating panicky fear." And from a dream, "Beasts are approaching people from the rear and biting off their heads. I could be both the bitee and the biter. With the bite, you could feel this occipital tension, and then it was gone and so was your head! It was like the twilight zone." (**DANGER**)

## Analysis of the Proving

It is important to reiterate that all that has been said about Maiasaura is conjecture. The real story is impossible to recreate accurately because it occurred so long ago; the evidence is severely obscured. Several aspects of the proving are also a mystery, such as the theme of **HEIGHTS/FLYING**; it seems, on the surface, to have no relationship to this dinosaur. However, by chance, as I was writing this, I read an article, *The Origin of Birds—Is There a Dinosaur Link?*, by Virginia Morell. It discussed the well-documented, paleontological theory that birds, *all birds*, are descended from dinosaurs. "Everywhere we look, from their skeletal features to their behaviors, to even the microstructure of their eggs, we see evidence that birds are descended from dinosaurs," says Paul Sereno, a paleontologist from The University of Chicago. Another paleontologist, Mark Norell, from the American Museum of Natural History states: "We don't even worry...or question...whether birds are dinosaurs; they are." Other theories postulate that the ancestors of birds were earlier reptiles known as archosaurs, which were older than dinosaurs. These creatures, who date from 230 million years ago, gave rise to dinosaurs. Could it be that this ancient connection came out in the dreams of the modern-day provers? It is an intriguing speculation.

Also the theme of **ACCIDENTS**, which came out so strongly in the proving (three provers were actually involved in accidents), is not clearly related to what we know of Maiasaura. If this dinosaur tripped and fell during a migration, did it lead to her being trampled? With 10,000, 30 foot-long creatures striding along, it seems possible. Or is this theme related to the meteor that hit the earth in the Yucatan and sent a cloud of dust so high that it obscured the sun for three years and set off the drastic climactic changes that meant the demise of the dinosaurs? Finally, **JOY/FUN/ECSTASY**. Despite tremendous hardships, did the Maiasaura enjoy her life? We may never know the answers to these questions, but it is stimulating to think about them.

## The Substance

The particular fossil used in this proving was discovered in southern New Mexico. It was found on a paleontological dig and professionally analyzed as to its content. The individual responsible for its discovery is Zachary Krug. He has been very generous in giving us a piece of his fossil for this proving. The fossil is a small, pinkish, rough piece that is not identifiable as to body part.

Science had demonstrated that when a substance became fossilized, it lost a great deal of its DNA, but it was not known how much. The latest research, however, has shown that a fossil retains up to seven percent of its DNA content. This has been verified in scientific analysis of dinosaur bones. Michael Quinn of Hahnemann Pharmacy made a 30C potency for this proving.

*Maiasaura Lapidea* **Themes**

*Fossilized Bone of the Dinosaur*

- *Apprehension*
- *Danger*
- *Accidents*
- *Helping/No One Helping*
- *Heights/Flying*
- *Joy/Fun/Ecstasy*
- *Decadent Sexuality*

## *Apprehension*

**#1** It came. I opened the bottle, felt I had opened Pandora's box, and I had a strong feeling I shouldn't take it. It felt dark, evil, sinister, powerful. I told myself I was being silly; I put five pellets in my mouth, then spit them out. Something very strong; a message not to do this told me, "Don't take this remedy." Washed my mouth out.

**#6** When I volunteered for the proving last month, I felt apprehension. I had promised to take it, so I resigned myself, and I had no ambivalence when it arrived.

**#7** My first proving—I felt apprehensive. I was concerned. I was afraid I'd be harmed.

**#4** I took the first dose with considerable apprehension.

**#1** I was debating whether or not to take the remedy. I didn't get the remedy until the 12th of July. I was relieved every day when it didn't come. I was getting a message from my guides not to take it. I felt an obligation to take the remedy because I said I was going to do it. Once before I ignored such a warning and took a drug. I nearly died.

# *Danger*

**#2** Dream: Beasts are approaching people from the rear and biting off their heads. I could be both the bitee and the biter. With the bite, you could feel this occipital tension, and then it was gone and so was your head! It was like the twilight zone.

**#1** I did a shamanistic journey to ask if I should take the remedy. I had a very strong message that I could lose my mind if I took it. The next day, I felt guilty about not taking the remedy so I inhaled the remedy. Felt safe to do it this way. I felt an immediate flush over my face. An hour later I was reading, got fasciculations all over my face. I wondered if it was a neurotoxin of some kind.

**#1** Woke in the night. Was trying to go over my dreams, and I suddenly thought about the remedy. I got a huge sense of fear, just a tremendous feeling of fear. It first came like a free-floating panicky fear. Then I had a fear that a robber would break in. I never worry about this. I always leave my house unlocked. It is very unusual for me to worry.

**#3** Dream: Next night, more sex and death. Murder and disgust. There was a mutilated body in a mangled car at the roadside. Some woman roughly examined the dead body. There was a hacksaw blade. Someone's son was killed. I had to find the body.

**#7** Dream: Challenging, dangerous, amusement park rides.

**#4** Dream: I was at a garden party. It was a large estate house. The party was very formal, maybe even black tie. Lots of people very dressed up. I was married to the daughter of the host. I was helping organize. I noticed a long, heavy-duty electrical cable that was tied in a knot and stuck in a bucket of water. It was leaking gas. It looked unsafe.

# Accidents

**#1** We had an accident. The car went off the road and looked mangled.

**#5** I had an auto accident during the time of the proving. Driving to San Francisco, a young person plowed into the side of my car. No one was hurt.

**#3** Someone driving my car smashed a fender. I almost had an accident. I became cautious. I almost hit a pedestrian.

**#7** Dream: My oldest son wanted me to bring an old car and other items to Tucson. I wanted to walk to town. I had done it before. It's very far. My old neighbor girlfriend was there, drove us in the old car. The car started to slide backwards. I screamed and ran after her to use the brake. Was terrified. It would not stop. I knew it would hit the house. It veered. I was afraid the brakes were no good. Car did not hit house. Everyone said to get in, that it's okay. I did get in the car but felt uncertain; there's something wrong here.

**#3** Dream: We left and were wandering around in the dark and came on the scene of an accident. There were people lying on the ground in the dark and the rain. They needed oxygen. One person had half their face blue. Something like the chase scene like in the movie, *The Client,* where a young boy observes a murder. The dreams were filled with darkness and danger.

# *Helping/No One Helping*

**#1** Dream: On way to California. In airport parking lot, a woman takes my car key for valet parking; I'm surprised there is valet parking. I go to the cashier to get change for valet's tip, and she is unfriendly. I want help. I feel it's O.K. I can make a tip out of loose change. The woman is not back yet, so I go to find her. I see an ambulance in parking lot where people are doing CPR on a man on a gurney. I don't go to help, it doesn't feel necessary.

**#7** Dream: I was walking outside in a desolate landscape, in a field, walking slowly, going somewhere. I arrived and someone was trying to lead a dog. She couldn't get the dog to go. I knew I could get it to go. So I did it by playing with the dog, by dragging its leash along the ground. It followed along and played with the leash. I felt a sense of satisfaction that I could do this.

**#6** Dream: I was in a tropical country working. Phone call from a woman in Berkeley asking for help in understanding an arcane poet's work. I had to bone up on it and tutor the woman. Another woman called and asked to be tutored in the same poet. I realized they were turning me into an expert so they could use me to come to this nice vacation spot and get their tutoring. I felt abused.

**#6** Dream: I came upon a premature baby sitting in dark city street. The amniotic sac was still intact. On the front part of the baby was a much smaller, nonviable dead twin, attached. It was a dark, damp night. People passing by paid no attention, except for me. I knew it needed help. I hovered around. Soon the sac fell away on its own. It was a little, black baby. I held it. It was alive and slowly responsive. It had straight blond hair and no eyes. There were two nonfunctional, blue eyes when I parted the blond hair. I turned the baby around and on the back of the head was a different face. It was blond and Caucasian and had two supernumerary blue eyes, maybe a third one higher up. They had flat lenses and couldn't see. The feeling: It needed help and nobody was helping. It was a shock.

# *Heights/Flying*

**#5** Dream: I was visiting a friend in a large house 160 feet over the ocean. 160 stuck in my mind. Steps up to the house. My friend has a fear of heights. A feeling of being very high and overlooking the ocean. A very pleasant dream.

**#2** Dream: I've never flown before in a dream. I was zooming, looking down at the world, seeing everything, at about 1,000 feet. Soaring, seeing things. Lots of fun.

**#6** Dream: A boy operating a remote control, mechanical bird.

**#2** Dream: I was flying with a lot of flapping and soaring. Then I became anxious about how to land.

# *Joy/Fun/Ecstasy*

**#1** I awake feeling joyful and refreshed, and the first thing I see is a rainbow, a morning rainbow; it felt magical. (This is very unusual in the morning in New Mexico.)

**#2** I was having two or three vivid dreams a night, like being at the movies. Not scary. Rich in affect. Lots of feeling. The imagery was not as important as the affect. It was fun.

**#3** I had an ecstatic experience. I was riding my bike and swimming in a lake, when thunder and lightening started. I watched the lake become alive with raindrops. A shaft of light came over my shoulder. And a rainbow came and arched at my feet! I laughed and cried. I was wet, and I took my bicycle around the lake. I was covered with mud and rain. An immersed, ecstatic experience.

**#4** Next day, Sunday, 5 p.m. I was in a jovial state. I noticed a manic energy to it. I wasn't hurried. A pressure to have fun. Pleasant. Urge to garden. I don't have a garden, so I rearranged potted plants on my deck.

**#4** Dream: A great dream. Dreamt of a lamp on my mother's bedside table in England. She had a fluorescent, long-life bulb in the lamp. I'm normally so skeptical about my mother that I felt she had installed it wrong, so I inspected it. I looked closely and saw it leaking a white liquid light, that was vivid, with beautiful white roses being created inside the lampshade. I told my mother about the bulb squirting liquid and roses. She was quite nonchalant. She reached in under the shade. The shade grew like a huge tent. The bulb became a nozzle on a hose. She had this beatific look on her face, and she squirted the roses with this white light, and they began to turn towards her to receive the nourishment.

**#7** Dream: That night I had a very peculiar dream. I dreamed of being in a wire cage. A group of us. Like an enormous cage. It was pretty and exciting. It was like a bridal shower. They had to fill the cage with whipped cream before the men got there. It was this happy exciting feeling like, "Oh, good, the men are coming now!" I woke up when the whipped cream came up to my neck.

## *Decadent Sexuality*

**#3** Dream: Two very assertive women in a long, white limousine with a black roof picked up me and the husband of a good friend of mine for hostages and for sexual torture. They were going to take us away as hostages. He said to me: "How do you feel about this?" I said: "Well, I feel shitty. I don't want to do this." But we agreed that we would be in on it together. Then we attempted to pick up other friends to be hostages with us!

**#4** Dream: I met my wife. We took the elevator upstairs. I ended up seducing my wife's sister. I'd just told my wife how much I loved her. Both women didn't have much clothing on.

**#7** Dream: We went back to a ranch we used to live on with my youngest daughter. The buyer of the ranch looked scruffy, unshaven, unkempt. They had added an ugly porch to our bedroom. He complained about having four homes. I said it must be a lot to keep up. He said it's good for his liaisons, looking matter-of-fact and decadent. It took me a couple of minutes to get what he meant. He said his wife used the houses for liaisons also.

**#3** Dream: Then there was some sexy sex in a sleeping bag. Quick and rough sex.... A man was staring at me in the shower through an eyeglass.

**MIND**

- ACCIDENTS, tendency to, car
- ADVENTUROUS
- *ANTICIPATION; impending evil, sensation of*
    - *unusual ordeal, of any*
- ANXIETY
    - anticipating
    - disagreeable, as if something was
    - duty, as if he had not done his
    - exaggerated
    - *foreboding, with gloom*
    - heart; about his
        - *evil was going to happen, as if something*
    - ill, as if he would be
    - oppressive
- CURSING, swearing; curses, desire to curse
- DAYDREAMING; tendency for
- DELUSIONS, imaginations
    - accidents
        - fatal, he will have a
        - sees
    - animals, of
        - devouring him
    - assaulted, is going to be
    - danger; of
        - life, to his
    - dark
    - faces, sees; closing eyes, on
    - hole; digging a big
        - freezing cold waterfall
    - insane; become, that she will
    - mutilated bodies; sees
    - odor, smells a bad
    - repulsive fantastic imaginations
    - robbed, is going to be
- DREAMS
    - abused; feeling over requests to tutor

DREAMS (cont.)
- *accidents, of*
  - *in car*
  - mutilated body in mangled car
- amorous
- amusement park rides; dangerous
- *animals, of*
  - *being bitten by*
  - dogs
    - leading a
  - *pursued by, of being*
  - puppies; chasing cat
- attacked from above
- *bitten; animals, by*
  - from the rear, heads off
- body, body parts
  - dead
  - face
    - half blue
  - eyes
    - having three
  - head
    - bitten off by animals
    - with two faces
- bowling in dark alley
- bus takes to wrong place
- cage; wire, with whipped cream to neck
- car; won't stop, brakes no good
- child, children; about;
  - babies
  - black with blond hair, three eyes
    - but couldn't see, needed help
  - found a living premature baby on city street
  - rescuing
  - something had happened to
- climbing over piles of manure
  - tall ladders
- coition, of
- danger
- darkness
- desert, seashells and cacti like seaweed
- disputes about money
- eating, of
- ecstatic

- eulogy for man died of AIDS
- exams, missed
    - friend didn't tell me about
- excrement
- family
- fantastic
- fights, of
    - fighting with men, no one hurt
- flowers, of
- flying
    - 1,000 feet, soaring, fun
    - flapping, anxious about landing
- gardens, of
- helping people
    - aversion to
- high places
- hostages, taken as, for sexual torture
- house
    - for sexual liaisons
- hunting of
- landscape; desolate
- language; of teacher incomprehensible
- lascivious, smutty
- limousine, white with black roof
- manure, of
- men
    - dragging boulder by ropes
    - excited about arrival of
    - man staring at women in the shower through eyeglass
    - rough, unshaven
- money
    - disputes over
    - fund-raising
    - stolen
- monsters
- mother
    - beatific look on her face
- murder
    - son killed
        - hacksaw blade, with
- mutilated bodies
- naked, nakedness
    - unashamed
- nightmares

DREAMS (cont.)
nurse, talking to a
obstacles, easily dealt with
occipital tension gone with head off
parties
pleasant
prisoner, being taken
punches men, blows not felt
*pursued*
quilt, beautiful brown
relatives
restaurant
cannot pay for meal
expensive, $1,329.63
venison, eating
rich in affect
riding
roses; white, beautiful
safari
sex
and death with disgust
in a sleeping bag, quick and rough
seduced wife's sister
sexual captivity, of
snorkeling on dry land
*stones, of*
terror
torture of
trains
troop train carrying money
unpleasant
unsafe electric cable in water
visits; making visits
water, of
weeping over love of the word of God
women; without much clothing
ECSTASY
as rainbow arches at her feet
joy, as after excessive
morning on waking

- FEAR
  - accidents, of
    - car, to
      - almost having
      - smashing
    - threatened by fatal, as if
  - causeless
  - *danger; impending, of*
  - *evil, of*
    - *forebodings of evil*
  - free-floating
  - groundless
  - *happen; something will; terrible, horrible*
  - insanity, of losing his reason
  - night
    - waking, after
  - panic attacks, overpowering; without cause
  - poisoned; being
  - robbers, of
  - tremendous
  - unaccountable, vague
  - violence, of
- INSANITY, madness; feeling of
- JOY
  - fits of, with bursts of laughter
  - seeing a rainbow
  - waking, on
- MAGIC; rainbow feels like
- MANIA, madness
  - laughing and gaiety, with
  - restless
  - spasmodic sensation, with
- ORDERLY manner; cannot perform anything in
- RELAXED feeling, letting go
- SADNESS, despondency, depression, melancholy; conscious of unnatural state of mind, because
- SPACED-OUT feeling
- THOUGHTS; hurried
  - instability of, unsettled
  - intrude and crowd around each other
  - rapid, quick
  - rush, flow of
- TRANQUILITY, serenity, calmness

**VERTIGO**

FLOATING, as if
    body feels

**HEAD**

ITCHING; Forehead
LIGHTNESS, sense of

**HEAD PAIN**

GENERAL; afternoon
        2 p.m.
    air; open; amel.
    intermittent pains
    irritability, from
    noon
    perspiration; with
        profuse
LOCALIZATION; Forehead
        pressure

**VISION**

FLASHES

**NOSE**

EPISTAXIS
    blood; bright
        fluid
    easily, which amel.
    left
    morning

**MOUTH**

APHTHAE; Gums

**FACE**

*DISCOLORATION; red*
HEAT; flushes of
ITCHING; whiskers

- PAIN; General; chin
  - prickling; jaw
    - lower
- TREMBLING
- TWITCHING
- VEINS distended
  - nevi, spider

### THROAT

- CHOKING, constricting
- PAIN
  - general; extending to; ear
      - swallowing, on
    - right
  - burning
    - Oesophagus
      - evening

### EXTERNAL THROAT

ITCHING

### STOMACH

- APPETITE; increased
- CHURNING
- ERUCTATIONS; food; feeling of
- WEAK feeling

### ABDOMEN

PAIN; burning

### RECTUM

ITCHING

### MALE

SEXUAL desire; increased

### FEMALE

MENSES; late, too

## LARYNX & TRACHEA

*SPASMS of glottis; vocal cords*

## SPEECH & VOICE

SPEECH; stammering
  excitement
  fast, talking, when
  quick, and

## COUGH

CHOKING
MUCUS; chest, in
  upper, in, agg.

## CHEST

CONGESTION
ITCHING; Axilla
  left
PAIN

## EXTREMITIES

ITCHING; Foot
  sole of; right

## EXTREMITY PAIN

JOINTS
UPPER LIMBS

## SLEEP

*SLEEPLESSNESS*
  heavy feeling in; limbs
  midnight; after; 5 a.m.; until
    3:30 a.m.; after

## PERSPIRATION

*PROFUSE*

## GENERALITIES

ENERGY, lots of

EDITOR'S NOTE: *Punctuation, abbreviations, and individual stylistic nuances of the original journal entries have been preserved wherever possible.*

**Prover #1 · Female · 49 years old**

I was debating whether or not to take the remedy because I had relapsed with my leg fracture, and I had an intense emotional situation coming up. I didn't get the remedy until the 12th of July. I was relieved every day when it didn't come. I was getting a message from my guides not to take it. I felt an obligation to take the remedy. I said I was going to do it. Once before I ignored such a warning and took a drug. I nearly died.

**Day 1**

◆ It came, I opened the bottle, felt I had opened Pandora's box, and I had a strong feeling I shouldn't take it. It felt, dark, evil, sinister, powerful. I told myself I was being silly, I put five pellets in my mouth, then spit them out. Something very strong; a message not to do this told me: don't take this remedy. Washed my mouth out. I went and sat to meditate on what I thought would happen if I took it. I felt a huge sadness in my heart. I felt an overwhelming sense of sadness. Intellectually, I thought I'd get a lot of pain in my limbs. I told myself I was being silly. I did a shamanistic journey to ask if I should take the remedy. I had a very strong message that I could lose my mind if I took it.

**Day 2**

◆ The next day I felt guilty about not taking the remedy so I inhaled the remedy. It felt safe to do it this way. I felt an immediate flush over my face. An hour later I was reading, and I got fasciculations all over my face. I wondered if it was a neurotoxin of some kind.
◆ I had some dreams, not sure if they are related to the proving. Dreamed of new puppy chasing the cat. When I told him to stop, he did; unlike in real life. Positive feeling in dream.

**Day 3**

◆ Nothing remarkable. Dreams calm.

**Day 4**

◆ Fell asleep in bathtub, first time I had ever done that. A positive dream. I took it to be because I had ended a relationship that needed to end.
◆ Dream: On my way to California in airport parking lot, woman takes my car key for valet parking. I'm surprised there is valet parking. I go to the cashier to get change for valet's tip and she is unfriendly. I want help. I feel it's O.K. I can make a tip out of loose

change. The woman is not back yet, so I go to find her. I see an ambulance in parking lot where people are doing CPR on man on a gurney. I don't go to help, it doesn't feel necessary. Then I can't find my truck but eventually do and use the hidden key to drive it. I realize that I am now too late to make an appointment; call to say I won't be there. I feel O.K. once I've decided how not to be rushed. Overall feeling: obstacles and delays, easily dealt with. Not overextending myself.

**Day 5**

◆ Calm and peaceful day, allowed myself time to just sit and be, very unusual for me. During night, woke to try to remember dreams. They were of trying to raise money for the clinic. While awake, I thought of the remedy and felt fear, paranoia; someone will break into the house. Slept again without trouble. In dream, was on a train to California. It stops in the desert. I stepped out naked onto the desert. There are a lot of stones mixed with seashells and cacti growing like seaweed. I am delighted and call to a young girl to come and see. It was like looking at the bottom of the sea, seashells. We are snorkeling on dry land. A delightful dream. People were showing up. I was naked but had no shame or embarrassment. I did put on a long T-shirt.

◆ Dream: I was in the community house. It was much too hot. Someone has turned the thermostat to 95 degrees F. I turned it down to save energy. I thought they could put on the quilt if they got cold. It was made of synthetic fabric, of poor quality and not warm. It had holes in it, shabby. I look at my bedroom and see there a beautiful quilt I had forgotten I had. It is warm, dark brown background with vivid color design. Thought I would redecorate my bedroom from pastels to this bold pattern. When I look again into bedroom, there are curtains that match quilt.

◆ I awake feeling joyful and refreshed and the first thing I see is a rainbow, a morning rainbow, it felt magical. (This is very unusual in the morning in New Mexico.)

**Day 6**

◆ Woke in the night. Was trying to go over my dreams, and I suddenly thought about the remedy. I got a huge sense of fear, just a tremendous feeling of fear. It first came like a free-floating panicky fear. Then I had a fear that a robber would break in. I never worry about this. I always leave my house unlocked. It is very unusual for me to worry.

◆ Today I noticed a different lesion on my left cheek. Looks like a spider nevi.

**Day 7**

◆ While sitting in a meeting, I had a nosebleed for the first time in my life. There was no reason that I was aware of at all. Bright red blood was pouring from my left nostril at 10:20 a.m. It stopped easily with pressure.

◆ Emotionally I did very well with this remedy. Better, in fact, than usual.

◆ We had an accident. The car went off the road and looked mangled.

**Prover #2 · Male · 44 years old**

**Day 2**

◆ Two days after the remedy, woke with headache over brow (I never get H/A's). Like a weight pushing down. Annoying headache. Accompanied with increased hunger and an irritability. I wanted to gnaw on things, like gnaw on people (irritability with the headache). It was intermittent.

◆ Increased perspiration, heat intolerance. Aversion to stuffy rooms. Drenching perspiration, easily dehydrated.

**Day 3**

◆ Dreams more active than in years. First dream: Beasts approaching people from the rear, biting off their heads. I could be the bitee and the biter. With the bite, you could feel this occipital tension gone, so was your head! It was like the twilight zone.

**Day 4**

◆ Dream: I've never flown before in a dream. I was zooming, looking down at the world, seeing everything, at about 1,000 feet. Soaring, seeing things. Lots of fun.

**Day 7**

◆ Dream: I was flying with a lot of flapping and soaring. Then I became anxious about how to land. I was having two or three vivid dreams a night, like being at the movies. Not scary. Rich in affect. Lots of feeling. The imagery was not as important as the affect. It was fun.

**Prover #3 · Female · 47 years old**

◆ I took the remedy July 6-7. My period came 10 days late.

◆ During the proving, I had persistent upper extremity joint pains.

◆ The first few days of this proving I had terrible dreams. I hated them. I repeated the remedy.

**Day 1**

◆ Someone driving my car smashed a fender. Almost had an accident. I became cautious. I almost hit a pedestrian.

◆ Dreams: In one we were at a conference in Hawaii. J was teaching from 5 a.m. to 7 p.m.! J was speaking another language and he was incomprehensible. N had cut her hair and had very short hair. Another teacher was like a dancer. It was a terrible conference. We left and were wandering around in the dark and came on the scene of an accident. There were people lying on the ground in the dark and the rain. They needed oxygen. One person had half their face blue. Something like the chase scene like in the movie, *The Client,* where a young boy observes a murder. The dreams were filled with darkness and danger.

◆ I ate chicken. I'm a vegetarian and usually averse to chicken. First time in six years that I had meat other than fish!

**Day 2**

◆ Dream: Next night more sex and death. Murder and disgust. There was a mutilated body in a mangled car at the roadside. Then there was some sexy sex in a sleeping bag. Quick and rough sex. Some woman roughly examined the dead body. There was a hacksaw blade. Someone's son was killed. I had to find the body. A man was staring at me in the shower through an eyeglass. I was in a park climbing over ladders, very tall ladders and piles of manure. Bowling in a dark bowling alley.

◆ A dream I've had before. In Berkeley Hills and I was trying to go one place but the bus took me to Oakland. Then two very assertive women in a long white limousine with a black roof picked up me and the husband of a good friend of mine for hostages, and for sexual torture. They were going to take us away as hostages. He said to me: "How do you feel about this?" I said: "Well, I feel shitty. I don't want to do this." But we agreed that we would be in on it together. Then we attempted to pick up other friends to be hostages with us!

◆ This has been an emotionally tumultuous time for me. I've been traveling. I did not like the dreams. I felt really unwilling to take these notes on my dreams while I was traveling.

**Day 3**

◆ I had an ecstatic experience. I was riding my bike and swimming in a lake when thunder and lightening started. I watched the lake become alive with raindrops. A shaft of light came over my shoulder. And a rainbow came and arched at my feet! I laughed and cried. I was wet and I took my bicycle around the lake. I was covered with mud and rain. An immersed, ecstatic experience.

### Prover #4 · Male · 39 years old

◆ I took several doses. I didn't get any great shakes. Normally I have vivid dreams, about three vivid dreams a week. Some physical stuff that may or may not be the remedy. Sunday, I had Mexican food, a dish I eat often. Had two Cokes instead of my usual one. Afterwards I had a sensation of floating. Lightheaded, mentally spacey feeling. Lasted a few hours.

◆ Another time, had breakfast 8:30, took remedy 9:20. 9:40 driving to office, got right-sided throat pain, dull, throbbing, out of the blue. Extended into my right ear. Worse swallowing. Lasted 15 minutes.

◆ Prior to taking the remedy I'd had some right SI pain for four weeks. It was diminishing by the time I took the remedy. After work I took a stroll with my wife, two miles. I got back pain in left SI area. I'd never had pain there.

◆ That night developed a cold sore on right upper gum.

◆ Dream: First night after I took the remedy I dreamt I was at a garden party. It was a large estate house. The party was very formal, maybe even black tie. Lots of people very dressed up. I was married to the daughter of the host. I was helping to organize. I noticed a long heavy-duty electrical cable that was tied in a knot and stuck in a bucket of water. It was leaking gas. It looked unsafe. I told my father-in-law. He put on diving gear and dealt with the situation by going into the swimming pool! I met my wife. We took the elevator upstairs. I ended up seducing my wife's sister. I'd just told my wife how much I loved her. Both women didn't have much clothing on.

◆ Next day, Sunday, 5 p.m. was in a jovial state. I noticed a manic energy to it. I wasn't hurried. A pressure to have fun. Pleasant. Urge to garden. I don't have a garden, so I rearranged potted plants on my deck. I got irritable in the evening.

◆ That night a great dream. Dreamt of a lamp on my mother's bedside table. She had a fluorescent long-life bulb in the lamp. I'm normally so skeptical about my mother that I felt she had installed it wrong, so I inspected it. I looked closely and saw it leaking a white liquid light, that was vivid, with beautiful white roses being created inside the lampshade. I told my mother about the bulb squirting liquid and roses. She was quite nonchalant. She reached in under the shade. The shade grew like a huge tent. The bulb became a nozzle on a hose. She had this beatific look on her face and she squirted the roses with this white light and they began to turn towards her to receive the nourishment.

◆ I'd taken six doses. I felt the remedy wasn't doing much. I took the first dose with considerable apprehension.

## Prover #5 · Male · 57 years old

I'm not sensitive to provings. I hoped something would happen, but not much did.

**Day 1**

◆ Nothing.

**Day 4**

◆ Repeated remedy. Had a dream. I was visiting a friend in a large house 160 feet over the ocean. 160 stuck in my mind. Steps up to the house. My friend has a fear of heights. A feeling of being very high and overlooking the ocean. A very pleasant dream.

**Day 5**

◆ Developed an itch in my left axilla. A minimal rash. My neck itched and beard hairline, also at head hairline. A persistent rectal itch.

**Day 6**

◆ Itch on both armpits.

**Day 8**

◆ Dream: I was physically fighting with a group of men, punches thrown. I was not hurt. A mass of people into physical interaction, but nothing physical felt. Blows were thrown, but I don't recall anyone being hurt. Another dream: a conversation with family members.

◆ Itch persisted in armpits. Itching under right foot 10 p.m.

**Day 11**

◆ All symptoms left and did not return. No itching since.

◆ I had an auto accident during the time. Driving to San Francisco, a young person plowed into side of my car. No one was hurt.

### Prover #6 · Male · 43 years old

◆ My first proving. When I volunteered for the proving last month, I felt apprehension. I had promised to take it, so I resigned myself and I had no ambivalence when it arrived.

◆ Some physical things I noticed: I was tolerant to more sweets than usual. I usually don't do well with sweets. I ate plenty and it didn't bother me.

◆ My energy in general was higher.

◆ Libido was higher.

◆ I was warmer. A generic type of remedy boost I get.

◆ Lots of thoughts intruding. Hard to concentrate.

◆ Daydreams coming in. I would push them out.

**Day 1**

◆ First night: Some sort of group feeling. Something needing to occur. Concern for the group.

**Day 2**

◆ Dream: I was chased. Another dream: I was at a large eulogy gathering, hundreds of people outdoors. A card passed around with a paper that told about the deceased man's life. He was young, perhaps died of AIDS. I took the paper to a hot tub. Later gave it back; lady was ticked it was wet and I was tardy returning it.

◆ Dream: I came upon a premature baby sitting in dark city street. The amniotic sac was still intact. On the front part of the baby was a much smaller nonviable dead twin, attached. It was a dark damp night. People passing by paid no attention except for me. I knew it needed help. I hovered around. Soon the sac fell away on its own. It was a little black baby. I held it. It was alive and slowly responsive. It had straight blond hair and no eyes. There were two nonfunctional blue eyes when I parted the blond hair. I turned the baby around and on the back of the head was a different face. It was blond and Caucasian and had two supernumerary blue eyes, maybe a third one higher up. They had flat lenses and couldn't see. The feeling: It needed help and nobody was helping. It was a shock.

◆ I felt less need for sleep.

**Day 3**

◆ I had a brief left chest pain. Worry about cardiac illness.

**Day 4**

◆ Again I had brief chest pain.

◆ Dream: I was in a tropical country working. Phone call from a woman in Berkeley asking for help in understanding an arcane poet's work. I had to bone up on it and tutor the woman. Another woman called and asked to be tutored in the same poet. I realized they were turning me into an expert so they could use me to come to this nice vacation spot and get their tutoring. I felt abused. I was preparing for a safari, talking to a nurse. Telling her how I love the word of God, and I was weeping.

**Day 8**

◆ Dream: I was on a troop-carrying train. I ran on without paying. Had to climb over file envelopes. They all contained money. After climbing through that, I was in a campsite with a lot of people. I ran back to the train because I forgot to pay. He said no big deal, to pay or not. He said $25. I gave him a tattered $20 bill I had stolen from the envelopes. I said to him that I knew his manager the US government and I didn't want to mess with him. Back to the campsite I passed the showers. A boy operating a remote control mechanical bird. Passed a huge boulder being chipped away by chains with motors that yanked the pole against the rock chipping it away. Passed a boulder being dragged down the road by men with ropes. They were all strange dreams. I was surprised.

◆ During the proving I decided to dig a pond, ripped out flower bed, started to dig a big hole in my yard. On a hike I went under a freezing cold waterfall.

**Prover #7 · Female · 55 years old**

**Day 1**

◆ My first proving: I felt apprehensive. I was concerned. I was afraid I'd be harmed. Woke 1:30 in laryngeal spasm, couldn't inhale.

◆ That night I had a very peculiar dream. I dreamed of being in a wire cage. A group of us. Like an enormous cage. It was pretty and exciting. It was like a bridal shower. They had to fill the cage with whipped cream before the men got there. It was this happy exciting feeling like: "Oh good, the men are coming now!" I woke up when the whipped cream came up to my neck.

◆ Throat burned. Weakness in stomach area.

◆ Dream: I was walking outside in a desolate landscape, in a field, walking slowly, going somewhere. I arrived and someone was trying to lead a dog. She couldn't get the dog to go. I knew I could get it to go. So I did it by playing with the dog, by dragging its leash along the ground. It followed along and played with the leash. I felt a sense of satisfaction that I could do this.

◆ Felt afraid, some burning pains in abdomen and cried because I did not want child to leave; felt sad.

**Day 2**

◆ Sad, wanted family around me. Daughter would be leaving end of month.

◆ Dream: We went back to ranch we used to live on with my youngest daughter. The buyer of the ranch looked scruffy, unshaven, unkempt. They had added an ugly porch to our bedroom. He complained about having four homes. I said it must be a lot to keep up. He said it's good for his liaisons, looking matter-of-fact and decadent. It took me a couple of minutes to get what he meant. He said his wife used the houses for liaisons, too. Daughter and I went outside, she called W by the wrong name, which saddened and embarrassed me. I realized she did not really have the experience of living on the ranch because she was so young when we left. It was time to leave. My oldest son wanted me to bring an old car and other items to Tucson. I wanted to walk to town. I had done it before. It's very far. My old neighbor girlfriend was there, drove us in the old car. The car started to slide backwards. I screamed and ran after her to use the brake. Was terrified. It would not stop. I knew it would hit the house. It veered. I was afraid the brakes were no good. Car did not hit house. Everyone said to get in, that it's okay. I did get in the car, but felt uncertain, there's something wrong here.

**Day 3**

◆ 10 a.m. sadness. Daydreaming. Didn't want children to leave, I am enjoying them here. I snuggled with my daughter. Wept. Want to be with children and husband. Had to call my husband at the office. Felt myself again in afternoon at 5 p.m.

◆ At 7:30 to 8 p.m. burning in esophagus, like reflux. Very unusual. At 8 p.m. feeling food wanting to come up my esophagus.

**Day 4**

◆ Seven-eight p.m. burning in esophagus. I only slept two hours and am not tired. Mind feels sped up. I feel pushed, somewhat anxious. I want to slow it down.

**Day 5**

◆ Felt like myself, positive, up. Took another dose.

◆ That night dreamed I was in school, exam time. I went two days. Third day didn't know where to go to take the exam, if I had exams, or where to go to find out. That afternoon at 3:00 I found old friend. Found I'd missed exams that day. I was concerned but did not have a clue how to find out if there was one that day.

◆ Dream fragment: Something about challenging dangerous amusement park rides.

**Day 6**

◆ Good energy. Muscle soreness right scapula. No Sadness.

**Day 7**

◆ Focused, lots of energy. Mind sped up. Mind quickly moved from thing to thing. If someone wanted my attention they weren't moving fast enough. Shooting, prickly pain in glands under my chin.

**Day 8**

◆ Woke with imaginary odor, smelled bad; husband said he smelled nothing.
Good energy focused.

**Day 9**

◆ Good energy.

◆ Felt shaky at 8 p.m. before dinner, weakness in stomach area.

◆ That night woke 2:40 a.m.; stayed awake until 3:14.

**Day 10**

◆ Felt choky and gaggy from chest mucous.

◆ Tired 12:30 p.m. needed a nap. Slept until 3:40. Annoyed and irritated at being awakened for appointment. Slept deeply.

◆ That night woke 2:40 a.m., couldn't sleep, got up and stayed awake, worked till 5 a.m.; slept until 7:55.

**Day 11**

◆ Stomach churned, felt like food would come up. It didn't. I never have this problem.

◆ Dream: Went to lunch with husband and another couple. Man said he couldn't pay. Was $1,329.63. The man thought it was only $329 and he couldn't pay it. He had eaten venison. They told us we had had the venison and that is why it was so expensive. We objected, there were no prices on the menu, how could we have known? We couldn't pay.

**Day 12**

◆ Headache noon, < 2:30 p.m.

**Day 13**

◆ After reading headache 5-6 p.m.

**Day 14**

◆ Headache noon and 3 p.m. Trouble reading. Stuttering. Thoughts coming quickly. Trouble getting out what I wanted to say. Tripping over words.

◆ I only slept two hours last night. Felt sore in places, heavy in bed. Flashes of light on closing eyes to fall asleep.

**Day 15**

◆ A few tiny light flashes in my visual field visual flashes, small punctuate. Anxiety 9-10 a.m.

# LIMENITIS BREDOWII

*Butterfly*

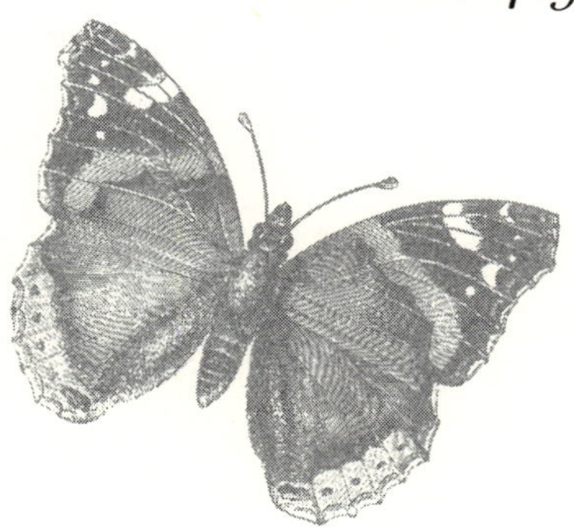

# LIMENITIS BREDOWII *Butterfly*

The butterfly is a mysterious and magical creature. It is beloved by humans and animals alike, but for very different reasons. Humans are in awe of its fleeting beauty. In fact, the ancient Greeks used the word, "butterfly," synonymously with the word, "soul." Animals find it a tasty and abundant source of food.

Butterflies made their place on the earth over 100 million years ago. The oldest-known, butterfly fossils date from the same time as the dinosaurs. They fly on all continents except Antarctica. They live in virtually every type of environment, from the frigid polar regions to the tropics—where they are the most prolific. The insect order, Lepidoptera (which includes butterflies, moths, and skippers), is noted for its abundance and variety. It is the second largest of the insect orders (beetle is first), with more than 100,000 species. There are over 700 species of butterfly in North America alone. Each species relies on a specific and often narrow food habitat. Thus, they are vulnerable to environmental modifications, especially ones that alter the availability of flowers. At the present time, in Europe alone, over 50 species are in danger of extinction.

It is said that butterflies can see many more colors than humans can (they prefer violet, purple, and blue); can taste more with their leg-positioned taste buds (the Milkweed butterfly has a taste sensitivity 2,408 times greater than that of man); and can smell the most subtle scent. (**BODY AWARENESS/SENSUALITY**) Thus, they are highly qualified as "nectar enthusiasts." They need abundant glucose to supply the energy required to move their wings constantly. Flowers, richly endowed with reservoirs of sweet, liquid nectar, meet all their needs. Most species of butterfly feed only on one specific flower, often one that grows in a particular setting—for example, a south-facing hillside with a loamy type of soil.

A few, rare butterfly species are carrion eaters and prefer rotten meat. If that is not available, they may turn to coprophagy, the eating of urine and feces. Fruit, especially if fermented, is the choice of yet another species of butterfly. Once this species drinks their fill, their abdomens protrude and they fly in drunken zigzag patterns.

The main eating apparatus of the butterfly is the long, straw-shaped proboscis. This is placed deep into the flower or liquefied food, and the juice is sucked out. While they are sucking the liquid, the butterfly is also aiding in the pollination of the plant by rubbing its body on the pollen and carrying it to the next plant. Next to the bee, the butterfly is the most active pollinator. One species, the Hawk Moth, is able to fertilize 100 flowers in approximately three minutes.

The butterfly itself makes a great meal for many other members of the animal world. Birds and bats especially relish this winged delicacy. Among its other predators are spiders, beetles, wasps, toads, lizards, and monkeys. Several species of butterfly have developed self-defense systems whereby they eat highly toxic plants, assimilate them, and then poison any creature that eats them. Predators soon learn to avoid them. Many other butterfly species imitate the coloring of this group, hoping to mimic the poisonous butterfly and confuse its enemies. Still other butterfly species have developed startling, large "eyes" on the two lower wings to frighten predators. The coloring on the wings helps to camouflage the butterfly and contributes to its great beauty.

The *Limenitis bredowii californica*, or "California Sister," used for this proving is a "regal butterfly of dignified demeanor and exclusive habits," says entomologist J.A. Comstock. It is a member of the largest and most diverse butterfly family, nymphalidae. The California, Oregon, and Nevada woodlands, where oak predominates in canyons and hillsides, is the native home of these beautiful creatures. When, with wings folded, they sit on branches or tree bark they are nearly invisible. The adult *Limenitis bredowii* has a large, orange spot at the tip of each forewing and a white band across the wings on a field of dark brown. The underside of the wing is a bluish-brown color, sometimes matching the hue and shape of a dead leaf.

The larvae of the *Limenitis bredowii* eat oak leaves and sequester in their bodies an alkaloid (the chemically active ingredient in a plant, like nicotine in Tobacco or cocaine in Coca), which it retains in the adult stage. These alkaloids are unpalatable to birds and thus serve as a protective agent for the California Sister. A unique difference between the Sister and most other adult butterflies is that they are seldom found among flowers, although they do get nectar from them. They prefer to fly around oak trees, mating and laying eggs, and approach flowers only when they need a quick supply of glucose. They also absorb minerals from streams and puddles.

The highly territorial males perch on high branches in sunlit gaps along the edges of the forest, to see what enemies may be encroaching. Their terrain, however small it may be (often just a tiny patch of light), is vigorously defended. They keep their wings partially open at all times while on guard, ready to chase other males away and fly towards females. (**SEXUALITY**) They are not nearly as aggressive, though, as the common Cabbage White or Swallowtail, which will chase anything that flies within their wide range of vision.

Butterflies have four stages in their life cycle: 1) egg; 2) caterpillar, also known as larvae; 3) pupa, also known as cocoon or chrysalis; and 4) adult butterfly, also known as imago. There are three generations in a year, with the caterpillar-larva stage representing the longest part of the life cycle. The first three stages might metaphorically be considered equivalent to infancy, childhood and adolescence in a human being. (**BEING A BABY, A CHILD, OR PARTICULARLY AN ADOLESCENT**)

Since most butterflies live only three to ten days, the first and foremost activity is finding a mate so as to reproduce quickly. On the day of their emergence from the cocoon, the males stake out a territory and the females find a partner. The females release pheromones (odorous substances) which attract the males. They then flutter together in a highly ritualized and graceful courtship dance. (**LOVING FEELINGS**) Each species has its own unique dance, which reduces the possibility of hybridization. The females fly to the trees and test the leaves by tapping their feet on them. If the leaves meet with their satisfaction, they will deposit an egg, then quickly depart. (**MOTHER/FATHER/FAMILY**) Unlike many other butterfly eggs, which are hidden in niches or covered over by the female, the eggs of the *Limenitis bredowii* are placed in the open. (**A CHILD FEELING UNPROTECTED BY ADULTS**) The eggs are then left in a completely vulnerable state. The larvae and pupae are camouflaged by their coloration, but this and their foul taste from the alkaloids are the only protection they have. The larvae, or caterpillars, build themselves a winter home of dried leaves called a "hibernaculum," a sort of "roll-your-own" tent that gives them protection from the cold. The larvae's main task is to eat, and they do so prodigiously. They increase their weight 10,000 fold during this period.

At the pupa-cocoon stage, *Limenitis bredowii* builds a silk house around itself and hangs there quietly, until its body disintegrates and magically transforms into that of the complete, adult butterfly. (**BUILDINGS**) It emerges by shaking off the old house, drying its new wings in the sun, and winging off to start the cycle again.

### Analysis of the Proving

After reading the journals and listening to the provers' reports at the group meeting, I have the impression that the essence of this remedy is the state of an unprotected adolescent. The adolescents have the feeling that their parents, though they love their children, do not think carefully enough about protecting them. In this situation, the children are without guidance and feel anxious.

Butterfly might also be helpful for parents who are unwilling or unable to set limits of safety for their children; parents who "don't want to think" about limits or rules who "just want to feel" their love for their children. (**EMOTIONS, NOT THE MIND**) J.C. Cooper, in *Symbolic and Mythological Animals,* says: "Butterflies can...symbolize a life of pleasure, irresponsibility, 'a butterfly existence,' or spiritedness."

A startling coincidence during the proving was the simultaneous news event which reported the tragedy of a seven-year-old girl who piloted a plane across the country with her father and flight instructor and fatally crashed in an icy rainstorm. She was the youngest ever to attempt such a feat. When reporters asked him, prior to the flight, why he allowed his daughter to fly an airplane at age seven when 16 was the minimum age for a pilot's license, the father explained: "My daughter requested it." The mother was asked before the flight if the weather might delay her daughter's takeoff. Her reply was: "The weather will move for her. It is not luck. It is the power of her being. There is something about Jessica that things move for her. She is just a wonderful being." Experts advised other parents after the accident to "tell their kids the truth, let them grieve, and assure them of their own safety."

An interesting theme in the proving was that of buildings. This reminds one of the cocoon stage, where the pupas are housed in "a beautifully decorated house" of silk. Silk has been obtained from the cocoon wrapping of the silkworm moth (*Bombyx mori*) since the fifth century B.C. The princess who discovered it was given the rank of divinity for her incredible find. Silk is regarded the world over as the most elegant and sensuous fabric.

The most significant symptom to emerge from the proving was the aversion and inability to think. As one prover put it: "It's as if the gears in my head are filled with a thick, gooey, viscous gunk and that they are not moving well and that they freeze." At the same time, there was a striking orientation towards loving emotions in this proving: "...interactions are full of love and mutual respect.... I felt really loving on an almost global level." It seems that the butterfly represents a state of emotional freedom and love without the "hindrances" of responsibility and thought processes.

### The Substance

This butterfly had an interesting history. It was found perched on a stone altar that was being used for a wedding ceremony in a meadow beside a creek in Nevada City, California. Many people commented on the odd, subdued behavior of this butterfly. It remained in this spot for four days, during which time one of the wedding guests received a phone call informing him of his mothers' sudden death. "In Asia," states Alain Eid in *Butterflies and Moths of the World*, "moths are held in special esteem; they are believed to be the manifestation of dead souls who have returned to protect the living." I had wanted to prove butterfly and decided that if this particular *Limenitis bredowii* remained quietly sitting on that altar one more day, I would take it and immortalize it as a remedy. Harianna Chilstrom identified it, and Hahnemann Pharmacy made up the entire butterfly into a 30C potency for this proving.

*Limenitis Bredowii*

# Themes

*Butterfly*

- *Being a Baby, a Child, or Particularly an Adolescent*
- *A Child Feeling Unprotected by Adults*
- *Emotions, Not the Mind*
- *Sexuality*
- *Body Awareness/Sensuality*
- *Loving Feelings*
- *Mother/Father/Family*
- *Buildings*

## *Being a Baby, a Child, or Particularly an Adolescent*

**#5** It was a long day at work; it was productive and good. I felt resentful that I had to be indoors working on such a beautiful day. I wished I was a kid.

**#5** Dreams of being an adolescent; realized adults didn't have all the answers. I felt anxious, unsettled.

**#2** Spent last night and today with a group of mothers and daughters from my sons class. It was very moving to hear girls express themselves. Tears came to my eyes several times, at the expression of pain and separation; wanted to be treated still as young girls but also wanting their freedom at the same time. There was a wave (in me) of desires and needs and missed communications, so poignant. I was so glad to be part of this sharing.

**#5** Dream: Of being with high school friends. We were going shopping for a couch. We kept trying out different couches and asking for advice, guidance from our parents and sales folk; we were looking to older people to make the decision.

**#6** Dream: I was with my children and three adopted adolescent boys who are mature and able. We are very attached and yet aware of their preoccupation with their loss. A large group of children from group homes convenes on us.

**#5** Dream: I was at a friend's ranch in Wyoming. There were a lot of young people there, teenagers. People told me I wasn't wearing the right clothes so I changed into pink high-tops and was thus dressed up like the others. Baggy, huge jeans and a pink striped, baggy T-shirt, with my hair pulled up, Latina gang style.

**#5** Overall feeling—the theme of adolescence and looking to adults for teaching and guidance. However, realizing that they were either not noticing or their answers were stupid or "full of shit." As an adolescent, I clearly realized that the adults didn't have all the answers. I felt anxious, restless, indignant, unsettled, about finding the right answer.

# A Child Feeling Unprotected by Adults

**#1** Dream: I have a child, maybe one year old, looked after most of the time by another woman, who has a family. It is brought to me to be fed regularly. I feel great love for it. It has little characteristics of speech and behavior that are very endearing and sweet. I suddenly realize it is a terrible thing it is not with me always. She is sitting in a little box, or behind a ledge. I reach over and pull her out—whilst doing so the back of her leg scrapes on the edge of the box. The back of her knee is bruised. I hug her and apologize. I take her home and somebody says, they can't imagine why I never did so before. That evening I go to see her, and she is dead. I cry so hard, it seems I can hear myself in my sleep. I am told it was an embolism in her heart, and it was probably due to the bruise I had caused. I am devastated.

**#5** Dream: ...Suddenly, we looked out to sea and a tidal wave was coming in slow-motion to shore, and we realized a hurricane was coming. It was very surreal; we could see a huge storm a mile or two out, yet it was calm and sunny where we were. We all started to move things indoors and looked for a safe place to go.... Than someone told me that the fire station was a safe place to go. I went there, and people were standing in lines outside, just waiting; I joined them. I had the thought that I am an adolescent, and here are the adults, having us wait outside! Don't they know it isn't safe out here?

**#3** Dream: Of a machine that pressed big sheets of glass into thin sheets of glass. It was in my parents backyard. One sheet of glass was very long, 40 (meters) spanning the back yard. My sister was running beside the machine, causing anxiety because the glass is very hot. I was very nervous for her. It was dangerous; I had a lot of anxiety for my sister. I tried to tell her not to do it. Suddenly, the machine was in the house on the kitchen table. My mother got too close to it and burned her hand. I was frustrated because I had just told her to be careful. I grabbed her and took her to the sink, to run the hand under cold water. I needed someone to find some aloe vera.

**#5** Dream: For my return length, the pool was being drained very quickly; the race was being finished in just a few feet of water. I remember seeing the coach walk alongside, encouraging the swimmer, and (I was) thinking, "Why doesn't he notice that the pool is draining, why doesn't he do something?" I did the wrong stroke. The pool was draining quickly. Wondered why the adults did not do anything about this.

**#1** Dream: Of a baby chopping up large bone in butcher shop.

**#5** Dream: For some reason there were several animals in boxes. If they were left there, they would die. There also was a small child in a box. We wanted to save a dog, or a bear. The man cut the claws off the bear; they looked like plastic, white and somewhat translucent, and we affixed them to the little girl; we left the girl there to die, I guess, and rescued the animals.

## *Emotions, Not the Mind*

**#1** I wanted to lie in bed and just think of emotional thoughts.... I felt that the head associations are just so mundane and limiting.... It feels so complicated and gross, where I am having to live from and it is so hard. I keep thinking, "I'm at the wrong sphere of the universe, internally and externally." I felt I was in the wrong place, I felt gross and materialistic, the work I had to do, I mean. I had to organize some things; it felt gross, I didn't want to be there. I felt I was beyond the material sphere, somewhere else.

**#1** I was seeing a patient, and as she was talking, I suddenly became aware that she was speaking with an accent. I then wondered, "How do I understand what she is saying? How can I understand any language at all?" I thought: "I will not be able to understand her at all—and that's because I am not making any mental effort at all to understand her." So my thought was that my mental faculty is likely to disappear. I went to sit in some woods; I felt in the wrong medium. I want to be in another state, either planted in silence in the earth or existing in space.... I want to dream in a mindless state.

**#6** I have the idea that life is fine without thinking.

**#1** The term, "losing my mind," takes on new significance.... Feeling divorced from the mental realm. I have longed to communicate from the heart.

**#5** Mentally, there was a feeling of dullness, and not wanting to do anything intellectual.

**#2** I feel I am an observer, compassionate and gentle, yet still an observer. I am concerned and at a loss for how to fix things, which usually I think I am good at. I focus in more clearly on the other person, and I really listen. My perceptions are so subtle, I sometimes think I am making them up. I often have thoughts of how I can give more to others, the need is so great. I have been given so much financially, emotionally, physically, and materially.

**#6** Visceral aliveness where I don't have to think. Irritated by having to give a thinking response or if someone wants to think about something.

**#5** This afternoon I tried studying a case, working on (the proving of) carbon dioxide, but I couldn't focus on anything longer than 5-10 minutes. It's hard to describe, but it feels like the gears in my head are covered with thick, gooey, viscous gunk, and they are not moving well and they freeze. When I'm thinking clearly, it is more like a Swiss watch, very clear, crisp, brisk, and an easy flow. I just take it for granted. It is not working that way now. This only applies to mental work. Otherwise, I am just going through the motions—cooking, cleaning, driving, shopping, etcetera. That's all fine.

**#1** The feeling of being divorced from the mental realm in some way "came up" for me. An ongoing wish to communicate and not being able to explain my feelings. In the place of my mind, there was a possibility that I could operate my life from my feelings rather than my head. I did not know how to do it, but interestingly there was a possibility of that now.... I can understand everything from my heart. I have longed to communicate from the heart. This is a somewhat unrealized and unexercised level of communicating for me.

# *Sexuality*

**#3** Dream: House plants and groups of people living in a large house. I was in bed with four other people. I knew these people only vaguely, we were vaguely sexual. I was not uncomfortable in this situation; it didn't appear to be very strange that there were men and women together in one bed.

**#4** Dream: There was a large orgy, not tender, more animal-like.

**#6** Increased sexual desire and also an aliveness and a way of meeting someone immediately.

**#2** Dream: I was talking to teacher about a father of an applicant. She alluded to a sexual contact she had with this man. In the dream, there was a feeling of mystery, drama, and sexuality.

# *Body Awareness/Sensuality*

**#1** I had clarity of smell as if having inhaled menthol; it was a cool, clear and unobstructed feeling.

**#1** The bronchial passages and windpipe felt clean and as if they were expanding.

**#1** Sensation of the heart chakra being very open.

**#2** Wanted to act, not just sit. Felt hyper-alert. Went outside, tried out different spaces.

**#2** I am aware that I am observing situations from behind my eyes, very much internally. I felt focused on others' eyes; I would look into their eyes with more attention.

**#2** No food cravings, I am feeling good in my body.

**#2** Dream: Of two men, one in wheelchair (paraplegic), the other standing in front of him on the road and talking to the man in the wheelchair. He is leaning over. The man in the wheelchair took some drug, and it obviously did not work right. Here is the fear of the remedy, the fear of incapacitation. (While doing the proving.)

**#2** Acute sense of smell. The flowers had smelled exceptionally fine; cat pee in the study, shampoo in shower, all are acute smells.

**#2** Acute sense of hearing.

**#2** Dream: I dig the nails of my left hand under the skin of his neck as hard as I can. I can feel the skin break and his blood. I lay into him hard. I am fighting for my life. It is totally graphic. I am enraged, impassioned, and wild.

**#4** Dream: Suddenly, we saw him swim in the river with great ease—in and out of the tumultuous currents that would surely have drowned most people. He was diving in and out of the water like a fish. He would go into the rapids. The woman with me said we'd have to jump in and do the same thing.

**#5** Dream: A "Michael Jackson dream." I was in some large house or studio; I was waiting to take a lesson from Michael Jackson, with a gymnastic, back flip harness.

I was intrigued by this contraption. I was impatient and tired of waiting, so I tried using it by myself. I was soon buckled into it and doing back flips. I was amazed at how easy it was. Then Michael Jackson showed up, and I was embarrassed that I had started without him. Suddenly, I was nervous and became clumsy and could not use the device correctly anymore.

**#6** Resentful of having to be inside in this weather. Wanting open air. Wanting to be very physically active. Wanting to move and connect with other people this way.

**#6** Strong sense of smell. And liked it, a way of connecting. (Smell) could almost take the place of ideas. When I smell my children or my wife, it is a savoring that percolates through my being. Aware of cat peeing in the wrong places.

**#6** Spontaneous shivering or shuddering quality through body as with rush of emotion but without fever. As though something is coming alive, spine tingling.

**#7** Dream: Teaching an exercise class and had a strong sense of the exercises I was doing, especially the deep plies. How easy it was to do extreme exercise.

# *Loving Feelings*

**#1** Sensation of the heart chakra being very open. Experienced a deep sense of compassion, feeling of real joy for other people's happiness. Very spontaneous feeling of pleasure. Felt really loving, on an almost global level.

**#2** Felt very present. Emotions right there in the forefront. Felt present and connected to whomever I am relating to. I saw a picture of my nephew, whom I don't see very often, and started crying, missing him. Emotions were right "on my sleeve." Feeling of being vulnerable yet calm, refreshing feeling.... Had a really good connection with several people; one-to-one relationships were everything. People and things were smooth. There was so much loving energy coming my way; I was giving out that same energy.

**#2** I have a feeling of heightened compassion and love in the world. I am receiving many compliments. I have smooth interactions with people that I usually "bump" into. Relationships seem so good and smooth, interactions are full of love and mutual respect.

**#3** Dream: My uncle was there, I was glad to see him, I had a feeling of love for him....

**#2** Felt incredible loving feelings towards my family, towards my kids and my husband. Really a delight, wonderful. Peaceful, happy, easygoing.

# *Mother/Father/Family*

**#1** Very deep missing of my mother, who died eight years ago. I feel very sad she is dead and almost a little angry that she does not appear to me somehow. I feel needful of her for no particular reason. I just want my mother, so I dig out an old cape of hers that I have in the cupboard and that still smells very strongly of her perfume, and I wrap myself up in it. I sleep with it around me all night.

**#2** Good connection with my kids, smooth, no friction. [a mother]

**#4** Strong desire to spend time with my family. I wrestled with my son, which he likes and I usually do not. [a mother]

**#7** Dream: Two other mothers and several children were in a car and we were taking (the children) to see animals at a home. We were locked in the car and trying to figure out how to get out, but we were all happy.

**#6** Dream: I am a nurturing father and I am enjoying it. A large group of children from group homes convenes on us, and I am surprised and wonder if we can step up to this. Still calm, I attempt to feed them all but feel overwhelmed by their neediness and their feral quality or wildness. My wife returns from her great adventure hike, and I am a little resentful, but then realize I have had fun.

# *Buildings*

**#4** Dream: I was walking through a beautifully decorated house. It was decorated in pastels and white and had flowing curtains.

**#5** Dream: A very strange dream! I was in basement of large, old, decrepit house from the late 1800's. A businessman was considering buying the property. The property consisted of two houses with large dorms. It was ill kept, falling down, but beautiful buildings. It seemed that it had been used as a school, maybe a homeopathic school.

**#6** Dream: Large, sprawling, semi-wooded, farmhouse setting....

**#1** Dream: Of...strange, dark cities. Of life around the gardens now in pain. Of lots of big structures. Of industry and dark, big, old, buildings.

**#7** Dream: Moved to a new house, big in the country with clinic attached. I said: "This is perfect. We love it here."

**#5** Dream: I was living in an East Coast city on the ocean side. The architecture was like 1940-50's era. I lived near the top floor of a twenty-story building, and I was having a picnic with composites of friends I knew in the past, on the rooftop. The strange thing was that some friend looked like one person I knew and talked like another. The building was near the beach, and we had an expansive view of the ocean because the buildings around were only two to three stories high.

## MIND

- ACCEPTANCE
- *AFFECTIONATE*
- ANGER, irascibility; tendency
  - alternating with; sadness; over mother who died eight years ago
- ANXIETY; free-floating
  - germs; will catch from others
- AWARENESS heightened
- *BENEVOLENCE*
- BUSINESS; averse to
  - incapacity for
  - neglects his
- *CHEERFULNESS, gaiety, happiness; tendency*
  - *gaiety, happiness; tendency; lightness, with feeling of*
- CHILDREN; nurture, desires to
- *COMMUNICATIVE, expansive*
  - *from the heart, desire to be*
- CONCENTRATION; active
  - *difficult, troublesome*
    - *studying, reading, while*
- CONFLICT between higher consciousness and worldly existence
- CONFUSION of concentrate the mind, on attempting to
  - conversation agg.
  - knows not where she is nor whenever came to objects around her
- CONTENTED
- COUNTRY, desire for, to go into the
- DELUSIONS, imaginations
  - alien, she is
  - insane; become, that she will
- DESIRES; company; deceased mother, of
  - mother who died eight years ago
- DREAMS
  - *adolescents*
    - disturbed by adults at critical time
    - wish to be an
  - animals, of
    - bats
    - bears
    - beetles

DREAMS, animals, of (cont.)
birds, of
bugs
lethally skitter on floor while she is barefoot
chickens
dogs
fish
lizards
moths
opossums
raccoons
rats
shellfish
suspended animation, in
wolves
beautiful movements; galloping up hill in moonlight
anxious
bathroom, cannot find
beach
bombs; bomb threat
blood transfusion
*buildings*
big and beautiful
dark and old
drab and decrepit
sacred temple made of gauze
cars
*child, children; about*
adopting them
babies
death of; due to embolism mother caused
great love for her child, yet cared for by another woman
neglected
taking care of endangered parents
wildness of
*danger*
*children feel unprotected by adults*
drowning, of
unnoticed by authority figures
dead; infants
people, of; relatives
beloved
death, of; child, of
difficulties; feats actually easy

discovery of secret for performing difficult trick
embarrassment
enraged, impassioned
evil, impending; coming in to the house
families, of
fights; for existence with man who caused deep offense
forest, of a
glass sheet, very hot and dangerous; mother burned hand on
*guidance or advice; asking parents for*
    receiving unsatisfactory
high school
house, houses
    large with flowing curtains
    old
hurricane approaches, yet sunny and calm
industry
injuries; mother's hand burned by hot glass sheet
interruptions; critical moment, during
jumping
jungles, tropical rainforest
    deep ravine, woman's lover is hiding in
men; older man is ally
metamorphosis, about
    bug or beetle to moth
    man to bat
music, songs
    Jamaican reggae
    lively even though people are poor
nakedness, about
nest; moving birds to a safe place
orgies
people, of; strange things, doing
performance of teacher, observed by adolescent, is inadequate
poverty
remorse, of
    death of child due to maternal carelessness, over
*responsibility, of*
    *children, for*
        *adults overwhelmed by*
rivers
school
secret; discovery of
snow; strange dark cities filled with
strange

DREAMS (cont.)
    teacher; seen to be incompetent by adolescent
    tidal waves
    torture, of
    water; swimming in
    weeping, tearful
        death of child, over
    wild
    women; pregnant woman screaming and hitting her
    youth, time of
*DULLNESS, sluggishness, difficulty of thinking and comprehending*
    *mental exertion; from*
*EMOTIONS; spontaneous and natural*
HAPPY
IRRITABILITY; driving a car, while
JOY
    happiness, at other's
    spontaneous feelings of pleasure
LANGUAGES, amazed she can understand
*LOVE; children, for*
        *without awareness of imminent danger*
        *yet naive about responsibilities*
    exalted
    family, for
    feelings; coming toward her and from her
        given and received
    husband, for
    overflowing, for humanity
MAGNETIZED; desires to be
MEDITATION; desire to be in
*MOTHER*
PLAY; desire to, playful
PLEASURE; spontaneous feelings of
POSITIVENESS
*PROSTRATION of mind, mental exhaustion, brain fag*
RELATIONSHIPS; focus of life, are
    good, sweet and smooth, are
RELAXED feeling, letting go
*RESPONSIBILITY; aversion to*
    wants to give up her
SADNESS, despondency, depression, melancholy
    grief; with
    loss, after; death of mother
    missing mother who died eight years ago

SENSITIVE, oversensitive
- pain, to; emotional, of others

SPACED-out feeling
- desire to have

SYMPATHETIC, compassionate
THEORIZING; philosophic, mind dwells on
THINKING; will disappear, ability for
- ailments, complaints, of; agg.
- alienation of mind, mental associations are so mundane
- aversion to
- desire for
- future, of
- *long, cannot think*
- mundane, is

THOUGHTS; expressing correctly, weakened power of
- obscurity, of
- one thought excludes all other
- rapid, quick
- speculative
- vanishing; attending business, while
- vacancy of

TRANQUILLITY, serenity, calmness
VULNERABLE, emotionally; emotions on sleeve
*WORK; aversion to mental*
- crazy, seems to drive him, in mental occupation, owing to the impotency of his mind
- fatigues
- accomplish, imagines she cannot

## HEAD

HEAVINESS, sensation of
*PRESSURE; behind eyes*

## HEAD PAIN

DULL, blunt
- lasting four days
- Temples
    - left

LOCALIZATION; Occiput
- exertion, after
- extending; back, down
    - neck, to
    - temples, to
- Temples; left

## EYE

*AWARENESS of*
BAND around the eyeballs, sensation of
*PAIN; pressing, pressure*
    backward
    inward
    left
*PRESSURE; sensation of*
  forenoon
  behind eyes
  motion of eyes amel.
TWITCHING

## VISION

ACCOMMODATION; defective
BLURRED
WAVERING

## EAR

PAIN; General; extending; gums, to
      left
    mouth, buccal mucosa
      left
    teeth, to
      left lower
  stitching, stabbing
    left
    noon

## NOSE

CATARRH; dry, chronic
COLDNESS; inside; as if had smelled menthol
*OBSTRUCTION*
OPEN; nostrils feel as if had smelled menthol

## SMELL

*ACUTE*
  flowers
  cat urine

## FACE

CRACKS; corners of mouth
ERUPTIONS; acne
        chin
HEAT, flushes of

## MOUTH

SWELLING; sensation of
    Palate; sensation of
    Tongue; sensation of

## THROAT

DRYNESS
PAIN; General; extending to; ear; swallowing, on
            left
        left; morning
        swallowing; on
            liquids; amel.; warm
        warm; drinks; amel.
PRICKLING
ROUGHNESS
SWELLING; sensation of

## STOMACH

*APPETITE; capricious, hunger, but knows not for what, or refuses things when offered*
    *increased, hunger in general*
    relish, without
*INDIGESTION*
JUMPING, sensation of
THIRSTLESSNESS
    night
UNEASINESS

## ABDOMEN

AWARENESS, of
*FLATULENCE*
    rolling
FULLNESS, sensation of
PAIN; General; afternoon; agg.; 5 p.m.
        ileo-caecal region
    cramping, griping

**STOOL**

COLOR; dark
FREQUENT
*LOOSE*
SMALL

**URETHRA**

PAIN; burning; urination; agg.; close, at

**MALE**

SEXUAL; desire; decreased
    increased

**LARYNX & TRACHEA**

WEAKNESS, weak feeling

**SPEECH & VOICE**

VOICE; weak
    whispering

**RESPIRATION**

ASTHMATIC
    night; sit up, must
        10 p.m.
EASY
WHEEZING; night

**CHEST**

CONVEX, sensation chest is
EXPANSION, sensation of; bronchi
    heart
FEATHERS or petals, sensation of; overlaying chest
OPEN, as if heart chakra
*PALPITATION heart*
    night; waking; him

## BACK

- PAIN; General; cervical region
    - extending; ear, to the; left, behind
  - left
    - aggravation bending left
    - pressure amel.
  - morning; waking, on
  - heat, with
  - aching; sacral region
    - afternoon
    - from long standing
  - pressing; sacral region
    - evening
- STIFFNESS; Cervical region
    - waking, on
  - Lumbar region
    - waking, on
- TENSION; Cervical region
  - Dorsal region

## EXTREMITIES

- DISLOCATION, sprains; Ankle; as if
  - Foot; ; as if
  - Hand; as if
  - Wrist; as if
- PARALYSIS; sensation of; night
- RESTLESSNESS
  - Leg
- STIFFNESS
  - Joints
  - Elbow, Knee, Ankle
    - morning
- TENSION; Foot
  - Hand
  - Wrist

## EXTREMITY PAIN

- DISLOCATION, feeling of; Ankle
  - Foot
  - Hand, joints of
  - Wrist
- *LOWER LIMBS; Knee; right*
    - walking amel.

## SLEEP

SLEEPINESS; afternoon
        4 p.m.
    driving, from
        air; open amel.
    evening
        8:30 p.m.
*WAKING; frequent*

## CHILL

CHILLINESS; headache; during

## FEVER

HEAT; EVENING; 6 p.m.
    INTERNAL heat; evening

## PERSPIRATION

CLAMMY
    evening

## SKIN

CICATRICES; painful
    red, become

## GENERALITIES

AIR; open; amel.
        *desire for*
EXERTION, physical; desires
FOOD and drinks; bacon; desires
        yet does not enjoy
    cold; drinks, water; desires cool
    fried food
    warm; drinks; desires
*HEAT; sensation of*
    as if fever
    internally
    on waking
SHUDDERING, nervous; emotions as if from
*WEAKNESS, enervation, exhaustion, prostration, infirmity; afternoon*
    *evening; agg.; 8:30 p.m.*

EDITOR'S NOTE: *Punctuation, abbreviations, and individual stylistic nuances of the original journal entries have been preserved wherever possible.*

**Prover #1 · Female · 49 years old**

**Day 1**

◆ When I first received the remedy, I didn't take it right away; I had a lot going on, so I started on 2/5/96. I held the bottle to see what would be my first impression, it was a sharp prickly sensation, then I had a picture of a lizard and then blossoms. Then I took the remedy.

◆ Afterwards my left eye felt like being compacted and pushed inwards; that was in the lower area of my face in the mouth area; it felt elongated.

◆ I had clarity of smell as if having inhaled menthol; it was a cool, clear and unobstructed feeling.

◆ The bronchial passages and wind pipe felt clean and as if they were expanding. Sensation of a convex chest. It felt like a bird's breast. Sensation of feathers or petals in chest area, some soft overlay feeling in that region.

Felt a click in chest area and bronchial passages, as of chest expanding.

Terrific ease of breathing. Noticeable that breathing felt easy. When lying in bed; arms felt as if I wanted to stretch them, but I couldn't move.

◆ Throat: A prickly feeling in my throat.

◆ Restless legs.

◆ Dream: Unremembered story. Of a baby chopping up a large bone in a butcher's shop. Like a European butcher shop. Doesn't remember more about baby.

◆ General sensations, recorded after the first day of taking the remedy: openness and expansion in chest, heart and solar plexus.

◆ Sleep: Did not sleep well. Woke up throughout the night. Waking with stiff elbows, knees, and neck.

**Day 2**

◆ Head: Pressing inwards in morning in late afternoon.

◆ Eyes: Felt jiggly and hard to focus.

◆ Sensation of the heart chakra being very open. Experienced a deep sense of compassion, feeling of real joy for other people's happiness. Very spontaneous feeling of pleasure. Very spacey. Felt really loving on an almost global level.

No mental energy, did not want to do anything involving mental outputs, did not want to do anything with my head. I thought the only way out of this feeling was to go home and lie on my bed and daydream. I just wanted to lie there and just think of things, especially emotional thoughts. I felt that the head associations are just so mundane and limiting.

◆ Sleep: I wanted to sleep. (4 p.m.) Waking in the afternoon. Woke feeling very hot as though I had a fever. Face flushed and burning.

◆ Stomach: Food felt stuck in stomach.

◆ Felt shaky and inner trembling.

◆ Dream: Of being tortured. A red-hot metal pole is hammered up my backside. Of coals stuck up me. It is scary but not painful. Other various tortures.

◆ Dream: I meet an ex-boyfriend, a short dark-haired woman comes raging out of the house; she is enormously pregnant, she is hitting me, screaming, shouting at me and crying, it is scary.

**Day 3**

◆ Chaotic day! Could not find anything in the house that I needed, everything seems a mess. There is no method to my work, no structure. I start doing ten things at once; and I follow none of them through. It's a tremendous effort to try to follow anything through. I just want to "space out" on another level of consciousness.

◆ It feels so complicated and gross, where I am having to live from and it is so hard. I keep thinking, "I'm at the wrong sphere of the universe, internally and externally." I felt I was in the wrong place, I felt gross and materialistic, the work I had to do I mean. I had to organize some things; it felt gross, I didn't want to be there. I felt I was beyond the material sphere, somewhere else.

◆ I was seeing a patient, and as she was talking, I suddenly became aware that she was talking in an accent. I then wondered, "How do I understand what she is saying? How can I understand any language at all?" I thought, "I will not be able to understand her at all—and that's because I am not making any mental effort at all to understand her." So my thought was that the mental faculty is likely to disappear.

◆ I went to sit in some woods. I felt in the wrong medium. I wanted to be in another state, either planted in silence in the earth or existing in space. I wanted to be in a relative quiet state that comes in meditation, that seems to be the state that part of me is in. I didn't want to be at a mundane level.

Similarly when driving along the road, I had a moment of panic; suddenly I did not know what road to drive on. "So Americans drive on the left side..."—very quick I needed to know "How do I know this?" There was confusion as to what side I was on.

◆ I don't feel competent in anything, I want to dream in a mindless state. "No!" I thought, I'm going nuts. I had just this feeling of, "Oh, am I losing my mind?" It was hard to be disciplined, to do mundane tasks, it was awful to deal with office work, it pulled me down, kept me submerged. I don't mind doing new things, reading new material when learning things that interest me. It is fine to apply myself. My heart is still open.

◆ Dream: I have a child, maybe one year old, looked after most of the time by another woman, who has family. It is brought to me to be fed regularly. I feel great love for it. It has little characteristics of speech and behavior that are very endearing and sweet. I suddenly realize it is a terrible thing it is not with me always. She is sitting in a little box, or behind a ledge. I reach over and pull her out—whilst doing so the back of her leg scrapes on the edge of the box. The back of her knee is bruised. I hug her and apologize. I take her home and somebody says, they can't imagine why I never did so before. That evening I go to see her and she is dead. I cry so hard, it seems I can hear myself in my sleep. I am told it was an embolism in her heart and it was probably due to the bruise I had caused. I am devastated.

◆ Dream: Of arranging to marry my ex-husband again, but when the baby dies I see no point and won't continue with the plans. Other people are upset.

◆ Dream of snow and ice in strange dark cities. Of life around the gardens now in pain. Of lots of big structures. Of industry and dark big old buildings, sense of having dreamed of family children and babies, nostalgia and anxiety and sadness.

◆ Confusion as to which side (of the street) I'm on. It is a momentary flash of fear. I just feel that I'm not quite on earth and it's a strange place. I don't feel competent to deal with it (life) totally, I feel a bit like an alien.

◆ I feel very tired, too tired to do anything with my ordinary mind, I want to dream, or just go into a mindless state, not to sleep, but yet not to be without intelligence either. The emotional and or psychic realms are where I am reaching for, or wanting to connect to.

◆ The term "losing my mind" takes on a new significance; it feels like that, but not in a disturbing or nutty sort of way. It is hard to be disciplined in regular work, there is a tremendous resistance. In mundane tasks, like washing up dishes or cleaning, or feeding the animals. It is awful to have to deal with business mail, returning or making telephone calls and office work. It feels as though it pulls me down and keeps me submerged in the material level.

◆ I don't mind reading or studying, where I am learning new things; i.e. my Buddhist study group or homeopathic books, that is nice, I can get absorbed in that.

◆ The area of the heart seems expanded, open physiologically and emotionally.

◆ Very deep missing of my mother, who died eight years ago. I feel very sad she is dead and almost a little angry that she does not appear to me somehow. I feel needful of her for no particular reason. I just want my mother, so I dig out an old cape of hers that I have in the cupboard and that still smells very strongly of her perfume and I wrap myself up in it. I sleep with it around me all night.

◆ The next day I woke up feeling absolutely back to my normal usual self. Felt very good. There seemed to be no trace of the proving, or unusual symptoms. I feel quite relieved, since I have much work to do, that had been impossible. I intend to take the remedy again if there are still no symptoms.

◆ I considered the remedy to be very sudden in its onset and short acting.

**Day 4**

◆ Woke in the morning completely covered with poison oak all over body. This poison oak could have been from the cape because I used to wear it in the woods. Woke up, my face is a bit itchy, looked in mirror and the left eye is very swollen, noticed spot on hand, hands and legs and then felt systematically chilly, shivering and hot at same time. More and more poison oak eruptions appeared. I could barely see. My eyes looked like two dots in marshmallow mountains, couldn't open my eyes in the morning.

The bottom, legs, tummy and sides felt really itchy, I felt really ill, took a bath, it helped

to lie in the bath with baking soda. Remedies did not help much; finally I took Pulsatilla which did not help the itching but helped me feel better in my self.
◆ Proving was discontinued on day four. Had to take other remedies because I felt really sick from the poison oak. The last week and a half I've been recovering.

Summary of the proving:
There seemed a lot around the feeling of expansiveness of the emotional center. Mothers and babies came up a lot.
The feeling of being divorced from the mental realm in some way "came up" for me. An ongoing wish to communicate and not being able to explain feelings. In the place of my mind there was a possibility that I could operate my life from my feelings rather than my head. I did not know how to do it, but interestingly there was a possibility of that now. If I could take the time to understand that it was something which was worth opening up to, then it was possible I would do it. There seemed to be a whole other place of interpreting language. I can understand everything from my heart. I have longed to communicate from the heart. This is a somewhat unrealized and unexercised level of communicating for me.

**Prover #2 · Female · 44 years old**

◆ This is the first time I have done a proving. It is so similar to the previous prover! I was "blown away" by the similarity of the account that she gave. I took the remedy at 8 a.m.
◆ At 9 a.m., felt heaviness around the eyes.
On Sunday 2/4/96 twitching for an hour. Felt a band around the eyes. Sensation behind the eyes as of an internal band, ability to focus impaired.
Pressure around the eyes stayed until midday. Ameliorated by movement.
Very aware of my eyes. Pressure in the head behind the eyes.
◆ Urge to keep my mind moving, wanted to keep shifting perspectives. Wanted to act, not just sit. Felt hyper-alert. Went outside, tried out different spaces. Felt incredible loving feelings towards my family, towards my kids and my husband. Really a delight, wonderful. Peaceful happy easygoing. By late afternoon felt fine, myself again.

**Day 2**
◆ Sound sleep. Waking easy.
◆ Stool not quite as soft as usual.
◆ 10.30 a.m.—pressure behind and around the eye sockets.
◆ Felt very present. Emotions right there in the forefront. Felt present and connected to whomever I am relating to.
◆ Drove the car pool, was late. Irritable in the car, another driver almost hit me.
I saw a picture of my nephew, whom I don't see very often, and started crying, missing him. Emotions were right "on my sleeve," feeling of being vulnerable yet calm, refreshing feeling.
◆ Had a really good connection with several people; one-to-one relationships were everything.

People and things were smooth. There was so much loving energy coming my way, I was giving out that same energy.
◆ 7:30 p.m. slight knee pain, inside of the right knee, as I walked, the pain went away.
◆ 3 p.m. in the afternoon, mild pain and pressure in eye sockets, in the bone.
◆ 5 p.m. sensation of mild pressure and pain in right sacral area, also in the lower right and front abdomen.
◆ 6 p.m. felt internally hot and clammy but calm and slow at the same time. Clammy head.
◆ I am receiving good energy and compliments from people, they tell me that I am beautiful.

**Day 3**
◆ Right lower back pain.
◆ I feel a fullness in pelvis, more gas, moving and rolling sensation. Awareness of that area.
◆ I am aware that I am observing situations from behind my eyes, very much internally. I felt focused on others' eyes; I would look into their eyes with more attention. Pressure behind the eyes continued.
◆ Relationships are the focus, things are going good, sweet and smooth. A neighbor called for help with her daughter, I went and helped her and I felt good and unruffled by the situation; felt in a neutral vantage point, not disconnected but mentally not engaged. There is a spacious acceptance of things. Very much heartfelt, the "edges are smooth." I feel like "not needing to fix things," critical thoughts have no power. Observing and positive.
◆ No food cravings, I am feeling good in my body.
◆ Dream: Of two men, one in wheelchair (paraplegic) the other standing in front of him on the road and talking to the man in the wheelchair. He is leaning over. The man in the wheelchair took some drug and it obviously did not work right. Here is the fear of the remedy, the fear of incapacitation. (While doing the proving.)
◆ Dream: I am sitting with friend on her bed, in Washington D.C. I am visiting her for two nights, it is so nice; they (her husband and she) are such good friends. She visited me, I am watching her husband J. read a story to my daughter and son. I have a warm feeling of love and gratitude for having friends.

**Day 4**
◆ Acute sense of smell. The flowers had smelled exceptionally fine, cat pee in the study, shampoo in shower, all are acute smells.
◆ Morning: No constriction or pressure around the eyes, yet I am still more aware of them than usual. 6.00 p.m. Increasing pain around the eyes, the insides of the sockets are dull and aching.
◆ My body feels good.
◆ I have a feeling of heightened compassion and love in the world. I am receiving many compliments. I have smooth interactions with people that I usually "bump" into. Relationships seem so good and smooth, interactions are full of love and mutual respect.
◆ Dream: I was talking to teacher about a father of an applicant. She alluded to a sexual contact she had with this man. In the dream there was a feeling of mystery, drama and sexuality.

**Day 5**

◆ Very mild awareness around my eyes. It sometimes rises to pain, then it subsides. Sometimes I forget about it, usually when I'm engaged in conversation, or at work.

◆ My body and emotions feel very normal to me, it seems the effects of the proving have waned.

◆ Some gas. Slightly darker stool than usual( at 2:00 in the afternoon).

◆ I'm starting to want the remedy again. I feel more easily irritated, got "on my son's case" about some sloppy homework. I noticed that all the loving feelings and the spacious feelings were slipping away.

**Day 6**

◆ I am feeling good.

◆ There is a mild awareness of my eyes.

◆ Late afternoon, aching in the lower back—have been standing all day on my feet.

◆ I am feeling a little more separate. I don't feel as spacious and loving as I did shortly after taking the remedy. I am moving in and out of these spaces. It feels like I am coming out of that loving space, a little more mind oriented.

**Day 7**

◆ Dream: I am observing a wolf, he is black with mottled gray. He is in the woods, running uphill and bounding down again. The wolf is wild but bushy, like a dog. It is nighttime. I am observing, as if I weren't there. My son is with me. We are awed by the agility and beauty of the animal. Then another wolf comes from the right, the first wolf bounds up to greet this one. They move to edge of woods into the moonlight and gallop up the open hill. In the shadows I see a man, also appearing from the right, running after them. My son and I run to a new spot near a tree to be ready to see them again upon their return. There is some fear of the wolves coming for us but mostly awe of the beauty of their movements.

◆ Spent last night and today with a group of mothers and daughters from my son's class. It was very moving to hear girls (13 years old) express themselves. Tears came to my eyes several times, at the expression of pain and separation, wanted to be treated still as young girls, but also wanting their freedom at the same time. There was a wave of desires and needs and missed communications, so poignant. I was so glad to be part of this sharing.

◆ I had a phone call, connected with work, I felt attacked, but I did not defend myself, I was at a loss about what to do, didn't know what to do with it, my edges coming up but different than usual.

◆ Slight band around my eyes.

◆ Stools are regular.

**Day 8**

◆ Feeling good. Spirits good.

◆ No sensation around the eyes.

**Day 9**

◆ Morning: I am feeling good.

◆ Evening: Had a bumpy phone call, doing enrollment work, it caught me by surprise, I couldn't find a way to be smooth. The "edges" are showing again. Nothing new.
◆ I am feeling attacked, not reacting, speechless. Yet below the surface the irritation or anger seem to be gone, I am not looking to fix things. I am more observant and thoughtful.
◆ Sensation around the eyes is gone.

**Day 10**
◆ Dream: Of a shellfish in water under waves, watching to see different kinds am standing in water near the beach, waves draw back and uncover fish, then wash over them again. I am observing the movement of the fish.
◆ Dream: There is a bug like a beetle a centipede and moth, all put together that has gotten loose in the kitchen. It is not my house, but I am there. Some guy is responsible for having let it in, I got it by mistake. It is lethal, if it stings or bites you. I realize that I am in bare feet, we see the bug skitter on his back, across the floor, then it turns over, and then it starts to fly, this is a big surprise to me and then we lose sight of it. I start slapping my clothing, hoping it is not in my pant leg. I leave in a car, still worried about where this critter is.
◆ Took 15 pellets of the remedy on Tuesday the 12th at 6:00 a.m.
◆ That evening fullness in nose. Fullness at the top of the nose. Stuffy.
◆ The same eye sensations as before, when taking the remedy at first, but not as strong the first time. Sensation of fullness, building awareness.
◆ Afternoon: 5 p.m. Relaxed eyes.
◆ Slight ache in lower right, which I had a week before taking the remedy. Familiar ache (old symptom).
Slightly clammy.
◆ Pain in lower right sacrum. Mild pointed pain.
◆ I am feeling smooth and observing and slightly paranoid. Started to feel more confused, things not as clear, more confused about what is old and what is new.
Smooth relaxation with kids.

**Day 11**
◆ Dream: I am in Jamaica (I have never been), with a woman friend. We are walking through town; I ask if this is shanty town, it is so poor here, the huts are monotone, dark built from mud. We seem to be looking for a friend or something. There is music playing, such great music, it is reggae music, so colorful and lively but I see everything in dark poor browns and grays. The music is so lively. I am feeling a sense of what it is like, living in that poverty and flatness and mud and contact with music that feels upbeat.
◆ Acute sense of smell.
◆ Acute sense of hearing.
◆ I feel a little confused, because things feel so smooth and then I bump, and then it is smooth again, feel a little detached, but very loving and in love with life. There is a strong heart feeling definitely present.
◆ It is Valentine's Day, I am so grateful to my husband, my boys and my friends. I am way more sensitized to pain, my own and other people's. I realize I have less of my own agenda.

I feel I am an observer, compassionate and gentle, yet still an observer. I am concerned and at a loss of how to fix things, which usually I think I am good at. I focus in more clearly on the other person, and I really listen. My perceptions are so subtle, I sometimes think I am making them up. Thoughts are often of how I can give more to others, the need is so great. I have been given so much financially, emotionally physically and materially.

**Day 12**

◆ My relationships are good, I had a good walk with my neighbors, had generous feelings towards them of attachment.

◆ So smooth. Couldn't catch my dreams, yet my sleep even though interrupted by cats coming in and out was smooth, calm and restful.

◆ 5 p.m. perspiration clammy and internally hot.

◆ Chocolate craving (usual pre-period symptom).

◆ Pain in lower right neck, radiating down to the shoulder. It makes me move with extra awareness. At 10:00 p.m. the neck is fine.

◆ Lower back stiff in the morning, fine by the afternoon.

◆ Pimple on my chin.

◆ Dream: This is strongest dream I ever had. In the dream I am a man wrestling with another man. I have dark hair, the other guy is blonde. Duality. At some point the other guy plays unfair, he does something that totally offends me (maybe this was done before we fight), so I attack this person. So graphic, I dig the nails of my left hand under the skin of his neck as hard as I can. I can feel the skin break and his blood. I lay into him hard. I am fighting for my life. It is totally graphic. I am enraged, impassioned and wild.

It is clear that I have finished, completed something—I go to my car sobbing, racked with tears. I am stunned by the passion and power of it. I go to my car, just sobbing. I back up the car into my driveway. A third guy, who feels like my friend and ally, helps me out of the car. (He must also have watched the car.) We go to house, into the kitchen where an older man is; he seems to understand what is happening. The blonde guy from the fight walks by outside the door. My friend and ally just goes and closes the door. I am still sobbing from my gut, I woke up in tears.

◆ To me the dream was about huge righteous anger, all boundaries have been disregarded, I am fighting for my existence—my moral existence, but I had an ally.

**Day 13**

◆ I am extremely tired—I think from the dream.

◆ Awareness of eyes. Awareness of neck.

**Prover #3 · Male · 33 years old**

**Day 1**

◆ This is my first proving. I took the first dose at 9:30 in p.m.

◆ Within the first half hour I had an asthma attack.

Wheezing rattle, > sitting upright.

The asthma is not necessarily different from the usual symptoms of asthma which I experience from time to time. Yet, I had not done anything to trigger an attack. I did have brand new sheets on the bed, though it may or may not have been those sheets.

◆ Dryness in the throat. This dryness happens occasionally after salty foods (didn't have any salty foods). Parched sensation. Sudden onset.

◆ Dull headache in left temple, soft round pain.

Direction: moving around to my right eye; managed to go to sleep.

**Day 2**

◆ Dream: Could not remember dreams. By the time I am fully awake I have forgotten them. That night had a snippet of a dream; I was dreaming of house plants and groups of people living in a large house. I was in bed with four other people, I knew these people only vaguely. We were vaguely sexual.

◆ I woke up thinking about that dream. The feeling in the dream was that people were friends. I don't know them well, but we are colleagues. I was not uncomfortable in this situation, it didn't appear to be very strange that there were men and women together in one bed.

◆ The next day was a weekend, had a somewhat lazy day. I had moderate physical and intellectual energy.

◆ Frequent bowel movements (four) over several hours. Loose stool.

**Day 3**

◆ Dream: I was going to the dentist in the shopping mall (not where any dentist really is). The dentist turned into my Ph.D. advisor and the office turned into a home office. There were no tools or equipment in the office. For a period of time I was naked, suddenly the dream seemed to turn into some kind of anxiety dream, I needed to get some clothes on. Then I had shorts and a T-shirt on. I was going to walk back to my house naked. I was not anxious at first, then I realized that this would be embarrassing. I went back to the dentist twice; on my second visit my advisor had forgotten to write my appointment down. My uncle was there, I was glad to see him. I had a feeling of love for him and no real other sensation other than that he was dead. (He died two years ago, from leukemia.) He was giving me advice. He gave me some computer equipment. It didn't seem to matter that he was dead.

◆ Dream: Of a bomb threat in a downtown city, dogs and the police trying to find the bomb. I was involved somehow. (Before bed I finished a book that ended with an anarchist trying to bomb a city's waterworks.)

◆ Overall slept well.

**Day 4**

◆ No noticeable symptoms.

**Day 5**

◆ Woke with neck and upper back pain. Pointed and sharp pain, down towards middle of back, hot quality. (Comes because of poor stretching at dance classes last night.)

◆ Tired and low energy by late afternoon. Very busy at work. Too little sleep. Too much to do.

**Day 6**

◆ No physical symptoms. Tired, but I've been working twelve hours a day, not much sexual energy, probably for the same reason.

◆ Dream: Of a machine that pressed big sheets of glass into thin sheets of glass. It was in my parents' backyard. One sheet of glass was very long, forty (meters) spanning the backyard; sister was running besides the machine, causing anxiety because the glass is very hot. I was very nervous for her. It was dangerous, I had a lot of anxiety for my sister. I tried to tell her not to do it. Suddenly the machine was in house on the kitchen table. My mother got too close to it and burned her hand. I was frustrated because I had just told her to be careful. I grabbed her and took her to the sink, to run the hand under cold water. I needed someone to find some aloe vera.

**Day 7**

◆ Throat a little rough.

◆ On waking, I don't feel like talking, do not have the energy to speak so I whisper. I feel like I don't want to push my vocal cords.

**Day 8**

◆ Work this week is wearing me down.

By 8.30 p.m. I feel winded like I had just run a race.

**Day 9**

◆ Tired but relaxed, no physical symptoms of note.

**Day 10**

◆ Had lots of dreams that I could only remember in snippets.

I know that I have dreams, even if I don't remember them fully.

◆ Dream: About needing a blood transfusion.

◆ Dream: About the president of my company. Anxious because I was driving my wife's car, and I was anxious because it was parked, so that it would block him.

◆ Dream: About cooking for lots of people, I was excited about it.

◆ For the most part, the dreams were not anxiety based but calm replays of events that have taken place over the last few days.

**Day 11**

◆ I woke up anxious about the coming work week.

◆ Woke with neck pain on left side, slightly painful behind the ear. Muscle pain up and down the neck, especially when tilted slightly towards the left shoulder. Pain feels better when pushed hard with fingers. Pain > pressure. It is a cool pain.

◆ Moderate energy level today.

◆ Repeated the remedy—took one more dose in the evening.
I did this due to the lack of dreams, and strong physical symptoms.

**Day 12**

◆ Pain fading.

◆ Could not remember any dreams. Once again, I've had several dreams, but I could not remember them upon waking. I know this because I always wake precisely at 5 a.m., just long enough to look at the clock, recognize I've had dreams, than fall back asleep. Usually I will remember one or two dreams, but maybe my mental exhaustion is stifling this.

◆ Bowel movements still irregular. I've had slightly smaller bowel movements, than usual, which I would attribute to recent intake of spicy food. Slightly more gas too.

◆ I am pushing my limits for multi-tasking, i.e. I can't handle too many more responsibilities, my present state is stressed.

**Day 13**

◆ Loose bowel movement.
Unsettled feeling in my stomach. "Jumpy." Mild cramps.

**Day 14**

◆ Woke with having to have bowel movement. Loose stool.

◆ Feeling of needing to whisper in the morning instead of talking.

**Day 15**

◆ Yesterday and last night feeling crummy in gut and noticed day before and today that I woke having to have a bowel movement, which was not particularly satisfying.

◆ Energy level is okay, considering that it is Friday.

◆ Again, I can't recall any dreams. I have a feeling that at least one dream had some theme of a sexual content.

**Day 16**

◆ Overall reflections: I have been in control of myself and with people. I've been "staying on top" despite demands. I've been doing good things in challenges.
I remember that I have had an increased desire for junk food, greasy fried food, wanted to get French fries, did not want to eat healthy food, wanted some intangible junk food.

◆ I did not notice anything physically "way out" of the normal.

**Prover #4 · Female · 31 years old**

**Day 1**

◆ Dream: The dream took place in a jungle with a very deep ravine and with a huge strong river flowing through it. A woman asked me to help find her lover who was hiding from either the law or a group of bad guys. We climbed up a tall pipe that crossed over the river to see if we could see him, and we looked down. It was very high and I began to panic. The only way down was to jump into the fast-moving current. We were up hundreds of feet in the air. I began grasping for the pipe with the attitude that I was sure to fall, almost wishing my worst fear of falling to come true. I said to myself: "Is this the way that 'Aurum' feels?" I desired to jump or let go. Then, suddenly, we saw him swim in the river with great ease, in and out of the tumultuous currents that would surely have drowned most people. He was diving in and out of the water like a fish. He would go into the rapids. The woman with me said we'd have to jump and do the same thing. Next we were in a house at the bottom of the ravine, it was a southern large grass house, and it had a verandah. The woman's lover comes to us in the form of a huge black bat. Being scared of bats I sprayed something in his face and he fell down, died; but I knew that her lover was very strong, indestructible and he would just take another form and come back to life. Came back as seven-foot man and he and his lover went off to dinner. Then there was a large orgy, not tender, more animal-like.

**Day 2**

◆ Sleep was overall unsettled. Less sound.
◆ Strong desire to spend time with my family. I wrestled with my son which he likes and I usually do not.
◆ Low energy. Sensation of heaviness, similar to a drug hangover.
Body temperature much warmer, markedly so.
◆ Appetite increased. Nausea at 10:20 p.m.
◆ Sexual desire strong.
◆ Repeated the remedy.
◆ Only minutes after taking the remedy I got strong heart palpitations, awareness of my chest.

**Day 3**

◆ Dream: I was walking through a beautifully decorated house. It was decorated in pastels and white, it had flowy curtains. I was on a road trip.
◆ Dream: A man gives me some computer parts.
◆ Sleep disturbed, not sound. Waking frequently.
◆ Heavy sensation in the head. Heavy sensation around the eyes, markedly so.
◆ Dullness of mind. Low energy. Physically stronger but mentally weaker.
◆ Heart palpitations and conscious of the chest region.
◆ Markedly less thirsty than usual especially at night.
Appetite markedly increased.
◆ Body temperature markedly warmer.

**Prover #5 · Female · 34 years old**

◆ I am aware of performance anxiety (as about to share experiences of the proving with 20 other provers).
◆ I took the first dose of the remedy on 2/1. 15 min. after taking the remedy, I had a marked return of sore throat. The pain was bilateral, < swallowing, > warm drinks.
◆ Dream: A "Michael Jackson dream." I was in some large house or studio, I was waiting to take a lesson from Michael Jackson, with a gymnastic back flip harness. I was intrigued by this contraption, I was impatient and tired of waiting so tried using it by myself. I was soon buckled into it and doing back flips. I was amazed at how easy it was. Then Michael Jackson showed up, and I was embarrassed that I had started without him. Suddenly I was nervous and became clumsy and could not use the device correctly anymore. The feeling was of being caught: feeling sheepish and as if I was doing something wrong and I felt inadequate in the presence of someone well-known. Also, there was a feeling of having discovered the hidden trick behind a technique. My attitude towards Michael Jackson is best described by the saying "The Emperor has no clothes." I realized it may be easier to do his thing than I formerly thought.
◆ Afraid I would catch germs from a patient.
◆ More tired in general.
◆ Two bowel movements in the day, loose stools.

**Day 3**
◆ Dream: I dreamed of being with high school friends. We were going shopping for a couch. We kept trying out different couches, and asking for advice, guidance from our parents and sales folk, we were looking to older people to make the decision. The feeling was somewhat lighthearted but there was apprehension about choosing the wrong couch. There was a definite tone: "This is no small decision—this is a big purchase—a major commitment!"
◆ Felt very shaky in the early afternoon, between 1:30-3:00 p.m. Felt anxious in the evening and could not stop eating pretzels. I am not sure "what is up;" normally, if I do feel anxious it is for a definite cause and this feeling is very generalized and free-floating.
◆ Less control to stop eating. Eating without relish.

**Day 4**
◆ Dream: Dreamed of the movie, "Dead Man Walking," the movie, which I had seen last night. Basically, it was just reexperiencing the movie, nothing different.
◆ Whilst eating breakfast of potatoes, sun-dried tomatoes and goat cheese I realized that my mouth and palate and tongue felt numb and swollen. My upper windpipe felt somewhat closed or rather narrower. I thought immediately that it must be an allergic reaction—and wondered if I should be worried, or/and go for an epi-shot in case I started to go into anaphylaxis. I never ever had anything like this in my life. (I eat potatoes, sun-dried tomatoes and goat cheese frequently.) I stopped eating and gradually my mouth and throat improved, and came back to normal.

◆ I didn't connect that reaction to the remedy until much later. I also remember, yesterday at dinner thinking about my father-in-law's peanut allergy while having peanuts in a Thai restaurant. I recalled the scene from the movie where Sean Penn received an antihistamine injection before his death from lethal injection. All these events didn't particularly affect me emotionally. I felt an almost clinical detachment.
◆ I remember thinking rationally: "I am only half a mile from an emergency room. And I could probably get there myself." Yet later at about 11 a.m. I felt emotional thinking about it and panic-stricken that it was probably the remedy and felt a fight and flight response/adrenaline rush. Felt more weak and shaky early noon, 12:30-2:00 p.m. That might have been some adrenaline leftover.
◆ Mentally there was a feeling of dullness, and not wanting to do anything intellectual.

**Day 5**
◆ Felt tired in the afternoon, 1:00-2:00. Had to drive to Berkeley, and felt snoozey in the car, wanted to pull over and nap. Felt better with the window open, > fresh air. Felt tired after dance class, which usually invigorates me, I was ready for bed by 9:30 p.m.

**Day 6**
◆ Slightly sore on first waking.
◆ It was long day at work, it was productive and good. I felt resentful that I had to be indoors working on such a beautiful day. I wished I was a kid.
◆ Thirst: I seem to be craving warm drinks especially mint tea, although I tend to finish drinking it normally when it's room temperature.
◆ Stool is loose.

**Day 7**
◆ Dream: About wishing I could be an adolescent again. I was at high school swim team, the team needed one more person to make it complete. It was a sidestroke event. They asked me to take part and I said yes. For some reason we were going off a low diving board to start each length. I was embarrassed because I dove in and practically made it to the other side before I came up for air. For my return length, the pool was being drained very quickly, the race was being finished in just a few feet of water. I remember seeing the coach walk along side encouraging the swimmer and thinking, "Why doesn't he notice that the pool is draining, why doesn't he do something?" I did the wrong stroke. The pool was draining quickly. Wondered why the adults did not do anything about this.
◆ Thirsty; craving warm drinks.
◆ Stool still loose.
◆ Extremely tired in p.m. Fell asleep reading at 8:30 p.m. I don't remember doing this for years.

**Day 8**
◆ Dream: I was living in an East Coast city on the ocean side, the architecture was like 1940-50's era. I lived near the top floor of a 20-story building and I was having a picnic with composites of friends I knew in the past, on the rooftop. The strange thing was that some friend looked like one person I knew, and talked like another. The building was

near the beach, and we had an expansive view of the ocean because the buildings around were only two to three stories high. Suddenly we looked out to sea and a tidal wave was coming in slow-motion to shore and we realized a hurricane was coming. It was very surreal, we could see a huge storm a mile or two out, yet it was calm and sunny where we were. We all started to move things indoors and looked for a safe place to go. I heard a tornado went towards Second Avenue, and I realized my car was parked in the tornado route. Than someone told me that the fire station was safe place to go. I went there and people were standing in lines outside, just waiting. I joined them. I had the thought that I am an adolescent, and here are the adults, having us wait outside! Don't they know it isn't safe out here?

◆ Dream: I was going to some lecture at University of Toronto and there was a charismatic lecturer. (I'm not sure on what topic.) I was walking around through this large building, upstairs and downstairs, trying to find the lecture hall. I did not recognize the campus or the building. There I was looking for a bathroom. First I could not find a bathroom. Then I saw two doors marked "men" and "women." I went into the women's, and it was a large dorm room with five beds in it. There was no one there. I thought maybe they'd let me use their bathroom, but there was none to be seen. Then I realized I'd better hurry, or I'd miss the lecture. All of a sudden I had a long glass cylinder of gas in a dolly that I was bringing with me; it seemed to belong to my husband. I found the lecture hall, but I couldn't bring the gas cylinder in. Somebody said: "Put it there!" But I didn't want to leave it because I thought it would be stolen. It again was the idea that the adults could not see the inappropriateness of the situation.

◆ Throat slightly sore on waking, left side. Pain radiates to the left ear on swallowing.

◆ Ear pain, stitching. Side; left. Started at 12:00 noon, lasting until early evening. Pain, pressure, occasionally winced from pain. Felt like an otitis media. I've not had one in years. Pain gone by dinnertime.

Some pain in left buccal mucosa and teeth, < lower teeth and gums. From ear ache.

**Day 9**

◆ Ear fine.

◆ This afternoon I tried studying a case, doing proving work for carbon dioxide, but I couldn't focus on anything longer than five to ten minutes. It's hard to describe, but it feels like the gears in my head are covered with thick gooey viscous gunk and they are not moving well and that they freeze. When I'm thinking clearly it is more like a Swiss watch, very clear, crisp, brisk and an easy flow. I just take it for granted. It is not working that way now, this only applies to mental work. Otherwise I am just going through the motions, cooking, cleaning, driving, shopping, etc. that's all fine.

**Day 10**

◆ Can't get myself to do mental work, I attempt to do so, but my mind seems dull. I feel lethargic, can't get into things.

◆ Thirst for cool water.

◆ Slight burning at close of urination. This is unusual, since I drank a lot of water. I have had this symptom in the past, but only if I'm really dehydrated.

**Day 11**

◆ Felt especially irritable and impatient at a meeting, though this was probably due to the facilitation.

◆ Dry coryza; stuffy, but can still breathe through.

◆ Indigestion, slight from a piece of pumpkin pie, uncomfortable feeling, lasted thirty minutes. Acid reflux. Ordered an omelet with bacon, it seemed like I really had to have bacon, but I did not enjoy it.

◆ Mild burning at the close of urination.

**Day 12**

◆ Catarrh, stuffy.

◆ Crack in the corner of mouth. Although it is not entirely unusual to get cheilosis for me, it only happens when I am under a lot of stress, and not taking care of myself. This was unusual, also it did not respond quickly to taking B-complex, which it usually does.

**Day 13**

◆ Dream: A very strange dream! I was in basement of large old decrepit house, from the late 1800's. A businessman was considering buying the property. The property consisted of two houses with large dorms. It was ill kept, falling down, but beautiful buildings. It seemed that it had been used as a school, maybe a homeopathic school. It had gone bankrupt forty or fifty years ago, and it had been empty all the time. All the people around really wanted this person to buy it, so that he would restore it. He decided it would be a money pit and said no. Then I was near a river that flowed through a natural tunnel for a short while, quarter of a mile or so, than exited through the other side. People were throwing rocks into the tunnel, which was dimly lit from each side, by the entrance and exit. I saw some large gulls inside, and a large white dog. I threw some dirt onto the dog, and I felt that the people around me thought badly of me, I only wanted to make a contrasting mark on him. I went down into the tunnel with some man I did not recognize. For some reason there were several animals in boxes. If they were left, there they would die. There also was a small child in a box. We wanted to save a dog, or a bear. The man cut the claws off the bear, they looked like plastic, white and somewhat translucent, and we affixed them to the little girl, we left the girl there to die I guess, and rescued the animals. Then we were back at the property from the start of the dream. There were myself and people I know from medical school. It seemed we were playing hide-and-seek. I was leading a group of people down a long hallway, and now it seemed a natural history museum. We were hiding behind an exhibit of a polar bear possibly. I am not sure what it was, everything was in a decrepit state. Then people found us. There was a feeling of fun and danger.

◆ Crack in the corner of mouth.

◆ Acid indigestion. Low-grade discomfort in chest.

**Day 14**

◆ Dream: My husband and I at a relative's house. It was some holiday, probably Thanksgiving and both parents were there. Lots of relatives were there of my husband's, at least they seemed related to him. I did not recognize them. I was supposed to be making the gravy and I was trying to, but people were interrupting me and asking me questions. I was younger like an adolescent. I felt annoyed internally, but tried to be pleasant. The kitchen was full of people milling around. I ended up burning the gravy and discovered a new twist on the saying: "Too many cooks spoil the broth." I had always thought it meant too many people adding ingredients, but here it meant too many interruptions, so you could not give full attention to something that needed care at a critical point.

◆ Still having a hard time focusing, tried for one and a half hours to study a case, and couldn't get my mind to kick in. Lots of distractions.

◆ Acid indigestion.

◆ Crack in the corner of mouth.

**Day 15**

◆ Dream: I was at a friend's ranch in Wyoming. There were a lot of young people there, teenagers. People told me I wasn't wearing the right clothes so I changed into pink high-tops and was thus dressed up like the others. Baggy huge jeans, and a pink striped baggy T-shirt, with my hair pulled up, Latina gang style. There was a birdhouse in the backyard, mounted on a fence. (I recently hung the same birdhouse up on our patio.) I looked inside, and there were a pair of purple martins nesting. I was concerned for them because the entrance had been damaged and the hole widened so much, it would be easy for a cat or squirrel to come up the fence and paw into the nest. I felt we need to do something about this. Suddenly a friend, who is an avid bird-watcher was there; she helped me move the birds to a safer nest, which was a semicircular nest with plastic wrapping. I had the feeling that I was being taught by her, and I was in some kind of relation to her, that she was a school teacher. I still was afraid that the birds would be harmed. Now I was afraid they would be suffocated, and again I had the feeling of an adult or authority figure who is doing wrong. Then my husband, my friend—who is the avid bird-watcher—and I were at an art show, perhaps the Sonoma County Fair. We were looking at art work and hoped to find some entries there, done by people we knew. We were looking at pictures with birds.

**Day 17**

◆ Overall feeling—the theme of adolescence and looking to adults for teaching and guidance. However, realizing that they were either not noticing or their answers were stupid or "full of shit." As an adolescent, I clearly realized that the adults didn't have all the answers. I felt anxious, restless, indignant, unsettled, about finding the right answer.

**Prover #6 · Male · 49 years old**

**Day 1**

◆ Within hours a feeling of lightness, relaxed, calm and joy, everything was just fine.

◆ Slept deeply but interrupted by five year old with stridor. Prescribed successfully. But I slept on the floor because he was in the bed.

◆ Crescendoing supra-orbital tightness and achiness. For 36 hours.

◆ Did not need or want to think very much, able to function from this calmness. The idea that life is fine without thinking.

◆ Dream: Like a Hollywood production. Large sprawling semi-wooded farmhouse setting and I was with my children and three adopted adolescent boys who are mature and able. We are very attached and yet aware of their preoccupation with their loss. I am a nurturing father and I am enjoying it. A large group of children from group homes convenes on us and I am surprised and wonder if we can step up to this. Still calm, I attempt to feed them all but feel overwhelmed by their neediness and their feral quality or wildness. My wife returns from her great adventure hike and I am a little resentful but then realize I have had fun.

◆ Feeling of lightness lasted. My son had a relapse and I treated him again. Good response.

◆ Spontaneous shivering or shuddering quality through body as with rush of emotion but without fever. As though something is coming alive, spine tingling.

◆ Strong sense of smell. And liked it, a way of connecting. Could almost take the place of ideas.

◆ Then second phase: marked by a lot of physical symptoms. Unpleasant.

Ankle and foot and wrist and hand complaints, tension, deforming and feeling of dislocation. Bilateral trapezius tension.

◆ Feeling on the hunt for something and just not satisfied, raiding the fridge, unsatisfied hunger.

◆ Then third phase: visceral aliveness where I do not have to think. I want to be viscerally present, just connected to people. Irritated by having to give a thinking response or if someone wants to think about something.

◆ Resentful of having to be inside in this weather. Image of seeing patients on a porch in my dream. Wanting open air. Wanting to be very physically active. Wanting to move and connect with other people this way.

◆ Increased sexual desire and also an aliveness and a way of meeting someone immediately.

◆ Sense of smell continues. When I smell my children or my wife it is a savoring that percolates through my being. Aware of cat peeing in the wrong places.

◆ Yesterday a dead opossum was outside the garage. Last night there was a large raccoon fight outside the house. Two unusual events.

**Prover #7 · Female · 42 years old**

**Day 1**

◆ Dream: Waiting for my children who were driving home and I was anxious about them and they came and surge of great joy.

◆ Dream: Two other mothers and several children in car driving to a home and we were taking them to see the animals at a home and we were locked in the car and trying to figure how to get out but we were all happy. Farm animals. Family moved to an apartment on a busy street from a large house. I had positive feelings. "This is a new experience" type of thing (feeling).

◆ Woke with good mood. Enjoyed family activities.

◆ I pulled into a parking lot and ran into a car. Aware of the car and watched myself drive into it. Depth perception seemed off.

◆ Spent the day with four of my children, relaxed and pleasant day. Taking weight-lifting class with my daughter, and with the second set, blinding occipital HA came on and so I stopped. Totally exhausted and fatigued and could hardly walk despite the lighter workout.

◆ Impression that the scar on my heel from four months ago was achy and uncomfortable and redder and more swollen.

◆ HA had moved to the temples more on the left. No longer debilitating.

◆ Mind not clear at this conference. Ski conference so I sat in my car to do some work and fell into a drugged-like sleep and could not wake up.

◆ Dream: We had moved to a perfect house in rural place. Overwhelmed by the physical beauty of it. A man drove up and wanted us to buy his house for almost nothing, but we had to agree to get rid of our chicken, and we could not have any animals. I realized he was drunk and tried to get him to stay and not drive. I was worried about him.

◆ Lots of concern for people.

◆ Slept poorly. Kept waking with my heart pounding, 120 beats.

◆ Fear of something evil that is coming into the house and trying to lock all the doors but could not find them all, there were too many, and no one would help me though I asked. Anxious feeling in bed and pulled slowly out of bed by something I could not see. I tried to call for help but sound would come out but no words. I thought my husband was nearby but he would not come.

◆ Mouth and nose very dry. (Sometimes normally happens.)

◆ Dream: About doing medical teaching on the beach, walking on the sand. Then teaching an exercise class and had a strong sense of the exercises I was doing especially the deep plies. How easy it was to do extreme exercise.

◆ Dull headache going into left neck into the trapezius and rhomboids. Stayed for four days.

◆ Chilled. (Other days warmer than I usually am.)

◆ Mild right knee pain. (Hasn't had in over a year.)

◆ Dream: Of trying to assess complicated older patients all at the same time. Could not find their charts. They all wanted me to write to other doctors. I was afraid I would forget before I could write it down.

◆ Dream: Grocery shopping with my husband and I left my wallet in the shopping cart and had thought I could go back for it and it was there but I never got around to check and make sure everything was there.

◆ Dream: Moved to new house, big in the country with clinic attached. I said: "This is perfect, we love it here." Several extra children were living with us. Everyone was taken care of. Relaxed, good interactions, happy, peaceful.

# LAC EQUINUM

*Milk of the Horse*

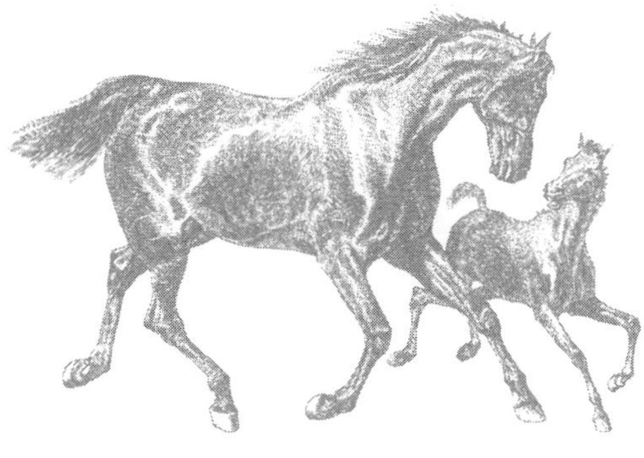

# LAC EQUINUM *Milk of the Horse*

Much to the surprise of most people involved with this proving, horses seem to be among the most unhappy and dissatisfied creatures on earth. To those who love them, this is an astonishing and heartbreaking statement. Yet if one takes an even cursory glance at the history of horses throughout the world, the cause of their suffering becomes immediately apparent.

One of the earliest uses of the noble beast was to drink his blood and eat his flesh. This was an essential part of the ancient Celtic ritual sacrifices. The horse was especially desirable for this because he was so important to the everyday life of the Celtic people. The Irish king even took a formal bath in horse soup at his inauguration ceremony.

The family of horse has been selectively bred and otherwise domesticated for about 6,000 years. A recently exhumed ancient grave in the Ukraine revealed horse bones whose teeth showed wear from a bit. The domesticated horse is literally a world apart from its wild and ancient ancestors. In fact, it is believed that there are no longer any true wild horses except for the Przewalski's horse from the steppes of Mongolia. It is the last of the wild stock of ancestral "proto-horses," close family descendants of the original horse. Horses were indigenous to the Americas but disappeared with the dinosaurs. In the 16th century, they were brought back in by the Spanish conquistadors.

Man has subjugated the horse and used it for a variety of horrendous tasks. The horse, first and foremost, has been used in battle. Everywhere, wars were fought on the backs of these unfortunate creatures, who died in untold numbers, without the slightest idea of what the screaming and shooting was all about. Next, the horse was used and abused on the farm. Day in and day out, horses pushed and pulled and carried heavy loads until they dropped from exhaustion. The final insult was that once their usefulness ended, they were sent to be killed and made into glue. The rodeo and racetrack provided other settings for horse suffering. Certainly they love to run, but spurring and whipping diminish the pleasure. The use of the term, "breaking," reveals a great deal about the relationship that man has had with the horse over the centuries.

How is it that horses find themselves in this terrible position? It is because of their naturally sociable and cooperative natures. The horse community in the wild is affectionate and herd-oriented. They have transferred these characteristics to their interactions with humans. They have a great desire to please and to bond with those who are their masters. Yet it seems that, however much they try, there is never an end to their labors or to the demands that are made on them. The following quotation from a prover seems to capture the state precisely: "Quicksand, a feeling of sinking. Crazy month. Struggling and struggling, but I am losing ground.... Sense of doing my duty, doing the things I have committed to and following through, but my life is crumbling around me. Felt desperate rather than sad.... Life is hard."

A wild horse herd can be as large as twenty-one or as small as three; the average size is about seven. It is typically made up of a mature stallion, his mares, and their offspring. The mares are extremely protective of their foals for the first year, but if the foals are males, they quickly become a threat to their father. Just as in a lion pride, the male wild horses are driven off at about 18 months old and learn to fend for themselves. They form a bachelor grouping out of which will eventually emerge a natural leader. This vigorous young stallion will gather fillies around him and force out the other males. In this fashion, a new band is established.

Another method for a young stallion in the wild to assume dominance is to overcome an established stallion and acquire his harem. This requires great strength and courage and is rarely accomplished unless the older horse is in some manner infirm. All this is remarkably similar to lion behavior, except for one major difference: The male lion taking over the pride will kill the vanquished male's offspring. This does not happen in the horse herd. In addition, the older stallion is basically just protecting his position when he defends the herd against another younger stallion. Most of the time, this is done with vocal threats and physical gestures, such as snorting and shoving and pawing the ground. (**CONFRONTATIONAL/CRITICAL/NASTY**) Only when he is unsuccessful in deterring the interloper, will the stallion behave more aggressively by striking or biting.

As with dolphins and lions, the horse family is basically run by the females. They make all the decisions about the herds' movement patterns. The stallion lags behind but not so far that he cannot watch over the females should they show interest in another, younger male. Studies show that when a horse was seen trailing the herd, 73 percent of the time it was the stallion.

A horse herd in a natural environment will have a large territory of 30 to 80 square miles. They do not defend this territory, however, nor do they become cantankerous if other horses use the watering holes and such. If two herds should encounter one another in the open, they both calmly go their own ways. Without fighting, they seem to work it out as to which herd belongs in which territory.

(**ORGANIZATION**) However, in a tight domestic pen, a horse may feel the need to defend his extraordinarily small home. Thus, when a new horse is put in the paddock, a horse already in the paddock may react with unrestrained and uncharacteristic violence. Suddenly the issue of who has the right to the space becomes very important. (**KILLING/VIOLENCE**)

When a horse is worked for farming, hauling or riding, the animal is submitting to the task, difficult as it may be, to please its master. Horses have a very strong and natural desire to cooperate and will do so under the most difficult conditions. They will remain loyal to the end of their lives. Only under seriously inhumane conditions will a horse give up and not respond to an owner's demands to make it perform. Then they may go into a depression and not do anything at all. (**APATHY/ENNUI**)

We tend to anthropomorphize horses more than we do any other animal. For example, many people believe, or want to believe, that the horse knows what is happening when it is put in a race. A racehorse is intentionally kept in a very small paddock so it develops an unnaturally intense state of pent-up energy. (**IMPATIENT**) (**IRRITABLE**) This energy is what is released when the horse is raced. He desires to run and will do so with great relish, for a short time, until the distance becomes too great, and then he is thoroughly exhausted. However, a horse in the wild runs a short distance for the joy of it and then cavorts on the grass and nibbles some fresh leaves; he never gallops full out for long distances unless he is running from a feared enemy. In this case, his brief galloping spurt would be fueled by panic. Desmond Morris, in *Horsewatching,* says; "Somewhere in a racehorse's mind there must be a fantasy, at least, of a pursuing killer.... (T)he pain of the whip is...reminiscent of the scratch of a feline claw.... (Thus,) the horse makes an extra effort to escape...as long as it has any strength left in its limbs."

The act of running itself, while it is natural to the horse, is a big strain on the horse's heart. Studies have revealed that there is an enormous increase in the heart rate from resting to galloping—from 25 beats per minute to 250. To race repeatedly at a forced pace for an unnaturally long distance causes great damage to the heart of the horse, as well as other organs. Added to this is the stress of feeling that he is being attacked by a lion, wolf, or dog. The animal is totally exhausted emotionally and physically at the end of these events. (**DIFFICULT ENCOUNTERS/FRUSTRATION**)

It is easy to catalogue the number of ways in which the beauty of horses running has prompted humans to abuse them. For example, in steeplechasing, horses are forced to jump over unnaturally high barriers, and they suffer frequent severe injuries when they fall. The Tennessee Walker show horse is naturally inclined towards a high-stepping style, but when the hoof is allowed to grow extra long and is trimmed in a distorted fashion, the horse is forced into a more exaggerated, high gait. Weights are put on the ankle and on the foot to further elaborate the gait.

The final insult to this faithful creature is for his master to behave as if the horse enjoys his "victory" should he win a race or competition. It is unfathomable to imagine that a horse knows what the finish line is, much less that he has crossed it. Racing competitively is not a natural behavior for horses. When they run from an enemy, they do so in groups to improve their chances of survival. The horse that gets caught is the one who stands out from the crowd by either being in front or behind the group. It is only by mistaking the whip for a claw that the horse can be induced to run ahead of the group. (**MISTAKES**)

**Analysis of the Proving**

This proving was a great surprise to all who were involved with it. No one realized that the state of the horse was so intensely unhappy. Most horse lovers took issue with this idea and felt it just could not be true. But the themes that came out seem to fit what many modern horse sympathizers are saying about the true-life experiences of most horses. Writers like Monty Roberts, who wrote *The Man Who Listens to Horses,* and Desmond Morris express revulsion at the manner in which horses are treated—from the breaking in, to the equipment used to ride them, and the whips and chains used to subdue them. Monty is a man with a lifelong experience training horses. He says: "I changed the nomenclature.... I called my method 'starting horses.' If traditional breaking was designed to generate fear in the horse, I wanted to create trust. If the old way involved ropes and tying horses' heads and legs, I wanted no part of that either. A significant moment came when I realized I could cause trust in a horse without pain or restraint.... Instead of telling young horses 'you must,' I wanted to ask them 'will you?' "

What the proving tells us is that this abuse aimed at horses has resulted in a central state of frustration. Nothing seems to go right. All that is attempted is thwarted. The horse (or the Lac equinum patient) struggles to do his duty but never gets a sense of satisfaction. This proving was an incredibly difficult experience for everyone involved with it. The initial provers found the state unbearable and were eager to end the proving. One prover said, "Felt frustrated and overwhelmed by everything. Wanted to quit school, quit work, get divorced, stay home and do nothing." Some provers had to take their constitutional remedy to get over the effects. Claire Green reported that after working on horse rubrics, she became so irritable, frustrated, restless, and dissatisfied, she could hardly work for the rest of the week. She said she felt like "running away from it all." Marianne Heger, M.D., of Deutsche Homeopathic Union, told of the incredible difficulties they had making up Lac equinum to 200C, 1M, and 10M. They had never experienced so many things going wrong at once—this from a company that is famous for organization and quality in the production of its remedies. Even the impatience of the horse being kept in the paddock was expressed by one prover: "I continue to be impatient and confrontational at almost every encounter. I am intolerant of any delay and will confront anyone whom I feel is to blame or is the cause of delay."

Thus, we must understand that the life of a Lac equinum patient is as hard as that of the typical, domesticated horse.

**The Substance**

The milk for this proving was obtained by Vicki Menear, M.D. She has been an avid horsewoman all her life, and she held the horse as the horse's owner milked it. The horse, named Patches, was an 18-year-old Appaloosa broodmare who had six prior foals. She was very desirable as a broodmare due to her beautiful white coat with big, black spots. Patches had been put out to pasture and was no longer required to do any work. She had not been ridden in several years. As far as we know, she had always been treated humanely, yet she was quite irritable with humans and did not seem to want their attention. She was a good mother, very attentive to her young, and seemed happy to be out to pasture. Her only physical problem was in her left hip, which showed signs of arthritis and caused a shortened stride.

I want to thank Vicki very much for obtaining this substance, one which resonates highly with the human condition and has and will continue to be the source of many cures.

For two years, I have been attempting to get the milk of a wild horse. I have access to a group of wild horses in California, but there are two problems. The first problem is that no horse is truly wild, except for the Przewalski's horse from the steppes of Mongolia. All the wild horses in the United States are descendants of domesticated horses. Problem two is that I am unable to physically obtain the milk of a wild horse because restraining the horse is quite difficult. Wild horses have been known to throw themselves off a cliff rather than be captured. The point of allowing the horse to remain wild is not to terrorize or traumatize it, which the mere act of capturing it would do. If the opportunity ever arises to obtain wild mare's milk, we could compare the natural state of this magnificent animal to the domesticated and unhappy state revealed in this proving.

*Lac Equinum* **Themes**

*Milk of the Horse*

- *Apathy/Ennui*
- *Difficult Encounters/Frustration*
- *Confrontational/Critical/Nasty*
- *Mistakes*
- *Organization*
- *Impatient*
- *Irritable*
- *Killing/Violence*

# *Apathy/Ennui*

**#4** Did not write anything this week. Was very low energy, apathetic.

**#6** Struggling and struggling, but I am losing ground.... Sense of doing my duty, doing the things I have committed to and following through, but my life is crumbling around me. Felt desperate rather than sad. Feeling of apathy, exhausted. I can't deal with this and I don't care. Hard to sort out what is what. Life is hard.

**#7** Feeling flaky, I don't give a shit. Depressed, hopeless angst about the world. Driving down the freeway thinking, "What is this whole thing about anyway?"

**#9** Not able to pay attention to remedy, not recording symptoms. Not very concerned. Just no ability to do it.

## *Difficult Encounters/Frustration*

**#4** Felt frustrated and overwhelmed by everything. Wanted to quit school, quit work, get divorced, stay home and do nothing. Finally took a 30C dose of my constitutional remedy and felt immediate improvement in mood, energy, sex drive.

**#6** In real life, there were some things not very important but felt compelled to do them. My priorities shifted, e.g. I had promised classmate a copy of notes, but I forgot until last minute. Got them together and trying to get to Fed Ex, but it snowed so could not go. I was trying to call his office, his house, but could not get a hold of him, but put a lot of effort into it, more than I probably should have. Fighting quality. Quicksand, a feeling of sinking. Crazy month.

**#5** Irritable: felt very irritated at a general business meeting conducted by Robert's Rules.... I have been to meetings like this before and never felt this way.... The meeting seemed very forced and constrained by artificial rules that did not facilitate the goal. I actually brought this up to the group, but the reply was that the state required that general business meetings be conducted this way. I felt left out by the majority rules process, frustrated, almost moved to tears and felt like getting up and leaving.

**#6** I'm on a rehabilitation team that gets together at weekly meeting. One therapist, who is somewhat domineering and smartass, brought up an issue about a patient who got Thorazine from another doctor. I had been so busy, I had not been going to the hospital early to check on charts, so I did not know about this yet. I had a feeling of embarrassment, and after the meeting, I yelled at her: "You were out of line!" I knew in my heart I was embarrassed; I had not done my job, and I was frustrated. Felt terrible later and realized it was mean and bad politically for the unit. Feeling of drowning in disorganization, feeling of sinking or drowning....

**#2** Dream: I was trying to buy the business office of a pharmacy to use as my homeopathy practice. They wanted to give it to me to use but talked about selling me the pharmacy instead. Not what I had in mind! Then I was trying to figure out remedies for people. Presented cases to a visiting expert. Went to bookstore, but the books were too expensive and elaborate, outdated. Feeling of mild frustration.

**#7** Dream: Driving down freeway, battery is going dead. I'm in a store returning a shirt; the salesperson says they don't sell this particular shirt. The shirt keeps turning different colors: green and red and blue. She shows it to everyone and tries to sell it. I'm impatient. I've driven a long way and want to complete the task. I walk out, and I am with my brother going back to the car with a now dead battery.

**#2** Dream: I hear noise outside the house, and I get up to look. Neighbor is also looking, and he sees me naked. I found out later oldest son was being sprayed with fluid by neighborhood youths. Feeling of frustration that I could not catch them.

## *Confrontational/Critical/Nasty*

**#1** Felt confrontational repeatedly. I needed to be first on the bus, first off the bus, first into the rental car office. I was feeling impatient, irritable; confronted the clerk as to why I was not the first person called, even though I was the first person in line. When clerk encouraged me to buy insurance, I told her I was a hard sale and asked her if she got a commission. I insisted she note every scratch and mark on the car and note exactly the gas gauge level. I had a competitive, impatient attitude toward people. I did not want people in front of me or in my way. Really annoyed with salesperson. This is not me. Usually I don't care, but this time, it seemed very important. If she is going to give me a hard time, I am going to give her a hard time—confrontational and competitive. When I got to motel, the front desk clerk was busy, and I commented how she was not attentive to her job. Very intolerant of delays....

**#2** Dream: I was not feeling well, and people were not helpful as I looked for a bathroom. Actually they were nasty.

**#2** Dream: Discussed the proving with the proving director. (I can't remember what we said.) People very critical, like junior high, nasty edge. I was cleaning a bathroom and doing dishes, and in both situations people made nasty, personal remarks. One person was at least pleasant and sympathetic but then turned negative. The proving director said Nitric acid was the remedy. Out-of-town stranger asks for directions, and I try to help and accompany him to dinner and a movie. In the middle of the movie he leaves me to join others.

**#4** Unpleasant day, things that usually make me happy just had a brief impact. I tended to dwell on the negative thoughts. Felt nasty when cut off by other drivers: "F— you!" feeling.

**#7** Dream: I got pulled over in my car by police. He was going to arrest me for making an illegal turn. I was pissed off, screaming, "You are unfair. Who the f— are you?"

# Mistakes

**#1** Secretary said I was making mistakes adding numbers; couldn't add simple figures.

**#2** I made major mistakes with people, e.g. there was a patient in waiting room, and I could not figure out who it was. Called a classmate by another classmate's name: confusions with names, used phrases differently, twisting numbers around. I am feeling like "I am not my mind or body." On a physical level, I understand that, but when I saw my mind going haywire, I thought to myself, "Wow, you are getting demented!" It was very unsettling. Simple things I always took for granted, like figuring out co-pay. Had trouble doing the calculation. I did my taxes, and conceptually, I did well, but addition was a problem. Forgetful, e.g. I didn't take the key off the computer, even though I thought to myself that I would and should. So some mental difficulty that was compensated (for) through increased neatness and efficiency.

**#2** More mistakes with confusing numbers. Memory not precise; only remembering parts of dreams and in waking hours parts of phrases.... Worked on tapes and accidentally deleted a computer program; otherwise more efficient and organized than usual.

**#3** Memory poor—forgetting things more than normal.

**#4** Increased trouble picking up phone numbers correctly from voice-mail messages; reversing numbers, not able to follow rapidly spoken numbers.

**#2** Continue to make mistakes with phone numbers. Had trouble calculating simple co-pay amount. Conscious of mind not working well. Thoughts of the play, *Flowers for Algernon*...and Alzheimer's disease.

# *Organization*

**#2** Much neater than usual, keeping things cleaner, more organized.

**#3** Stayed late at work, cleared off desk completely; felt the need to organize; bothered by clutter and mess. It had been piled with paper and things I could not quite throw away for three months.

**#5** Felt very motivated and energetic in the evening: got a lot accomplished—cleaning, sewing, typing—things I had been putting off for months. Getting organized.

**#5** Dream: A very clear dream of anatomy lab—dissection of the brachioplexus with a feeling of precision, fastidiousness, teamwork. We were also cleaning out the bins the body parts are kept in.

# Impatient

**#1** Continue to be impatient and confrontational at almost every encounter. I am intolerant of any delay and will confront anyone whom I feel is to blame or is the cause of delay.

**#1** Mental state continues: very irritable, impatient, confrontational.

**#3** Impatient with my patients, with unhelpful salespeople. A feeling of impatience.

**#7** Urination frequent; nine times out of ten, the bathroom at work was already occupied. I was impatient and outraged, pounding on the door, "C'mon!!"

## *Irritable*

**#1** Went to restaurant with friends, and they told the waiter to put shrimp in a doggie bag, and the waiter tossed it. I wanted to go to the owner and make a scene; I was looking forward to it. I liked the feeling. When feeling just impatient and annoyed, it was not a good feeling; but when confrontational, I liked it. When at the rental car place, I said, "You people just can't run this show, can you?" Every situation was like that except at school. I began to realize this was my current state, and I began to enjoy it, but the gut level state was irritation.

**#4** I feel a bit more moody today—got real cranky when hungry and snapped at husband.

**#5** Dream: I was living in a loft space with my husband. A large, loft-like space with partitions/walls built in it to make separate rooms. I came home one day to find several college-age kids had moved in with us—they had torn down the partitions to make it open space again. They did not seem concerned that we had already been living there and did not want any roommates. I was very annoyed at our landlord. How could he? Indignant and irritated. However, I was also intrigued by the people moving in and interested in their personalities, belongings, energy, art, and music (Hip hop stuff, graffiti, MTV stuff.)

**#1** Mental state continues: very irritable, impatient, confrontational.

**#5** Irritable: I felt very irritated at a general business meeting conducted by Robert's Rules.... Impatient yet bored. I have been to meetings like this before and never felt this way....

# Killing/Violence

**#2** Dream: A creature from outer space, like a Jell-O mold. It had psychic powers and could cause things to happen. I was involved in some group project, and I had to kill it by pouring pepper on it and using a big cookie-cutter to help break it up. An attorney was involved, and he screwed the group over. Exciting dream, kind of fun, but I did not like the idea of killing the alien.

**#2** Dream: ...A woman who was coming there was accidentally shot. She turned into a sort of rag doll, actually a stuffed bird with the sawdust fill coming out of the neck. Someone disposed of it like trash. I was struck by the disregard and demoralization. I felt a certain callousness of the will to do that, which was upsetting.

**#2** Dream: Like *Pulp Fiction.* I and another guy are two henchmen harassing a man. I'm telling the man what a week I've had: two close calls of almost being hurt. My partner pulls a gun on the victim. I am shocked, and then he points the gun at me, and it is apparent that it is me he wants to shoot. I don't know why.

**#6** Dream: Intense nightmare: multiple beings or people against me. Violent interaction with multiple other animals and beings, fighting for my life. People and extra-terrestrials of some sort. Fighting with my hands. They're trying to kill me.

**#7** Dream: In a restaurant eating with my brother. A couple nearby having an argument. I look at them, and the man gets upset. There is an exchange of words, and my brother gets up and physically "manhandles" him by striking him. Next, somehow I end up in a fight with this guy—we are all over the place. I have some kind of metal stick in one hand and a wooden stick in the other. I strike him over and over again, but this guy will not stop. He just keeps on coming; he is very crazed—like "Rocky." He won't hurt me and take me down. I'm afraid and I don't want to kill him, but I see no other option. I hit him on his head and ribs over and over. "I want peace!" He won't stop! I strike and strike and strike. He falls downstairs and climbs back again. He is bloody and beaten up but won't die.

**#7** Dream: On a large ship with terrorist-type, Middle Eastern men. I'm in great danger of being murdered. There are other people on the ship in a similar situation. I am trying to be amiable. I'm looking for a place to hide from these dangerous people. Next, I am hiding in a large room behind columns to avoid contact with these men.

## MIND

- AMBITIOUS
- *ANGER*
  - in traffic
  - touched, when
- ANSWERS; disconnected
  - inappropriate
- *ANXIETY*
  - *anticipating*
  - breathing
    - suffocative
  - conscience, of
  - expected of him, when anything is
  - health, about
  - lemonade; amel.
  - menses; after
  - morning; menses; after
    - **waking, on**
  - pursued, as if
  - safety of family, for
  - secrets revealed, from
  - time is set, if a
- ASSERTIVE
- ATTENTION; enjoys
- BITING
- BUSY
- CENSORIOUS, critical
- CHILDREN; beautiful; loves profoundly
- COMPETITIVE
- *COMPLAINING*
- **CONCENTRATION; difficult**
- *CONFIDENCE, want of self*
- *CONFUSION of mind*
- CURSING, swearing; curses, desire to curse
- DELUSIONS, imaginations
  - contraction, constiction; everything is
  - drowning; disorganization, in
  - duty; overdo, compelled to

DELUSIONS (cont.)
fail, everything will
hard, everything is
hardship, life is
*hearing, talk seems loud*
*hindered*
house; surrounded, is
*insane; become, that she will*
*insulted, he or she is:*
*neglected; duty, his*
*neglected; duty, his; indifferent to*
noise, hears
noise; seems exaggerated, loud
running out of control, she is
sinking, he is
sinking, he is; quicksand, in
stalked, he is
time; earlier, is
exaggeration of
*trapped, he is*
DESPAIR
DICTATORIAL, domineering, dogmatic, despotic
DISCONTENTED, displeased, dissatisfied
*DISHARMONY in the family; agg.*
DREAMS
accidents, of; car, with
hit and run
adolescence, time of
adventurous
alien from outer space; killing him, trying to
psychic
amiable; murdered; to keep from being
amorous
anger
animals, of
bears
*cats*
vicious
**horses**
marmots
rabbits
restrained by collars
apologizing
appearance; concern about

- bathroom, looking for
- beaten, being
- beautiful; earth is
- beauty; awe with
- betrayed, having been
- *body, body parts; breasts*
    - eyes; size; disparity in pupil
    - shrunk and enlarged; device, by
    - stuffed doll, turns into
    - toe cut off
        - child's; found in truck
- bombs
- bored; people are
- buildings
    - falling apart, as if earthquake split
- business
- calm
- child, children, about
    - mutilated
    - precocious and arrogant
- coition; observed
- competition
- confidence; breach of
    - increased; to get things done
- dead; bodies; dissecting
- disgusting
- earthquakes; houses, buildings falling
- embarrassment
- *escape, of*
- escape, of; danger, from
- exciting
- family
- fantastic
- fights
- flowers
- foreigners
- friends
- frightful
- **frustration**
- groups
    - screwed over by attorney
    - *working well together*
- guilt
- happy; alive, to be

shooting; shot, of being; woman is accidentally
*singing*
sorting, organizing
sports, of
bicycling, of
bowling, of; metal platter, with
football, of
sunlight, of
superhero, of
*teaching, of*
*teamwork*
thrown away; body into the trash
traffic
trees
chopping down
unremembered
unsuccessful efforts
to do various things
vexatious
*violence*
striking with a stick
vivid; remember; could not
weeping
women
beautiful
work
DULLNESS
DWELLS on; unpleasant, disagreeable things
EATING; bingeing; food, on
*EFFICIENT, organized*
clutter; bothered by
mental confusion; compensation for; must be
EMBARRASSMENT; poor job performance, of
*ENNUI, boredom*
ESCAPE, desire to
family and children, from her
ESTRANGED; family, from her
FASTIDIOUS
*FEAR; Alzheimer's, of*
cancer, of
dark, of
disease, of; impending
happen; something will
horrible, terrible
*insanity, of*
motoring; snow, in

FIGHT, wants to
FORGETFULNESS
    purchases, of, goes off and leaves them
**FRUSTRATION; at unsuccessful or thwarted attempts**
    bears her teeth with frustration (child)
    *efforts to accomplish her desires*
    *in her/his ability to help family*
    sexual desire
**FUZZY, unfocused**
    waking, on
HANDLE things anymore, cannot, overwhelmed by stress
HOME; desires to; leave
**HORSEBACK riding; amel.**
HURRY, haste; tendency
IMPATIENCE
    boredom, with
    people, unhelpful; with
IMPULSIVE
    secrets; must blurt out
INDIFFERENCE, apathy
INDIGNATION
INDUSTRIOUS, mania for work
INJUSTICE, cannot support
INTOLERANCE; ambiguity, of
    hindrance, of; inflexible rules, of
IRRITABILITY
    business; proceed fast, when does not
    hungry, when
    menses; before
LOQUACITY
LOSES possessions
LOVE; profound; daughter, for; but limited in expression of
MEDITATION; difficult
MEMORY; weakness, loss of:
        names, for proper
*MISTAKES, makes; calculating, in:*
        *adding*
    computer; deletes program
    writing, in; transposing; letters
OBSTINATE, stubborn
OFFENDED easily
OPTIMISTIC
QUARRELSOMENESS, scolding
RAGE

RELAXED feeling, letting go
REMORSE
*RESPONSIBILITY; takes*
*too much*
REST; cannot, when things are not in proper place
*RESTLESSNESS, nervousness; tendency*
*meditation, during*
anxious
disorganization agg.
fresh air amel.
noise agg.
REVEALS secrets
impulsively, her own
SADNESS, despondency, depression, melancholy
menses; after
climacteric period, during
SENSITIVE, oversensitive; noise, to
*SHRIEKING, screaming, shouting*
*anger in*
*SIGHING*
STARING
STRIKING
children, in
STRUGGLE; everything is
SUICIDAL thoughts
THEORIZING
proving substance, about the
THOUGHTS; wandering
TIMID, shy
TOUCHED, aversion to being
TRAVEL; desire to
TRIFLES; important, seem
no attention for
UNCONSCIOUSNESS
when unable to mediate between loved ones

### VERTIGO

VERTIGO; morning; waking, on

### HEAD

CONSTRICTION
HAIR; falling

**HEAD PAIN**

LOCALIZATION; forehead
evening
20 hour
reading
temples
GNAWING
PRESSING; temples

**EYES**

DRYNESS
PAIN; stinging

**NOSE**

CORYZA; air, in open, cold
ameliorates

**FACE**

ERUPTIONS; acne
herpes
mouth; corners
PAIN; Jaw; articulation
extending into teeth

**MOUTH**

*APHTHAE*
palate
BLEEDING; gums; easily

**TASTE**

PUTRID

**THROAT**

PAIN; sore

**EXTERNAL THROAT**

CONSTRICTION
TOUCH; agg.
UNCOVERING throat amel.

## STOMACH

ANXIETY
AVERSION; chocolate
DESIRE for; lemonade
*DISORDERED*
    *emotions, from*
DISTENTION
    menses, with
ERUCTATIONS
    dinner, after
*HICCOUGH*
    *while eating*
    *after eating*
NAUSEA
THIRST; decreased
PAIN; burning
        night; 3-5 a.m.

## ABDOMEN

DISTENTION
    night; midnight, after
    flatus, from
ENLARGED; liver
FLATULENCE; after eating
PAIN; liver
    cramping; symphysis; eating, after
        6 p.m.
    pressure

## RECTUM

CONSTIPATION; ineffectual
    insufficient
FLATUS
    afternoon
    evening
    stool, during
    dinner, after
    eating, after
INVOLUNTARY stool
    elderly, in

### STOOL

FLATULENT
MUCOUS
*LOOSE*

### BLADDER

URINATION; frequent
    night

### MALE

SEXUAL; passion; diminished

### FEMALE

MENSES, early
PAIN; menses, during
  ovary; alternating sides; after menses
    left; after menses
SEXUAL; passion; diminished
    increased
      after menses
TINGLING, voluptuous; ovary; left; after menses

### RESPIRATION

ASTHMATIC
DIFFICULT
IMPEDED; constriction; throat, of
  oppression, from; epigastrium
WHEEZING

### COUGH

DRY

### CHEST

PAIN; General; mammae; menses; before
    respiration

## BACK

- ERUPTIONS; pimples
- PAIN; lumbar region
    - rising; seat, from a
  - aching; lumbar region
      - rising up; on

## EXTREMITIES

- COLDNESS; foot
- CRAMPS; Hand
  - Leg
- SHAKING; Hand
- DISCOLORATION; blotches
  - Upper limbs
    - black
    - blue
  - Toenails
    - black
- ERUPTIONS; forearm
    - desquamation
    - urticaria
  - itching
- HEAVINESS; walking, while
  - lower limbs
    - night
- NUMBNESS; hand; right
    - thumb; right
- RESTLESSNESS
  - hand
    - right
  - feet
- SHAKING; hand
- STIFFNESS; knee
    - morning; rising, on
    - ascending stairs
- WEAKNESS; hand; right; writing, while

**EXTREMITY PAIN**

UPPER LIMBS; Shoulder
        right
LOWER LIMBS; hip; right side; walking
            after rising from a seat
            extending to knee
        alternating sides
LOWER LIMBS; Foot; sole
SORE; knee
        morning; rising, on
        ascending stairs

**SLEEP**

BAD
RESTLESS
*SLEEPLESSNESS; after midnight*
        *3 a.m.*
        *3-5 a.m.*
    *full moon*
WAKING; frequent
    12-1 a.m.
    2 a.m.
    *3 or 4 a.m.*
    fright, as from
*UNREFRESHING*

**PERSPIRATION**

PERSPIRATION; PROFUSE

**SKIN**

DISCOLORATION; blackish
        bluish
ERUPTIONS; circinate
    herpetic
    itching
    pimples

## GENERALITIES

*EVENING or twilight; amel.*
CONVULSIONS
  right side of body
  children, in
  clonic
  heat, during the
  paralysis, followed by
  tonic
  waking, on
*CLOTHES; intolerance of*
*FATIGUE*
*FOOD; alcohol aggrav.*
*PULSE, frequent, motion aggrav.*
TENSION; muscles, of
WEAKNESS; bathing; warm; after
  weather; warm; from
  menses, after

EDITOR'S NOTE: *Punctuation, abbreviations, and individual stylistic nuances of the original journal entries have been preserved wherever possible.*

**Prover #1 · Male · 45 years old**

**Day 1**

◆ Difficulty taking a deep breath.
◆ There is an awareness of the epigastric area, the breath stops there. Pressure, a feeling of pressure at the epigastric area.
◆ Feet feel very cold.
◆ Soreness in throat. All these symptoms passed in about two hours.
◆ Difficult to meditate, mind wandering.
◆ Slept deeply, no dreams.
◆ Secretary noticed I was adding numbers wrong but I had blown that off.

**Day 2**

◆ Again soreness in throat, which resolved quickly otherwise unremarkable. No dreams.

**Day 3**

◆ Dose taken late next morning, early flight to Los Angeles to teach for a week.
◆ No dreams.

**Day 4**

◆ Feeling competitive, impatient, disliked people getting ahead of me, and being delayed. Felt confrontational repeatedly. I needed to be first on the bus, first off the bus, first into the rental car office. I was feeling impatient, irritable; confronted the clerk as to why I was not the first person called, even though I was the first person in line. When clerk encouraged me to buy insurance, I told her I was a hard sale and asked her if she got a commission. I insisted she note every scratch and mark on the car and note exactly the gas gauge level. I had a competitive, impatient attitude toward people. I did not want people in front of me or in my way. Really annoyed with salesperson. This is not me. Usually I don't care, but this time it seemed very important. If she is going to give me a hard time, I am going to give her a hard time, confrontational and competitive. When I got to motel, the front desk clerk was busy, and I commented how she was not attentive to her job. Very intolerant of delays; competitive, confrontational.
◆ Had feeling of having had dreams I could not quite grasp. I remember awakening and thinking: I'll remember this dream, but next morning I could not.

**Day 5**

◆ I find it difficult to meditate, too many thoughts, no depth or connection, very restless mind.

◆ Continue to be impatient and confrontational at almost every encounter. I am intolerant of any delay and will confront anyone whom I feel is to blame or is the cause of delay.

◆ Wake early 4:30 a.m.

◆ Urge to stool, insufficient results.

**Day 6**

◆ Dream: I am in a big cave lit by a fire with a Native American Shaman (short hair, medium build, modern appearance). I am telling him everything about myself: who I am, what motivates me, etc. I am very animated and verbose, he turns his head and I feel rejected. I felt I had to convey this information to him, it was very important that I do so. When he turned away, I felt as if he did not understand what I was saying or I was talking too much. Did not feel rejected in dream, only on next morning when awoke and thought about the dream. Had to let him know about myself.

◆ Waking, 4:30 a.m. up for the day, not tired.

◆ Mental state continues: very irritable, impatient, confrontational.

◆ Herpetic eruption of corner of mouth, right side.

◆ Meditation still not good, mind restless.

◆ Bowel function seems incomplete.

**Day 7**

◆ Herpetic eruption resolves by next day.

◆ Mental and emotional state remains. Still impatient and confrontational.

◆ Restless mentally with difficulty meditating.

◆ Waking, early.

**Day 8**

◆ Mental state remains.

◆ Sleeping better.

**Day 9**

◆ Flight home was delayed. Exposed to strong odors of phenol or formaldehyde in anatomy lab. I believe the remedy to be antidoted.

◆ Secretary said I was making mistakes adding numbers, couldn't add simple figures.

◆ Went to restaurant with friends and they told the waiter to put the leftover shrimp in a doggie bag, and the waiter tossed it. I wanted to go to the owner and make a scene, I was looking forward to it. I liked the feeling. When feeling just impatient and annoyed, it was not a good feeling; but when confrontational I liked it. When at the rental car place I said, "You people just can't run this show can you?" Every situation was like that except at school. I began to realize this was my current state, and I began to enjoy it, but the gut level state was irritation.

## Prover #2 · Male · 47 years old

◆ Overall impression: Much neater than usual, keeping things cleaner, more organized.
◆ Yet made major mistakes with people, e.g. there was a patient in waiting room, and I could not figure out who they were. Called a classmate by another classmate's name: confusion with names, used phrases differently, twisting numbers around. I am feeling like "I am not my mind or body." On a physical level I understand that, but when I saw my mind going haywire, I thought to myself, "Wow, you are getting demented!" It was very unsettling. Simple things I take for granted, like figuring out a co-pay. Had trouble doing the calculation. I did my taxes and conceptually I did well, but addition was a problem. Forgetful, e.g. I didn't take the key off the computer, even though I thought to myself that I would and should. So, some mental difficulty that was compensated through increased neatness and efficiency.

**Day 1** (Took remedy at 9 p.m. evening before.)
◆ As I took the remedy I pictured turning into a creature like Hunkra (Boopsie's channeled spirit in Doonesbury comic strip). Moments after taking the remedy, my wife said, "No horns or tail!"
◆ Slept fairly well. Got up at 12:45 am to urinate and woke again at 3:45 am. I usually wake up 0-1 times a night.
◆ Dream fragment: remarkable for feeling of taking things in stride and not getting uptight like I usually would, e.g. lost a wallet but traded with the person who picked it up by mistake (I had theirs); did not have credit cards but got to make a purchase through clerk anyway.
◆ Dream: Football players without pads: theme of human-ness and vulnerability; only humans seeing human-ness and vulnerabilities of others.
◆ Woke feeling relaxed and mellow.
◆ Very productive day. My wife and I went for a walk and my wife remarked I was more relaxed and did not have my usual "edge."
◆ She also noted I only blew my nose once. Usually it runs a lot in the cold.
◆ Around 6:25 to 6:30 p.m. suprapubic pain shortly after eating. Sharp, colicky.
◆ Slight gurgle once meditating. Pain > meditation.
◆ Bowels—increased gas and mucous with stool.

**Day 2**
◆ Good sleep.
◆ Dream: Driving in truck in bad sector of India. There was a child lying near the edge of the street, and as we passed by there, the truck bumped the child's head. The mother of the child ignored it. I said to the person driving that we should leave, but I was also thinking to myself that this is hit-and-run; we should not do that. Later some cops went by, but they were not looking for us. The feeling on waking was of shame and guilt that I would leave the scene of an accident. (A dream fragment related to part on TV show with a mother not caring for her child with asthma. The doctor helps her out by buying some medicine.)

◆ The theme of pursuit and trying to escape the consequences of things. Partly ashamed of the whole thing. Conflict between those two things. Feeling was disconcerting, I did not want to write it down later. But rationalized: "Hey, lots of things happen in dreams."
◆ Two regular bowel movements.
◆ Events: talked with a psychiatrist for two hours. She is interested in homeopathy and private practice. She is affiliated with Native Americans and wants homeopathic treatment.

**Day 3**
◆ Dream: About two Native American groups: one tried to coerce me into action (I don't remember what) but delivered violent beating. Other group was friendly and much nicer. Socially advanced with other groups. Ended on an upbeat note.
◆ Dream: Taking class and working at a clinic. Having trouble getting an ambulance authorized for patient. Drove to class, supposed to teach some other students. Trouble getting to class, stuck in a factory but eventually got there. Helped clean up a mess in huge tub (sense of community).
◆ Eventful day. Worked on tapes and accidentally deleted a computer program, otherwise more efficient and organized than usual.
◆ Noted no physical symptoms. Took second dose of remedy.

**Day 4**
◆ Dream: A structure or building falling apart as if an earthquake had split the building. I had been discussing homeopathy books in the library with the librarian. They wanted to remove the books from the library.
◆ Dream: Trying to get money to buy a new house. It would take a lot of work but felt like I could do it. Increased confidence in getting things done.

**Day 5**
◆ Dream: Two boys and I are being pursued by some guy. We are looking down on him from a mountain. He is chopping down trees and spots us. We cannot climb the mountain but we go inside the mountain which was actually just an artificial structure.
◆ Dream: A creature from outer space like a Jell-O mold. It had psychic powers and could cause things to happen. I was involved in some group project, and I had to kill it by pouring pepper on it and using a big cookie-cutter to help break it up. An attorney was involved, and he screwed the group over. Exciting dream, kind of fun, but I did not like the idea of killing the alien.
◆ Increased trouble remembering patients' faces, other facts, even the security code. It reminded me of patient with CFIDS whose case I took today. She had marked forgetfulness.

**Day 6**
◆ Worked on dinner clean-up crew, and this seemed to influence my dream.
◆ Dream: Theme of class working on project. Some competition (e.g. who could get upstairs first), but later the group was working well together.
◆ Felt relaxed on waking. Unremarkable day.
◆ Took one more dose of remedy.

**Day 7**

◆ Cannot really recall dream.
◆ Dizzy on getting up, gone in two or three minutes.
◆ Felt more assertive than usual and volunteered to run office meeting.
◆ Analyzed cases in p.m.

**Day 8**

◆ Dream: I was requested by co-worker to see a couple for couple's counseling, but I did not want to. Saw a tough case of a very precocious child who arrogantly says, "you don't get it," (possibly influenced by a television show about a bright murderer). Asked by prestigious clinic to help out in coverage. I was supposed to help in a stress management, so told joke about money and recommended a trip. The head doctor laughed.
◆ I felt good on awaking, but I wondered if I was not resonating with case of Sulphur I analyzed yesterday. I also wonder if cognitive problems with confusing or forgetting numbers related to the case of chronic fatigue I analyzed earlier in the week.
◆ Numbers: had difficulty picking up phone numbers correctly from voice mail; reversing numbers, not able to follow rapidly spoken numbers.

**Day 9**

◆ Dream: I was not feeling well and people were not helpful as I looked for a bathroom. Actually they were nasty.
◆ Dream: Discussed the proving with the proving director. (I can't remember what we said.) People very critical, like junior high, nasty edge. I was cleaning a bathroom and doing dishes, and in both situations people made nasty personal remarks. One person was at least pleasant and sympathetic but then turned negative. The proving director said Nitric acid was the remedy. Out-of-town stranger asks for directions, and I try to help and accompany him to dinner and a movie. In the middle of the movie he leaves me to join others.
◆ Continue to wake two times during the night, once around 1 a.m. another a little before 4 a.m.
◆ Today at 4 a.m. lower abdominal bloating and discomfort.
◆ Loud eructations about an hour after a large lunch.

**Day 10**

◆ Dream: A woman confides in me about money problems, and I discuss it in front of another. She feels that I have violated confidence. Later I am discussing a case with another student (it is a presentation), but we are so quiet no one else can really hear. I note they must be bored. My cat has the equivalent of a broken ankle and it is going to be cast. General immobilization occurs after much discussion about what it means. Also a device to shrink and enlarge people is used by people I know. No hostile intent, playful. I found the dream interesting, and especially towards the end, it seemed like an adventure. Last thing I talked about with my wife before going to bed was money.
◆ Woke at 4 a.m.

**Day 11**

◆ Dream: A bowling alley with no bowling balls. I had to use metal platter to bowl with, and it was not easy to bowl. It is a very well-to-do bowling alley, everyone owns their own ball. Earlier, I was at a very upscale abortion clinic waiting for a friend of a friend to help them with the wait. The clinic was like mall and a station stop on a subway, as well. A woman who was coming there was accidentally shot. She turned into a sort of rag doll, actually a stuffed bird with the sawdust fill coming out of the neck. Someone disposed of it like trash. I was struck by the disregard and demoralization. I felt a certain callousness of the will to do that, which was upsetting.

**Day 12**

◆ Dream: I was trying to buy the business office of a pharmacy to use as my homeopathy practice. They wanted to give it to me to use but talked about selling me the pharmacy instead. Not what I had in mind! Then I was trying to figure out remedies for people. Presented cases to a visiting expert. Went to bookstore, but the books were too expensive and elaborate, outdated. Feeling of mild frustration.

◆ More mistakes with confusing numbers. Memory not precise, only remembering parts of dreams and, in waking hours, parts of phrases.

**Day 13**

◆ Dream fragments: bunch of friends over for a Super Bowl game. I'm just dressed in bathrobe and pajamas...unusual for me. Problem with shoe falling apart. Friend tells me how to fix it. I thank him, not embarrassed. A little girl's sister appears; we find parts of her toes in the back of a pickup truck. Could a racist or cannibal group be responsible? We thought a pedophile was responsible before. Shock and disgust with both of these possibilities.

◆ I note a pattern of concern about feet, occurred in another dream.

◆ Dream: Work themes, getting remedies.

◆ 8-9 p.m. Right frontal, achy headache that I feel was brought on by being overtired and reading.

◆ Continue to make mistakes with phone numbers. Had trouble calculating simple co-pay amount. Conscious of mind not working well. Thoughts of the play, *Flowers for Algernon* (about Alzheimer's), and Alzheimer's disease.

**Day 14** Nothing noted.

**Day 15**

◆ Dream: Trying to get through traffic to destination. Along the way I stop at a restaurant and tease a doctor in a white coat: "Are you a busboy?" Perhaps related to *New York Times* article about idea that residents should not be called doctors. Usual theme of not uptight, theme of being more laid-back.

◆ Increased flatulence in afternoon and evening with stool.

**Day 16**

◆ I don't remember first dream, I recall it being bland, but the second dream makes up for it.

◆ Dream: Like *Pulp Fiction*. I and another guy are two henchmen harassing a man. I'm telling the man what a week I've had: two close calls of almost being hurt. My partner pulls a gun on the victim. I am shocked, and then he points the gun at me, and it is apparent that it is me he wants to shoot. I don't know why. He directs me out of the room. He knocks on the bedroom door and says, "Dad?" He walks in and two young people are in bed having sex. As he is caught up in that, I escape. Change of scene: We are analyzing a case and the woman who took the case is taken aback when colleague informs her that the person had a serious lung disease that she missed because she did not do a physical exam. Scene shift: Have to treat the patient, a young woman who is inappropriate and seductive. I have to set limits.
◆ Wake up feeling mildly anxious. I am struck by the contrasts: blandness vs. sex and violence, also my mental confusion and difficulties, yet in some ways more organized and conscious. I felt the dream drew on a law and order show I had seen and the lunch I had with a family practice doctor who is interested in homeopathy.
◆ Eructations half hour after lunch.

**Day 17**
◆ Dream: I am a character who has some talent. I am playing with jigsaw puzzles later on after a dissolute life. Burned out. Go back to puzzles, but they are just plain gray paper pieces, no color. Feeling of a sense of waste and lost opportunity. Scene shift: in a big seminar with female homeopaths dominant. They are sensitive, yet one gets an emergency call but essentially sloughs it off. Scene shift: evaluating ADD (Attention Deficit Disorder) children. Upset that child's history revealed clear problems several years earlier. When I woke up had feelings of lost opportunities. Interestingly my group may bid on contract for ADD screening.
◆ Increased flatulence after noon meal.
◆ Nose ran clear mucous—small amount while cleaning car off in the snow.
◆ Continue to make word and number mistakes.

**Day 18**
◆ Dream: I am working at new agency, very efficient and good, but homeopathy is not going so well. Patient is missing, and finding the remedy helps find the patient. Not clear how but nurse practitioner was also looking for this same patient. She asks me a favor. I forget what. Somehow, a sign on brass plate or doorknob indicated the missing person. Although I don't remember how, it felt like some things were resolved.

**Day 19**
◆ Dream: I took a course with P. I read about in the Similimum. He analyzed a case that a colleague and I had treated. We had prescribed allopathic medicines for back pain and depression. We discussed the case. Suddenly in a restaurant. Someone had disparity in pupil size. Someone commented that we were lucky to have an ophthalmologist there, as this patient had a very rare condition. (I felt this was a reflection of some of my concerns about being more of a generalist.)
◆ Dream: I hear noise outside the house and I get up to look. Neighbor is also looking

and he sees me naked. I found out later oldest son was being sprayed with fluid by neighborhood youths. Feeling of frustration that I could not catch them.
◆ Able to do simple calculating better than I had.

**Day 20**
◆ Dream: An alternative medicine clinic with Native American spirit of cooperation. Everyone working well together. Brief segment before woke up: Spiderman throws a time bomb into a truck. He lifts his mask so they will know who he is before they die. The bomb does not blow up and one of the men goes out of the truck. I think about how ego got Spiderman in trouble with hiding identity.

**Day 21**
◆ Dream: Recurring images of CD's with reading matter imbedded between them. Also was getting mail—magazines with other labels of magazines I did not get. I feel this dream represented concerns about incorporation papers. Important thing missing, etc. (The evening before this dream I attended business meeting about incorporating the group. I feel the review of our legal documents may have influenced the dream.)

## Prover #3 · Female · 38 years old

**Day 1** Nothing noted.

**Day 2**
◆ Stayed late at work, cleared off desk completely; felt the need to organize; bothered by clutter and mess. It had been piled with paper and things I could not quite throw away for three months.

**Day 3**
◆ I had two secrets that I had previously decided to keep silent about. I suddenly and impulsively could not keep them but had to share them with a close friend. I blurted them out, abruptly and with little forethought. The sensation inside was that I simply could not restrain myself. It was two things: a strong feeling from within, though not explosive—more overwhelming, coupled with no longer having any gate of restraint to hold it in. "I don't believe I am saying this," but a drive to do it. Less restraint. *This was a big deal.*
◆ Things seem more black and white, less gray. Not comfortable in the gray zone.
◆ After discussion, very worried, anxious. After telling the secrets, felt anxious about what I had done, would they still like me? Easily imagined the worst, imagination took off.

**Day 4**
◆ More driven in work, more driven to accomplish. Not just today—overall in the last week.
◆ Walked into a conference, greeted everyone and enjoyed briefly being in the limelight. More comfortable having attention on me.

◆ Restless, difficult to meditate.

**Day 6**
◆ Anxious about being late. Feel that I am late a lot, even though I am not. Feels hard to get somewhere on time. Not just today, but a pattern since the proving, but noticed it now. Feeling hurried.

**Day 9**
◆ Less tolerant of ambiguity.
◆ Overall note increased tendency for my mind to jump ahead and worry over the worst. Anticipatory anxiety.

**Day 10**
◆ Dream of work, needing to do something, sensation of being late.
◆ Had a massage and noticed tissues felt different: tighter, more rigid, less responsive, less resilient.

**Day 11**
◆ Insight from within: This remedy seems like a metal to me, silver comes to mind.
◆ Increased acne noted.
◆ Memory poor—forgetting things more than normal.

**Days 12, 13** Nothing noted.

**Day 14**
◆ Numbness, hands, falling asleep more.
Snowstorm today and I canceled my patients, afraid to drive in the snow, more so than normal.
◆ Constipation, some bloating.

**Day 15**
◆ Had to drive to work today in the snow, and I imagined a semi-truck hitting my car, and I could not control it or avoid an accident. Imagined it as though it were real. When coming home, I left the chains on too long and they broke. I was fearful that there might be ice up ahead, though the road I was on was dry. I would rather break the chains and be safe. Too fearful to pull over and take them off. More fearful than usual. Imagining the worst and it feels very real.

**Day 16**
◆ Impatient with my patients, with unhelpful salespeople. A feeling of impatience.
◆ Distention with flatulence.

**Prover #4 · Female · 39 years old**

**Day 1**

◆ Took the first dose just before bed. On lying down a few minutes later, I felt my lower legs to be extremely heavy and had the feeling they were paralyzed. Woke up later to urinate, and my body had the same sensation of great density while I was up walking. Had numerous brief wakings during the night.

**Day 2**

◆ Active dreaming during the night—didn't make notes but one had horses in it: racing horses on racetrack, I was a spectator, feeling was of excitement and fun. (Another was) about bicycle riding: I was riding with funny shorts. Just before waking I dreamed of my breasts. The arteries and veins were visible beneath the skin as great florescent red stripes radiating out from my nipples superiorly and green stripes inferiorly. I wished for the first time that I would reach menopause soon so they would recede.

◆ No symptoms during the day, generally pleasant and calm.

◆ Eruption, wheal and flare skin reaction brief on right forearm after shower.

**Day 3**

◆ Basically feeling O.K. Lots of dreams more vivid than usual, but no specific dreams recalled.

◆ Eruption, wheal and flare left arm two small areas.

**Day 4**

◆ No new symptoms. Remedy repeated before bed.

◆ Again, more vivid dreams, all on old themes.

**Day 5**

◆ I feel a bit more moody today—got real cranky when hungry and snapped at husband.

**Day 6**

◆ Unpleasant day, things that usually make me happy just had a brief impact. I tended to dwell on the negative thoughts. Very sensitive to noise. Felt like bingeing—actually did have a piece of candy in midafternoon (very unusual for me to snack between meals). Sex drive (which had been high for several weeks previous to taking the remedy) was depressed. Orgasm delayed. Felt nasty when cut off by other drivers: "F— you!" feeling.

◆ Feeling of lower abdominal bloating; had normal stool yesterday but now feel constipated. Haven't been drinking as much as usual.

**Day 7**

◆ Continued relatively thirstless but had a normal stool. No bloating.

◆ Still have low sex drive but in every other way better; not so irritable or sensitive to noise.

◆ Have noticed for last three days pulse rate more reactive to activity than normal.

◆ I'm aware of tachycardia with mild exercise, and then it very quickly returns to normal.

◆ Less dreaming last two nights.

**Day 8**

◆ Pretty much back to normal—no problems with constipation, mood or palpitations. Sex drive still low.

**Day 9** No change.

**Day 10**

◆ Fine all day. Sex drive better.

◆ Took third dose shortly before bed. Noticed a slight headache immediately. It cleared and returned a few minutes later—again very brief; slight pressure bi-temporally.

**Days 11-18**

◆ Did not write anything this week. Was very low energy, apathetic. Felt frustrated and overwhelmed by everything. Wanted to quit school, quit work, get divorced, stay home and do nothing. Finally took a 30C dose of my constitutional remedy and felt immediate improvement in mood, energy, sex drive.

◆ Increased trouble picking up phone numbers correctly from voice-mail messages, reversing numbers, not able to follow rapidly spoken numbers.

◆ Skipped morning meditation many times.

◆ Menses, spotted for one week mid cycle (very unusual).

## Prover #5 · Female · 33 years old

**Day 1**

◆ Took first dose before bed and within a few seconds, felt a band-like sensation around neck like a ribbon choker pulled too tight. Very uncomfortable, I had the feeling of suffocation, not being able to breathe well. I had to pull the blankets and loose hair away from my neck. Within 20-30 minutes, it gradually faded and I fell asleep.

**Day 2**

◆ Didn't remember any dreams. Mood good, nothing unusual.

◆ Feeling very sleepy—but haven't gotten caught up on sleep from two nights ago when only had four hours sleep.

**Day 3**

◆ Dream: I was living in a loft space with my husband. A large, loft-like space with partitions/walls built in it to make separate rooms. I came home one day to find several college-age kids had moved in with us—they had torn down the partitions to make it open space again. They did not seem concerned that we had already been living there and did not want any roommates. I was very annoyed at our landlord. How could he?

Indignant and irritated. However, I was also intrigued by the people moving in and interested in their personalities, belongings, energy, art and music (Hip hop stuff, graffiti, MTV stuff.)

**Day 4**
◆ Dream: At birthday party for a friend, we were all baking a strawberry shortcake together. A very sunny, light, spring-like feeling.
Pain, stiff, sore knees on first waking, climbing stairs.

**Day 5**
◆ No real dreams—only four hours sleep and surprisingly energetic for lack of sleep.
◆ Knees—stiff, sore.
◆ Eruptions, scaly, rough, patchy round patch size of nickel left forearm dorsal aspect. Patch on arm size of quarter, when scratched, a few scales scrape off with pinpoint bleeding underneath.
◆ Haven't noticed much change so took second dose before bed.

**Day 6**
◆ Don't remember dream. Busy morning. Knees stiff. Felt very tired, probably from lack of sleep two nights before.

**Day 7**
◆ Slight headache on waking in forehead > after eating breakfast (gave blood the night before).
◆ Skin continues to be rough, not itchy.

**Day 8** Overslept—don't remember dreams.

**Day 9**
◆ Dream: A garden of poppies, pansies, just an impression on waking; more a fragment than a real dream. I had planted some flowers a few days before in real life.

**Day 10-12**
◆ Have been very busy, getting up extra early in order to drive husband to work—don't recall any dreams.
◆ Flatulence, painless, odorless, some distention, probably from garbanzo bean curry yesterday that was undercooked.
◆ Patch of dry, scaly skin larger—quarter sized.

**Day 13**
◆ Tired in late morning about 11 a.m. I wish I could take a nap.
◆ Felt very motivated and energetic in the evening: got a lot accomplished—cleaning, sewing, typing—things I had been putting off for months.
◆ Getting organized, clearing away the clutter and accumulated piles.
◆ Took third dose this evening.

**Day 14**

◆ Dream: My pet rabbit with a shaven belly and scar (in real life we just had our rabbit fixed). No real feeling.

◆ Dream: Driving in a car over the hills while singing, very pleasant feeling. Beautiful spring scene in Sonoma County, blue sky and green pastures, blooming daffodils and plum trees. Intensely beautiful and happy to be alive feeling and awed at how beautiful the earth was.

◆ Irritable: I felt very irritated at a general business meeting conducted by Robert's Rules. The whole rules process was unhelpful and felt like an artificial constraint, a hindrance. Impatient, yet bored. I have been to meetings like this before and never felt this way. Perhaps it was partly due to attending a meeting the day before that was run by group process and consensus decision making: a very team oriented effort that ran smoothly. This meeting seemed very forced and constrained by artificial rules that did not facilitate the goal. I actually brought this up to the group, but the reply was that the state required that general business meetings be conducted this way. I felt left out by the majority rules process, frustrated, almost moved to tears and felt like getting up and leaving. But I felt trapped, thwarted and very restless there. I so desperately wanted to leave, but I had to stick it out.

**Day 15**

◆ Dream: Of the Emeryville Co-housing Project that I had visited two days ago: a cooperative residential development, warm fuzzy feeling about living in co-housing.

◆ Knees stiff.

**Day 16**

◆ Bleeding gums with tooth brushing for one week; a lot of blood, it frightened me.

**Day 17**

◆ Mouth: bleeding gums.

◆ Nausea, felt a little nauseous while standing in line at the bank this a.m. The bank was very crowded and it was a long wait; felt impatient. Took charcoal capsules and Echinacea and felt better within two hours.

**Day 18**

◆ Dream: A very clear dream of anatomy lab—dissection of the brachioplexus with a feeling of precision, fastidiousness, teamwork. We were also cleaning out the bins the body parts are kept in. Lots of sunlight which was unusual, since my real life experience with dissection lab years ago was of a rainy, overcast mood. Smell of formalin.

**Prover #6 · Male · 43 years old**

◆ Took the proving book out on the plane this morning and the book vanished! So no journal entries, only what I can recall.
◆ Unusual month circumstantially. My roommate was very ill, so had extra responsibilities. Also did four presentations in ten days, so doing a lot of late night preparations work.
◆ Burning pain in epigastrium after taking the remedy.
◆ Prolonged episodes of hiccoughing.
◆ Couldn't get it together, not able to keep things organized. Papers everywhere. I saw myself gong down same track, losing my mind feeling. Father is getting more disorganized. And I saw myself going down the same track. Fearful feeling.
◆ I'm on a rehabilitation team that gets together at weekly meeting. One therapist who is somewhat domineering and smartass brought up an issue about a patient who got Thorazine from another doctor. I had been so busy I had not been going to the hospital early to check on charts, so I did not know about this yet. I had a feeling of embarrassment, and after the meeting I yelled at her, "You were out of line!" I knew in my heart I was embarrassed I had not done my job and I was frustrated. Felt terrible later and realized it was mean and bad politically for the unit. Feeling of drowning in disorganization, feeling of sinking or drowning; I could not get a hold of her. I finally got to talk to her, and it all ended up fine.
◆ Compressed and pressurized, got a lot of work done, presentations went really well. Even though one night woke up at two and not able to go back to sleep.
◆ Dreams unremembered: Felt I was neglecting duty.
◆ Dream: Intense nightmare: multiple beings or people against me. Violent interaction with multiple other animals and beings, fighting for my life. People and extra-terrestrials of some sort. Fighting with my hands. They're trying to kill me.
◆ In real life there were some things not very important but felt compelled to do them. My priorities shifted, e.g. I had promised classmate a copy of notes, but I forgot until last minute. Got them together and trying to get to Fed Ex, but it snowed so could not go. I was trying to call his office and his house, but could not get a hold of him, but put a lot of effort into it, more than I probably should have. Fighting quality. Quicksand, a feeling of sinking. Crazy month. Struggling and struggling, but I am losing ground. But everything has worked out fine Sense of doing my duty, doing the things I have committed to and following through, but my life is crumbling around me. Felt desperate rather than sad. Feeling of apathy, exhausted. I can't deal with this and I don't care. Hard to sort out what is what. Life is hard.

**Summary of experience:**
◆ Was supportive of partner.
◆ Loosing ground, though struggling. Do your duty but life is crumbling.
◆ Desperate. Apathy. Life is hard feeling.
◆ Losing track of things. Can't get things done, like Sisyphus rolling boulder uphill. Drowning in disorganization. Fear of losing notebook.

◆ Pursued details instead of priorities. Effort without results. Fighting quality but sinking like quicksand.
◆ Not remembering dreams, feeling neglectful of duty.
◆ Pressured, compressed feeling.
◆ Insomnia: woke at 2 a.m., unable to sleep.
◆ Hiccoughs: four episodes in a single day.
◆ Lower sex drive.

## Prover #7 · Male · 34 years old

### Day 1

◆ Dream: In a restaurant eating with my brother. A couple nearby having an argument. I look at them, and the man gets upset. There is an exchange of words, and my brother gets up and physically "manhandles" him by striking him. Next, somehow I end up in a fight with this guy—we are all over the place. I have some kind of metal stick in one hand and a wooden stick in the other. I strike him over and over again, but this guy will not stop. He just keeps on coming; he is very crazed—like "Rocky." He won't hurt me and take me down. I'm afraid and I don't want to kill him, but I see no other option. I hit him on his head and ribs over and over. "I want peace." He won't stop!! I strike and strike and strike. He falls downstairs and climbs back again. He is bloody and beaten up but won't die. I'm apologizing to his wife. Finally he goes away and promises he will redeem himself by getting back at me. I feel frightened but very much want to live and survive myself. Next I'm with my family; my brother's face looks like that of an East Indian man. Someone hands me the phone and it is Phylis Diller—she wants to know about Homeopathy. My mom is there and I want to tell her about this terrible fight that happened. I'm crying, she seems to not understand and says, "Did you stain your suit?" I say, no, she will not hear me or understand me.
◆ Dream: Driving down freeway, battery is going dead. I'm in a store returning a shirt; the salesperson says they don't sell this particular shirt. The shirt keeps turning different colors: green and red and blue. She shows it to everyone and tries to sell it. I'm impatient. I've driven a long way and want to complete the task. I walk out, and I am with my brother going back to the car with a now dead battery. On the way, I'm in a field, and there are cats that have surrounded a marmot and are attacking it. I try to scare the cats away. I'm a little afraid, they are vicious cats.
◆ Dream: Going fishing. I have to walk down a large mountain and as I come to the river I see that it is dry. I look farther upstream and see the lake is dry. I am sad.
◆ Pain, aching in lower back < rising from a seat; hard to straighten up.

### Day 2

◆ Dream: I am seduced by a woman I don't know. I have a strong sexual desire for her. She makes a request that she wants me to pull her nipples very hard. I do it with the feeling of: "Who is this woman and why am I here?" A bit guilty, like: "My wife wouldn't be pleased about this."

◆ Dream: I'm touching a beautiful woman sexually; she is very beautiful. I realize it is my friend's wife, although it does not look like her. I am embarrassed and guilty but was so connected to the person. I say I'm sorry to my friend for betraying him. I can see he is shocked and angry. He is crying and starts to kiss me passionately—it is very weird and uncomfortable . I awaken with a strange feeling.
◆ Dream: I got pulled over in my car by police. He was going to arrest me for making an illegal turn. I was pissed off, screaming, "You are unfair. Who the f— are you?!"

**Day 3**
◆ Feeling flaky, I don't give a shit. Depressed, hopeless angst about the world. Driving down the freeway thinking, "What is this whole thing about anyway?"
◆ Urination frequent, nine times out of ten the bathroom at work was already occupied. I was impatient and outraged, pounding on the door: " C'mon!!"
◆ Sitting with my daughter, she was wearing a soft pink dress, her eyes looked so blue. She was exquisitely beautiful, I was profoundly in love with her. It was an unusually deep feeling with her. Realized how limited I am in expressing my love for her.

**Day 4**
◆ Waking, with a terrified feeling. I felt someone was stalking the house, my son jumps out of bed and sleepwalks, moaning. He gets into bed with us. Then the phone rings and nobody is there when I answer. Fantasized about how I would protect my family and myself. I kept hearing a noise outside. My dog was growling.

**Day 5**
◆ Dream: On a large ship with terrorist-type Middle-Eastern men. I'm in great danger of being murdered. There are other people on the ship in a similar situation. I am trying to be amiable. I'm looking for a place to hide from these dangerous people. Next, I am hiding in a large room behind columns to avoid contact with these men.
◆ Dream: I was with a friend, who was walking backwards teaching a woman how to sing.
◆ Impatient with others.

### Prover #8 · Female · 40 years old

◆ Dream: Of a bear, seemed important but couldn't remember details.
◆ Felt bad because I did not take good notes.

**Prover #9 · Female · 36 years old**

Hard to pay attention to the remedy, kept no record, no account, but O.K.
◆ After taking the remedy everything got constricted.
◆ Felt on the edge of getting sinus infection, not sick but tomorrow I could be, but I don't get sick. Feels irritated by it. I knew not to take the remedy.
◆ Dreams: Running naked with breasts exposed.
◆ Eyes dry and stingy.
◆ Feels like I have been drinking coffee, heart racing, etc. It is not steady but occasionally feels tension in head, like I get from coffee. A gnawing.
◆ Increased sensitivity to noise, street noise, husband's voice, kids' noise all very loud. Difficulty sleeping, very restless. Usually sleep very well.
◆ I know I am dreaming but can't remember them. Frustrating. In a fuzzy state on waking but no dream details come. Overall fuzziness, but I feel clear, it does not make sense. It is a state of being. The angels drove me here today. Consistent all week. Usually pay close attention to details, but I have not opened my calendar book all week, I am showing up where I need to be without actually paying attention to it. I feel I have moments of brilliance, but then it is gone. The fuzziness is peaceful, like moving through honey. Things are slowed down.
◆ Had a body work session and conversed for an hour, and then the session was up. Therapist asked: "Are you O.K. with not getting body work?" I was furious when left, actually that is too strong a word. I thought, "Oh, I just missed out on an hour of body work." Not that terrible because in the conversation we had, we were timeless and otherworldly in our conversations. Feel somehow buffered.
◆ Had a repulsion towards chocolate. Just seeing it, had no interest.
◆ Not able to pay attention to the remedy, not recording symptoms. Not very concerned. Just no ability to do it. Knew it would be O.K. Fighting to hold onto other state of openness (from Lac delphinum). Taking the remedy made me contract and that feeling of contraction is not good.

## BIBLIOGRAPHY


Beckett, Jamie. "Tragedy Ends Girl's Quest." *San Francisco Chronicle*, 12 April 1996.

Benyus, Janine M. *Beastly Behaviors*. New York: Addison-Wesley, 1992.

Blow, Richard. "dr. dolphin: Why Does Swimming with Dolphins Help Humans Heal? A Computer-Wielding Neurohacker May Have Found the Answer." *Mother Jones* 20 (January/February 1995): 28-31,82.

Burns, John F. "Killer Wolves Terrify Villagers in Indian Province." *San Francisco Chronicle*, n.d. First published in the *New York Times*, n.d.

Chellam, Ravi. "Lions of the Gir Forest." *Wildlife Conservation* 99 (June 1996): 40-43.

Christensen, James R. *Butterflies of the Pacific Northwest.* A Northwest Naturalist's Book. N.p.: University Press of Idaho, 1981.

Comstock, J.A. *Butterflies of California.* Los Angeles: n.p., 1927.

Cooper, J.C. *Dictionary of Symbolic and Mythological Animals.* London, San Francisco: Thorsons An Imprint of HarperCollins Publishers, 1995.

Dornfeld, Ernst T. *The Butterflies of Oregon.* Timber Grove, Oregon: Timber Press, n.d.

Eid, Alain. *Butterflies and Moths of the World.* Photographed by Michel Viard. New York: Chartwell Book, 1997.

Farlow, James O., and M.K. Brett-Surman, eds. *The Complete Dinosaur.* Bloomington and Indianapolis: Indiana University Press, 1997.

Fonseca, Isabel. *Bury Me Standing.* New York: Random House, 1996.

Fox, Susan. *Rats*. Neptune City, New Jersey: T.F.H. Publications, Inc., 1988.

Gaffney, Eugene S. *Dinosaurs*. Illustrated by John D. Dawson. New York: Golden Press, 1990.

Generic-Trost, C. "Born to Lose." *Wall Street Journal*, 18 July 1989.

Joubert, Dereck. "Lions of Darkness." *National Geographic* 186 (August 1994): 35-53.

Klots, Alexander B., and Elsie B. Klots. *1001 Questions Answered About Insects.* New York: Dover Publications, Inc., 1977.

Lambert, David. *The Ultimate Dinosaur Book.* With a foreword by John H. Ostrom, Ph.D. London: DK Publishing in association with the Natural History Museum, 1993.

Lawrence, R.D. *In Praise of Wolves.* New York: Ballantine Books, 1986.

Locke, Michelle. "How Do You Milk An Elephant?" *Star Tribune*, 3 March 1996.

Mann, A.T., and Jane Lyle. *Sacred Sexuality.* Rockport, Mass.: Element Books, Ltd., 1995.

Masson, Jeffrey Moussaieff, and Susan McCarthy. *When Elephants Weep: The Emotional Lives of Animals.* New York: Delacorte Press, Bantam Doubleday Dell Publishing Group, Inc., 1995.

Morris, Desmond. *Horsewatching.* New York: Crown Publishers, Inc., 1988.

Morell, Virginia. "The Origin of Birds: The Dinosaur Debate." *Audubon* 99 (March/April 1997): 36-45.

Norris, Kenneth S. "Dolphins in Crisis." *National Geographic* 182 (September 1992): 2-35.

Roberts, Monty. *The Man Who Listens to Horses.* New York: Random House, 1997.

Rojas, Aurelio. "Return of the Native." *San Francisco Chronicle*, n.d.

Rowen, Andrew N. "The Benefits and Ethics of Animal Research." *Scientific American* 277 (February 1997): 79-93.

Ryan, Joan. "Children Often Pay the Price for Parents' Dreams." *San Francisco Chronicle*, 12 April 1996.

Schwartz, Andrew. "Elegy for an Elephant." *San Francisco Chronicle*, 19 January 1997.

Williams, Terry. "Voices from the Tunnels: Deep Under Manhattan, Life Goes On." *Utne Reader*, no. 71 (September/October 1995): 92-101.

Woodman, Marion, and Elinor Dickson. *Dancing in the Flames: The Dark Goddess in the Transformation of Consciousness.* Boston and London: Shambhala, 1996.

## RESOURCES

There are two pharmacies which carry the remedies made as a result of the provings in this book, as well as other remedies newly proven by Nancy Herrick.

From **Deutsche Homöopathie Union** in Germany, the following remedies are available. Practitioners should request that their remedy vials be labeled "for research" when ordering. The remedies available are:

Lac delphinum (Milk of the Dolphin)
Lac equinum (Milk of the Horse)
Lac leoninum (Milk of the Lion)
Lac lupinum (Milk of the Wolf)
Buteo jam (Red Tail Hawk)
Rosa gallicia (Yellow rose)

These are available to all homeopaths in 12c, 30c, 200c, 1M, and 10M potencies. Orders should be sent to:

DHU - ARZNEIMITTEL
GMBH & CO. KG
Ottostrasse 24
D-76227 Karlsruhe-Germany

Phone 011 49 721 4093-230
Fax 011 49 721 4093-244

**From Hahnemann Pharmacy:**
Sanguis soricis (Blood of the Rat)
Limenitis bredowii (Butterfly)
Maiasaura lapidea (Dinosaur)
Lac loxodonta (Milk of the Elephant)
Lac delphinum (Milk of the Dolphin)
Lac equinum (Milk of the Horse)
Lac leoninum (Milk of the Lion)
Lac lupinum (Milk of the Wolf)
Buteo jam (Red Tail Hawk)
Rosa gallicia (Yellow rose)
Ginseng (American and Korean)
Ayahuasca
Nilumbo nucifera (Lotus)

Call Pharmacy for available potencies and prices. **1-888-ACONITE**

## A METHODOLOGY FOR CREATING RUBRICS

The creation of rubrics is the step in the proving process that yields to the practice of homeopathy the gifts of the proving material. But it is, without question, the most tedious part of the endeavor. Only the awareness of its importance sustained us.

In our particular process, the initial step in gathering rubrics included the provers themselves. Each prover was invited to attend a rubrics meeting, hopefully to reexperience the state created during the proving and to express the feelings of that state in repertory language. This meeting helped to clarify the journal entries and to focus the central feelings brought out by the proving.

From that point, the raw data was further shaped into actual rubrics. In creating mental rubrics, we used the language of the prover whenever possible. Using word search tools provided by MacRepertory, exploring the repertory for the prover's words or synonyms became easy. Our preference was to utilize existing rubrics where appropriate rather than to create entirely new rubrics. We also gave careful consideration to cross-references as possible choices.

However, we felt that creating new sub-rubrics was fitting; the primary goal was to capture as precisely as possible the feeling expressed by the prover. For example, a journal entry read: "I had an impulse to shoplift." The rubric, "KLEPTOMANIA, stealing," is already in the repertory. However, the prover did not actually steal anything; she only had the impulse. When we did a search for "shoplift," there were no occurrences of that word, and a search for "steal" yielded only "dreams stealing." This did not quite capture the feeling either because it was more of an impulse. Doing a search among existing rubrics for "impulse" yielded: "MIND; IMPULSE, morbid" and "MIND; STRANGE; things, impulse to do." Here, we felt it would be appropriate to create a sub-rubric regarding shoplifting or stealing. The new sub-rubrics became: "MIND; IMPULSE, morbid; shoplift, to" or "MIND; STRANGE; things, impulse to do; shoplift, to." This was more reflective of the prover's experience than "KLEPTOMANIA" and preferable to creating a new rubric, "Shoplifting, impulse to."

If there was no existing rubric to cover the feeling/experience of a prover—and we knew that the feeling was a common one—the creation of a new rubric seemed justifiable. As an example, there is no occurrence of "COMPETITION" in the repertory. It is now a new rubric from the Lac equinum proving because the theme of competitiveness was so strongly expressed.

### Dreams

As for dream rubrics, we largely followed the protocol already observed by the repertory. The sub-rubrics under "MIND; dreams" can be roughly divided into three categories: the noun/subject of the dream (e.g. books, animals, houses); the adjective that is descriptive of the dream or emotion (e.g. vivid, impressive, unremembered, humiliation, anxious); the verb/action of the dream (usually a gerund e.g. reading, swimming, feasting).

We chose again to use existing dream sub-rubrics first. However, we also created several others in order to adequately cover the feeling of the dream, especially if the dream was highly significant to the main feeling/themes of the proving. For example, a prover wrote: “Dream: I was sympathizing with a group of people who were mourning a friend who was moving.” This became four separate sub-rubrics: “MIND; DREAMS; friends; mourning the departure of;” “MIND; DREAMS; groups; mourning departure of friend;” “MIND; DREAMS; sympathetic;” and “MIND; DREAMS; sympathetic; with those mourning a friend’s departure.”

The creation of physical rubrics was more straightforward. The symptoms of provers were broken down into their appropriate components as per repertory categorization. For the most part, the rubrics were taken word for word from the repertory.

– Claire Green, N.D.

**BOOK ORDER FORM**

| To order additional copies of *Animal Mind, Human Voices,* please complete this form. |
|---|

Please send ______ copies of *Animal Mind, Human Voices* to:

Name________________________________Phone______________________

Street_________________________________________________________

City_________________________________State_____Zip______________

Enclose for Each Book: $39.95
CA Residents Add Tax: $3.30 (CA only)
Shipping and Handling (US): $4.25
Shipping and Handling Foreign: Ground $10.00, Air $15.00

____books @ $39.95 ________

Tax (CA only) @ $3.30 ________ (CA only)

US Shipping and Handling ($4.25) ________

Foreign S/H @ $10 or $15 ________

**Total Enclosed:** ________

Please send check or money order, payable to **Hahnemann Clinic Publishing.**

Mail to:
**Hahnemann Clinic Publishing**
**19775 New Rome Road**
**Nevada City, California 95959**
Telephone and facsimile 530-265-3856

Allow two weeks for US delivery.
Foreign surface: six weeks.
Foreign air: twelve days.